M. R. Parwaresch

The Human Blood Basophil

Morphology, Origin, Kinetics Function and Pathology

With a Foreword by K. Lennert

With 58 Partly Colored Figures

Springer-Verlag
Berlin · Heidelberg · New York 1976

PD Dr. M. R. PARWARESCH, Pathologisches Institut
der Universität Kiel, Hospitalstr. 42, D 2300 Kiel

ISBN-13: 978-3-642-66331-4 e-ISBN-13: 978-3-642-66329-1
DOI: 10.1007/978-3-642-66329-1

Library of Congress Cataloging in Publication Data. Parwaresch, M. R. 1940–.
The human blood basophil. Includes bibliographies. 1. Basophil leucocyte. I. Title.
QP95.P37. 612'.112. 76–4110.

Softcover reprint of the hardcover 1st edition 1976

Dedicated to my Parents
Mahi and Mahmoud Parwaresch

Foreword

The blood basophils lead a shadowy existence in the field of hematology, even now, 100 years after their discovery by PAUL EHRLICH.

In clinical medicine they were hardly noticed for many decades, since they occur in such small numbers in the blood that small and moderate variations in the basophil count were not detectable with common counting methods. This situation has changed since the introduction of direct counting methods. It was noticed, for example, that the blood basophil count is increased in hyperlipemia.

In the field of pathology the blood basophil was practically overlooked until recently. This was due to the fact that with common fixations in aqueous solutions the granules dissolve, so that the cells can no longer be stained specifically and therefore escape observation. This problem was solved through special fixing solutions. However, interest in the blood basophils remained confined to only a few research groups.

Dr. PARWARESCH belongs to such a group. With great initiative, he took over the studies started by the undersigned and devoted himself to the whole problem of the blood basophils. Dr. PARWARESCH attended to the cytological and cytochemical demonstration of blood basophils. He also investigated their kinetic features and their development in man and rabbits. Furthermore, he observed the quantitative and cytochemical behavior of blood basophils under functional stress (postprandial hyperlipemia) and studied the morphology, cytochemistry, and electron microscopy of blood basophils in myeloproliferative diseases, especially in basophilic leukemia. All of these investigations provided important new findings that considerably enriched our knowledge of the morphology, pathology, and function of the blood basophils.

The studies performed by Dr. PARWARESCH represent the framework supporting the findings on blood basophils scattered in the literature. The result is a monograph presenting the first comprehensive report on our current knowledge of the blood basophils and integrating it into a meaningful whole on the basis of the author's rich experience. Almost all previous larger papers on this subject suffered from the fallacy that blood basophils and mast cells are variants of the same type of cell. Those who are still in doubt should be easy to enlighten through the morphological, cytochemical, and kinetic proof that blood basophils are derived from corresponding precursor cells of the bone marrow.

This monograph therefore closes a gap, which would not have been possible merely by compiling literature. Clinical hematologists and pathologists are the main beneficiaries of the author's Herculean labors. However, experimental immunologists, who have become increasingly fascinated in blood basophils in recent years, will also be thankful for this reference book. I wish Dr. PARWARESCH widespread circulation of his work, not only to provide information, but above all to arouse interest in and to stimulate further study of this previously neglected cell.

Kiel, April 1976 KARL LENNERT

Preface

PAUL EHRLICH recognized the blood mast cells as being an independent type of leukocyte almost 100 years ago, in 1879, and distinguished them from tissue mast cells. Blood basophils have been referred to in the literature as mast leukocytes, blood mast cells, basophil granulocytes, and myelogenous mast cells.

The chemical nature and biological significance of the cytoplasmic constituents of basophils, especially heparin and histamine are well established. The literature on these substances is now almost too bulky to assimilate, yet blood basophils, which synthesize, store, and liberate them, and constantly circulate throughout the body in the blood, have received far less attention than tissue mast cells. This is because of the rarity of basophils in human blood and the technical difficulties of the research involved. Nevertheless, there has recently been an upsurge of original work, and the resulting reports on the human blood basophil have necessitated a new, integrating approach.

An impressive array of talent has been devoted to the study of tissue mast cells and blood basophils, as may be seen from the exhaustive bibliography, which impressively reflects the magnitude of the interest this cell system has aroused in investigators over a broad spectrum of medical and bilogical disciplines. Both old and new views have been scrutinized and their present significance critically evaluated. The author's aim was to develop within the framework of the present book a comprehensive concept of the role of human blood basophils, based on a survey of their morphology, origin, kinetics, physiology, and pathology.

This monograph was planned so that each chapter should present a complete treatment of a particular sector of basophil research and can thus be used as a more or less independent entity, with the references listed at the end of related sections or chapters, as set out below.

Chapter A, Sections I to IV, is devoted mainly to the occurrence, enumeration, and cytomorphology of human blood basophils with special reference to their light-, phase-contrast, and electron-microscopic features.

Chapter A, Section V, gives a detailed analysis of the cytochemistry of basophils with special reference to enzyme activities and the cytochemistry of the glycosaminoglycans that occur in basophil granules.

Chapter A, Section VI, is devoted to comparative morphologic studies. In preparing this section much use was made of the classic monograph on mast cells by N. A. MICHELS, published in 1938 and reprinted in 1963 by the New York Academy of Science.

Chapter B, Section II, is concerned with the detection of the basophilic cell line in human bone marrow. The derivation of mature circulating basophils from a nonspecific promyelocyte is traced and discussed in detail in Section III.

Chapter C, Sections I and II, discusses the functional and biochemical features of basophils and their granule constituents, heparin and histamine. Special reference is made to the hypersensitivity phenomenon, as well as to serum lipolysis.

Chapter C, Section III, deals first with the mechanism relating to granule discharge by blood basophils. In this context, an extensive review of tissue mast cells proved essential. There follows a report on experimental findings on the cytokinetics of tritium-labeled basophils in rabbits and man.

The subject of Chapter D is a study of the malignant variants that occur in various myeloproliferative diseases. This yields a set of reliable criteria for distinguishing pathologic basophils from normal basophils. Finally, a synthesizing view of the myeloid leukemias is put forward.

The compilation of this monograph would have exceeded the author's capabilities had he not enjoyed the sincere support and critical suggestions of Professor KARL LENNERT, Head of the Department of Pathology, University of Kiel.

The author gratefully acknowledges the unflagging assistance of Miss CHRISTIANE MÄDER.

The German Research Foundation, Deutsche Forschungsgemeinschaft, generously supported the experiments on which this work is based.

Kiel, Spring 1976 M. R. PARWARESCH

Contents

A. Basophils of the Peripheral Blood

I. Basophil Count

Basophils represent the least common type of granulocytes in human blood. Their rarity and the solubility of their granules have made it difficult to determine their biological significance. Considerable technical sophistication is necessary for determining the quantitative changes that occur in blood basophils.

1. Normal Values; Counting Procedures

As with other leukocytes, the basophil count varies according to the technique used. As a rule, somewhat lower values are obtained with differential counts (indirect counting) than with a direct counting method. Statistically supported assertions require not less than 1000 leukocytes (FREDRICK and MOLONEY, 1959). Fairly sensitive methods are currently available for the direct counting of basophils in chambers. If an indirect counting method is chosen, one must be aware of possible sources of error. Smears must be prepared immediately after sampling; satisfactory fixation is essential for reliable results. The usual panoptic stains reveal most of the basophils, but they are not suitable for determining the total population. Basic dyes like toluidine blue will selectively stain basophils, but do not permit efficient examination of other leukocytes. We use a special staining technique which makes it easy to identify and count the basophils, even at low magnification.

Low magnification is preferred for microscopic investigations as large areas of a smear can be scanned and random samples taken from regions with different leukocyte distributions. In our hands the following method has proved highly advantageous for a quick survey of basophils in blood and bone marrow smears.

Staining Procedure. Air-dried smears are fixed in a mixture of absolute methanol and formalin (9 : 1 v/v) for 5 min and stained for 30 min in a 0.5% solution of basic aldehyde fuchsin in 80% ethyl alcohol to which 1 ml paraldehyde and 1 ml concentrated hydrochloric acid have been added (GOMORI, 1950). The slides are rinsed in a solution of 0.5% borax ($Na_2B_4O_7 \cdot 10\ H_2O$) in 80% ethyl alcohol, differentiated in 70% ethyl alcohol, counterstained for 30 sec in a 1% solution of light green dye (National Aniline No. 594) in 70% ethyl alcohol, then rinsed with tap water.

Erythrocytes stain green and basophils red to deep purple (Fig. 1).

The distribution of basophils in a well-defined smear is fairly characteristic, the majority being regularly found in the marginal areas of a slide. Allowing for possible errors, a positive correlation with absolute values can

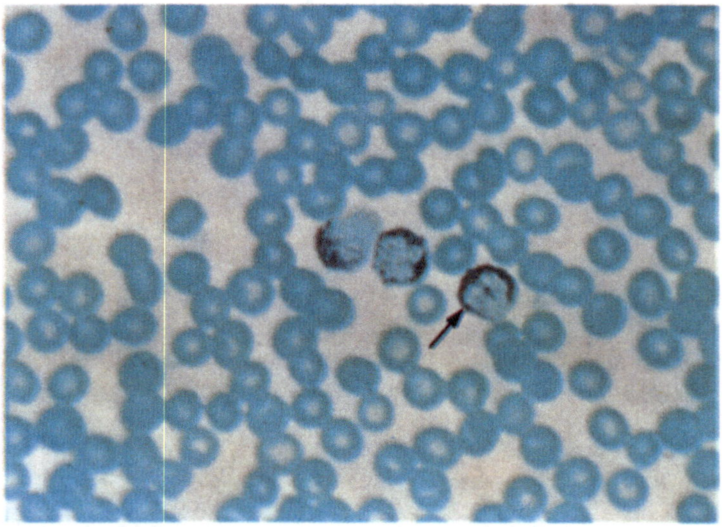

Fig. 1. Normal blood basophils (*arrow*). Aldehyde-fuchsin and light-green staining; ×400

only be obtained on the basis of differentiation of more than 4000 leukocytes (Moore and James, 1953).

It is not feasible to make a direct determination of blood basophils in counting chambers by means of suspension media and dilutions, as used for counting leukocytes. The solutions used must in addition to adequate elimination of erythrocytes by hemolysis, also ensure effective preservation of the basophil granules. Acetic acid and other inorganic acids will destroy erythrocytes, but they also dissolve the water-soluble basophil granules. Basic compounds like propylene glycol (Moore and James, 1953) are powerful hemolytic agents but fail to stabilize the blood basophil granules sufficiently. The use of ethylene glycol, digitonosid, or detergents like Tween 80 also proved inadequate for routine studies.

The first attempts to count blood basophils in chambers were made by Moore and James (1953) and James *et al.* (1955). They reported counts for men of 46.7 ± 18.9, for newborns of 43 ± 26, and for children under 2 years of age an average of below 21. These differences were not statistically significant. The technique of Moore and James (1953) was modified by Osada (1956), who reported a diurnal variation in basophil counts.

Inagaki (1957), using a 10% basic lead acetate solution as fixative, found 35.3 ± 10.3 (min 12, max 101) basophils per mm^3 blood for 53 adult men, and 29.7 ± 13.9 for 42 women. Braunsteiner and Thumb (1958), using a further modification, obtained a value of 28.03 ± 13.2 basophils per mm^3. Using Nageotte chambers ($v = 1.25\ mm^3$), Piette and Piette (1962) reported 40 basophils per mm^3 in peripheral blood. A method for determining eosinophils and basophils simultaneously was developed by Kovacs (1961). Rorsman (1957; 1962) affirmed that the biological variation in basophil counts was ± 3.5, hence somewhat less than that of the method. He reported that the standard deviation for a random population was ± 5.0 for high values (over 40/mm³), ± 3.3 for medium values (about 30/mm³), and ± 3.0 for low values (under 25/mm³). This author found no difference due to sex, but somewhat higher counts for the age group between 40 and 59 years.

Contrary to the results of DUNÉR and PERNOW (1958), RORSMAN (1962), and KARVONEN and KUNAS (1953) found no significant change in the basophil population after hard physical work. Some authors have pointed out that local irritation during blood sampling can result in an artificial increase (GRAF and SVENSSON, 1950; HARMS, 1954). However, under normal circumstances, even long-term catheterization of a vein does not induce a false basophil count, as maintained by RORSMAN (1962).

Views differ on the diurnal variation in the basophil count. Some authors found a rise in the morning (LABENDZINSKI, 1956), at 10.00 a.m. (GRABENER, 1967), at noon (SUNDBERG and WASASTJERNA, 1953), in the afternoon (BOSEILA, 1959), or at 10.00 p.m. (OSADA, 1956).

Since the description of the earliest technique by MOORE and JAMES (1953) numerous modifications have been introduced without achieving a satisfactory result. Even the use of lead acetate as fixative (INAGAKI, 1957; FRICK, 1966) or of neutral red as a supravital dye (SHELLEY *et al.*, 1965) brought no decisive advantages.

The introduction of substances long used for the precipitation of glycosaminoglycans in analytical chemistry was a step forward in the study of the basophils. Quaternary N compounds like N-cetylpyridinium chloride or cetyltrimethylammonium bromide (SCOTT, 1960; LINDAHL, 1969) allow optimal preservation of basophil granules and enhance their ability to absorb dyes while hemolyzing the red blood corpuscles. The best of the techniques known to us is that of COOPER and CRUICKSHANK (1966). The addition of aluminium sulfate as well as N-cetylpyridinium chloride is recommended to bind the dye to the granules. A 0.1% disodium-EDTA in saline solution is used as an anticoagulant. This technique, which we have been using since 1967, has several advantages: it is very easy to use, readily reproducible and gives a selective delineation of blood basophils without precipitation artifacts. Furthermore, blood samples treated with the working solution can be stored for a long time at room temperature and counted later. Normal values amount to 40 ± 3.2 basophils per mm³ blood. The technical error of ± 2.3 is mostly due to pipette errors.

Technical Procedure. Add 20 µl of free flowing blood to 80 µl of 0.1% disodium-EDTA in saline and mix by gentle shaking. Add 100 µl filtered dye solution and fill Fuchs-Rosenthal chambers. Allow cells to settle prior to counting. The dye solution consists of 25 ml of distilled water and 20 ml of 0.8% toluidine blue solution in 5% aluminium sulfate.

Basophils stain metachromatically purple to red, whereas other cells remain unstained. Recently a new method, using alcian blue, has been developed by GILBERT and ORNSTEIN (1975) which reveals excellent results.

On the basis of a total blood volume of 5 liters and of a total leukocyte count of 7000 per mm³, the total number of circulating blood basophils would be about 180×10^6. This does not include other pool systems (bone-marrow, marginal, lungs and spleen).

To sum up: the number of basophils in the blood is relatively constant. Their frequencies describe a Gaussian distribution (GRABENER, 1967). Their quantitative variations move between the extremes of 20 and 45 cells per mm³ blood. The mean value is 40 and the standard deviation of the mean is ± 3.2 with a 2.3 margin of error. Some authors claim the value differs with sex (CAMERADA and LEO, 1955; RORSMAN, 1957; BOSEILA, 1959), others disagree (MOORE and JAMES, 1953; ANGELI *et al.*, 1954; INAGAKI, 1957). Basophilia exists at values of over 50 basophils per mm³ of blood, and basopenia at values of under 20 basophils per mm³.

2. Basophil Leukocytosis and Basopenia

A reactive rise of at least 15% in the basophil count is referred to as basophil leukocytosis or blood basophilia, while a similar fall is called basophil leukopenia.

The number of blood basophils is influenced by various exogenous and endogenous factors. The majority of hormones, or their equivalents, act as depressants upon the number of circulating basophils. The actions of various hormones upon the basophil count are detailed below. While most of the counting procedures in use have considerable technical inadequacies, so that quantitative results need confirmation, the effects of many hormones upon the blood basophil count are recorded with sufficient certainty. This is especially true where similar results are reported by different research teams. Observations made on patients with diseases caused by hypo- or hyperactivity of a particular endocrine gland can provide further confirmation of the experimental results.

a) Thyroid Hormone

Thyroid hormones exert a pronounced depressing effect upon the basophil count. TURIN (1910), NAEGELI (1920) and NOMURA (1928) noticed this phenomenon and tried to use it as an indicator of thyroid function. Later, THONNARD-NEUMANN (1954), CAMERADA and LEO (1955), INAGAKI (1957), BRAUNSTEINER and THUMB (1958) and GRABENER (1967) worked on this problem using the direct enumeration method. Their results were in agreement and demonstrated the dependence of the count on the functional activity of the thyroid gland. In these investigations similar but much more pronounced reaction was observed with eosinophils. The infuence of thyroid hormones on basophil count could also be shown in experimental animals (BOSEILA and MOLTKE, 1958). Dried thyroid gland extract and L-thyroxine have been found to be as effective as D-thyroxine, leading to a basophil decrease even after one single application (INAGAKI 1957, TEDESCHI and CAVAZUTTI, 1959).

A direct depressive effect of thyrotrophin on the basophil count has been repeatedly discussed. CAVAZUTTI *et al.* (1959) and TEDESCHI and CAVAZUTTI (1959) observed a decrease in the basophil count following thyrotrophin application. D-thyroxine has a weak metabolic activity in man, its inhibitory effect on the pituitary being about half of that of L-thyroxine. At appropriate doses of D-thyroxine, clear inhibition of the pituitary system occurs with minimal peripheral activity (no significant changes in protein-bound iodine). After repeated doses of D-thyroxine the blood basophil count rose. Under similar trial conditions and with half as much L-thyroxine a significant rise was observed in the protein-bound iodine whereas the number of basophils changed insignificantly. On the basis of these observations, BOSEILA (1963) concluded that the effect of TSH on basophil counts is due to the hormonal activity of the thyroid gland.

To some extent the basophil count seems to reflect the functional condition of the thyroid gland. Treatment with thyroid extract, thyroxine, and triiodothyronine causes the basophils to decrease. This tendency to decrease indicates a reverse check on the other parameters of the thyroid function, for example, protein-bound iodine and basal metabolic rate (INAGAKI, 1957; CAVAZUTTI *et al.*, 1959; TEDESCHI *et al.*, 1959; GRABENER 1967). Thyrostatic treatment of a hyperactive thyroid gland with basophilic leukopenia correspondingly leads to an increase in the basophil count. The basophil count increases while the basal metabolic rate and the protein-bound iodine decrease. The type of thyrostatic therapy (potassium perchlorate, radioactive iodine, partial thyroidectomy, etc.) has no influence upon the quantitative depression of the basophils.

The depressive effect of thyroid upon blood basophils, which has been confirmed in later reports (THONNARD-NEUMANN, 1961; PETROVA, 1966; ARASE, 1969), must be considered as well-established. The mechanisms by which thyroxine acts on these cells, however, remain obscure.

b) Pituitary and Adrenal Hormones

Corticosterones cause a fall in basophil count, as shown by CODE *et al.* (1954) following oral administration of 200 mg cortisone for 3 days. A single application of 400 mg cortisone produced the same result. In all 8 cases, the decrease in eosinophils was markedly greater than the drop in basophil counts. OSADA (1954) reported similar results with ACTH. KELEMAN and BIKICH (1956) using 200 to 250 mg cortisone found a 90 to 100% fall in eosinophils whereas basophils fell to 50% of the initial value.

THONNARD-NEUMANN (1958) injected 10 healthy women with 20 – 40 I. U. depot zinc-ACTH and found within 24 h a significant decrease in basophils. The suppressive effect of ACTH in this experiment, however, could not be attributed to its direct effect on the basophils, for the same treatment failed to influence the blood basophil count in two female patients with adrenal insufficiency (BOSEILA, 1958 a, b). In this respect, rabbits (BOSEILA, 1958 a, b) react like man (TATAI and OSADA, 1957; BOSEILA and UHRBRAND, 1958; GRABENER, 1966; 1967).

The suppressive effect of corticosteroids upon the basophil count is a good experimental model for the study of the peripheral kinetics of these cells. Basopenia is especially pronounced 4 h after a single injection of ACTH; this state lasts for about 8 h, and 24 h after the injection the initial value is again reached. To maintain low values for a long time, depot forms have to be given (PADAWER and GORDON, 1954; HAMMERSTONE *et al.*, 1956; LABENDZINSKI and BROZOZOWSKA, 1957; BOSEILA, 1958; THONNARD-NEUMANN, 1958; 1961; TEDESCHI and CAVAZUTTI, 1959; BOSEILA, 1963; FRICK and KONRAD, 1963; 1964; PETROVA, 1966; SHELLEY and PARNES, 1965).

The level of histamine in the blood falls as basopenia occurs (CODE, 1956; KELEMAN and BIKICH, 1956; CODE and MITCHELL, 1957). In contrast to these findings in healthy persons, ACTH and glucocorticosteroids fail to exert any effect on basophils and blood histamine in patients with myeloproliferative diseases.

c) Sex Hormones

Very few studies have been carried out on the effect of sex hormones on blood basophils. Some authors believe that women have a higher basophil count than men; others deny this. A fall in blood basophils was observed by ALBRITTON (1953), POTUZHEK *et al.* (1959) and BOSEILA (1963) during pregnancy in women, and BOSEILA (1959) reported similar findings in pregnant rabbits. THONNARD-NEUMANN (1954; 1958) reported that basophil counts tended to increase in the last premenstrual week and fell rapidly at the time of ovulation. Estrogens are reported to evoke a marked rise in the basophil count whereas progesterone should induce basophil leukopenia. The number of blood basophils showed good correlation with an increase in the exfoliative tendency of the superficial cells in the vaginal smears. This finding is in agreement with the results of BOSEILA (1959) and POTUZHEK *et al.*, (1959).

A drop in the blood basophil count has been reported 12 h after copulation in rabbits and is assumed by some authors to be a sign of successful ovulation (THONNARD-NEUMANN, 1958; BOSEILA, 1959 a, b; ZACHARIAE, *et al.*, 1958). They claim that at this time there is a strong migration of blood basophils from the oviduct vessels into the surrounding tissue of the recently ruptured ovarian follicles with consequent accumulation in the corpus luteum. We were unable to confirm these results. According to POTUZHEK *et al.* (1959), testosterone does not influence the blood basophil count.

d) Insulin

A significant fall in basophil count was observed several hours after a subcutaneous or intravenous injection of insulin in rabbits (YANAGIHARA, 1958; BOSEILA, 1963). The blood basophil count has been reported to be significantly higher in people with diabetes mellitus than in normal people (BRAUNSTEINER and THUMB, 1958 a, b). This, however, may not necessarily be due to the direct effect of insulin, but rather secondary to the altered metabolic situation.

e) Other Factors

Changes in the number of basophils can be due to other causes besides hormonal effects. Some diseases have been found to be accompanied by basophil leukocytosis or basopenia. In such cases, even if a direct relationship between the disease and the hormonal balance cannot always be established, a pathogenetic connection is quite likely.

Basophil leukocytosis has been described in the chronic phase of drug and food allergies, erythroderma, psoriasis arthropathica, and spondylarthritis ankylopoetica (Shelley and Parnes, 1965; Westerhoff, 1966), colitis ulcerosa (Juhlin, 1963), and chronic tuberculosis (Fossati, 1950). The same is said to occur just before the onset of an attack of bronchial asthma (Kimura *et al.,*). Thrombocytopenia, possibly induced by a hyperimmune mechanism, is also reported to be associated with an increase in the basophil count (Braunsteiner and Thumb, 1958). In the acute eruptive phase of allergic urticaria, a massive decrease in blood basophils has been observed (Rorsman, 1957; Rorsman and Rosengren, 1958; Bersani, 1959; Meneghini and Levi, 1958; 1959).

Stress and shock, apart from any underlying pathogenetic mechanisms, also induce a fall in basophil count, as has been observed in the acute phase of infectious diseases, in myocardial infarction, after massive radiation, in circulatory failure caused by massive bleeding, in cases of acute pancreatitis, and in sterile inflammations after operations (Morelle, 1931; Frick and Konrad, 1963; Frick and Frick, 1966; Thonnard-Neumann *et al.,* 1969; Charton, 1969).

A marked increase in basophil count has been claimed to occur with hyperlipidemia (Braunsteiner *et al.,* 1965; Kehnscherper and Blau, 1966;

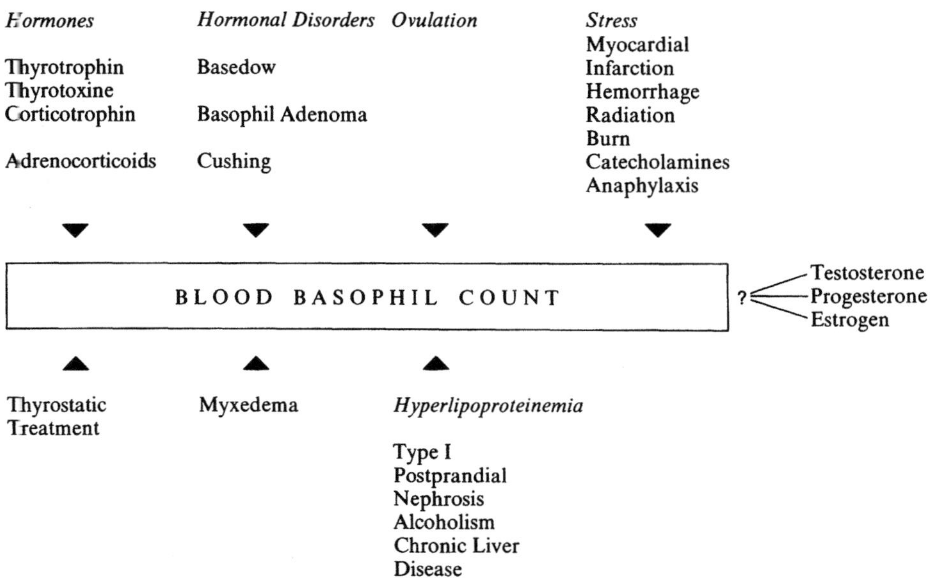

Fig. 2. Survey of factors influencing peripheral basophil count

LENNERT and PARWARESCH, 1970). According to these authors, the underlying mechanism giving rise to basophilia in such disorders as myxedema, diabetes mellitus, nephrotic syndrome, and gout, is the associated hyperlipidemia. A schematic survey of the factors influencing peripheral basophil count is presented in Fig. 2.

II. Light-Microscopic Morphology

In blood smears from normal subjects, stained with the usual panoptic techniques like PAPPENHEIM, GIEMSA, LEISHMAN, and WRIGHT, the blood basophils appear as coarsely granulated leukocytes, 14 to 18 μ in diameter. FREDRICK and MOLONEY (1959) referred to them as the smallest of all granulocytes. LENNERT (1961) stated that human basophils attain an average diameter of 8 to 14 μ.

The measured size of blood basophils as reported in the literature cannot be accepted without reservation. The size of blood basophils, as of other myelogenous blood cells, depends upon their adhesiveness as well as upon the thickness of the smear. In relatively thin blood smears on defatted slides, fairly spread out basophils with a diameter of 18 μ and more are observed. Thick blood smears, or smears prepared on a siliconized slide, show significantly smaller blood basophils, rounded and spherical, embedded in a thick serum emulsion. The basophil nucleus is poorly segmented and appears to be partially covered with granules or even completely submerged. This is especially so in the case of rounded cells in a thick smear. ARNETH (1920 a, b) described the nucleus as S- or K-shaped and divided the blood basophils into 4 different types according to the extent of the segmentations of their nuclei. LENNERT (1961) described the nucleus of the blood basophil as being irregularly segmented, resembling a clover leaf. In our experience, mature blood basophils display a heavily twisted nucleus with a small closed knot and a large open knot, resembling a figure of 8. In poorly spread cells the nucleus takes on a clover-leaf shape, consisting of three segments. Blood basophils with pronounced nuclear segmentation, as described by ROHR for other granulocytes, however, seldom occur. The chromatin is somewhat looser in texture than in neutrophil nuclei. The intensity of the nucleus staining with basic dyes rarely equals that of other granulocytes. Nucleoli very rarely appear in mature blood basophils. Semi-thin sections stained with the usual basic dyes are suitable for judging basophil nuclei in respect to shape and chromatin density. If toluidine blue solution are used, basophil nuclei are only distinguishable in blood smears stained in buffered dye solutions of pH over 4. The intensity of the nucleus coloration increases at higher pH values. A reduction of the nuclear coloration by panoptic staining, for example, for the selective discernment of granules or for autoradiographic examination, can be effected by pretreating the preparation with various organic solvents and diluted detergents such as a concentrated solution of N-cetylpyridinium chloride, which in addition serves as a potent fixative for the water-soluble basophil granules.

The striking feature of the blood basophil, on which all authors agree, as highly typical, is the metachromatic coloration of its granules to which blood basophils owe their discovery. Because of their high affinity for basic dyes, EHRLICH (1879) called them gamma granules in contrast to the acidophilic alpha and neutrophilic beta granules.

The literature is in agreement over the shape, size and numbers of granules. Most authors describe them as rounded (MAXIMOW, 1906; FERRATA and GOLINELLI, 1910; MICHELS, 1938) or oval (MISSMAHL, 1965) and finely reticular in structure. All three forms may appear in the same cell. The sharply defined rounded or oval granules display highly compact structures. In comparison with eosinophil granules they are quite irregularly distributed. Often the compact, round-to-oval granules appear in the periphery of the cytoplasm and the reticular structures in the immediate vicinity of the nucleus. Their size is given in the literature as 0.3 to 0.8 μ (ACKERMAN and BELLIOS, 1955) or 0.2 to 1 μ (BESSIS, 1973). It varies according to the quality of the fixative used. In properly fixed smears the middle-sized, compact granules predominate. Inferior preparations show basophils with few granules or with single, unsharply defined ones. In such cases the cytoplasmic background takes on a diffuse, pale reddish colour.

The smear technique itself, as well as the time span between the blood sampling and the completion of the smear – which must be as short as possible – are decisive factors in these morphological variations. Characteristic artifacts are seen in smears obtained from stored blood samples. Fine filamentous metachromatic structures in the area around the blood basophils are frequently observed in such smears. Typically, the direction of their spreading corresponds to the direction in which the smear has been established. We often observe this in smears of leukocyte concentrations.

Ever since the discovery of blood basophils by PAUL EHRLICH in 1879 the question of the solubility of their granular contents has been the subject of lively discussion. EHRLICH (1879), WESTPHAL (1891), MICHAELIS (1902), MAXIMOW (1906), and TOUKÉ (1929) in their fundamental works repeatedly referred to the solubility of basophil granules in water.

UNDRITZ (1946) maintained that basophil granules are more readily soluble in methanol than in water. LENNERT (1952) and LENNERT and SCHUBERT (1960) were unable to reproduce the granulolytic effect of methanol on smears and tissue sections and therefore concluded that the granulolytic action of commercially available methanol is due to traces of water. Today it is generally accepted that the granules of human basophils are extremely water-soluble. This is due to a genuine solubility principle and is not the consequence of a hypoosmolar treatment. If unfixed, air-dried blood smears are treated with sodium chloride solutions of increasing osmolarity, e.g. with concentrations of 0.2 to 2.0%, basophils in all smears undergo total granulolysis. In addition, variations in pH do not interfere with the granulolytic effect of water (PARWARESCH and LENNERT, 1967).

In our experience immature blood basophils contain extremely water-soluble granules, but only under normal conditions. Leukemic blood basophils and their immature forms may sometimes contain water-resistant granule variants (LENNERT, 1961). The contradictory reports in the literature might be explained by the fact that some investigators, having studied leukemic blood basophils, also drew conclusions from them about normal blood basophils.

Blood basophils lacking metachromatic granules can hardly be reliably recognized, so that adequate preservation of these cells must precede staining. We studied a number of common fixatives with regard to their capability of stabilizing the metachromatic basophil structures. Along with SELYE (1965), our criterion for a useful fixative is the absolute water resistance of the metachromatic substances. To test the degree of stability obtained, the fixed blood smears were either placed for 1 h under running tap water or put in a jar with water overnight. While this precaution may seem superfluous for routine histochemical procedures, it is essential in special instances, for example, in radioautography. We use for the preparation of metachromatic basophil granules and testing various fixing solutions 3-day-old, air-dried blood smears from basophil-rich leukocyte concentrations (PARWARESCH, 1968). Osmium tetroxide, formaldehyde, and diluted or commercial ethyl and methyl alcohols, as well as the fixation solutions given

Table 1. Effect of different fixatives on human blood basophils

Fixatives	Degree of granule preservation
Osmium tetroxide:	
solution 0.5 – 2%	±
vapor 4%	–
Formaldehyde:	
dilute	–
vapor	–
Ethyl and methyl alcohol:	
80 – 98%	–
freshly distilled	+
Methanol-formaldehyde (v/v):	
2 : 1 (SCHAFFER, 1908)	–
4 : 1 (SELYE, 1965)	±
9 : 1 (KAPLOW, 1950; SCHUBERT, 1958)	+ +
Lead acetate (4%, aqueous) (HOLMGREN, 1937; SYLVEN *et al.*, 1956, LENNERT and SCHUBERT, 1960)	+ +
Fixatives described by:	
MOTA *et al.* (1954)	+ +
PARWARESCH (1967)	+ +
Cetyltrimethylammonium bromide or Cetylpyridinium chloride	
1% aqueous	+ +
1% in methanol-formaldehyde (9 : 1) (PARWARESCH, 1972)	+ + +
5-aminoacridine hydrochloride	
0.4% in 50% ethanol	+ + +

by MÜLLER, ORTH and SCHRIDDE, ZENKER, FLEMMING, HELLY, MAXIMOW and CARNOY, and the fresh fixation described by WEIDENREICH (1905) all proved unsatisfactory for the fixation of human blood basophils. The best results were achieved by using N-cetylpyridinium chloride or 5-aminoacridine hydrochloride as dilute solutions (Table 1). Fixation time was 10 to 30 min.

III. Phase-Contrast Microscopic Morphology

Phase-contrast microscopic investigation of blood basophils has been carried out by a number of authors (FERRATA and GOLINELLI, 1910; JOLLY, 1928; WEIDENREICH, 1929; CUNNINGHAM and TOMPKIN, 1930; ACKERMAN and BELLIOS, 1955; RIND, 1958; ACKERMAN, 1963; MISSMAHL, 1964 a, c, 1965 a, b; SHIBATA *et al.*, 1966; BESSIS, 1973).

Identification of blood basophils in live observation with a phase-contrast microscope presents certain difficulties, as their granules display no clear anisotrophy and their scant numbers make them extremely difficult to spot. With respect to their morphology – especially as regards the shape and size of the nuclei and the distribution of granules – the results largely confirm those obtained by light microscopy. The nucleus is seen to be segmented, bearing coarse chromatin clumps. No nucleoli are observed. The cytoplasm appears as a narrow, coarsely granulated rim. Other cell organelles like mitochondria are regularly present. They appear predominantly as oblong or oval isotropic structures about 0.2 to 0.4 μ in length.

The blood basophils show very characteristic movements (JOLLY, 1928; MAXIMOW, 1929; ACKERMAN and BELLIOS, 1955). Under the phase-contrast microscope, living basophils differ from the other granulocytes in that they move very slowly. The nucleus – or part of it – surrounded by a hard-to-distinguish plasma rim, precedes the other parts of the cell (ACKERMAN and BELLIOS, 1955; WOLF-JÜRGENSEN 1968). The speed of this directed movement is nearly 12 μ/min according to SHIBATA *et al.* (1966) or about half that of the neutrophils.

The capability of blood basophils for phagocytosis has not been systematically investigated. RINGOEN (1923) could obsere only very slight phagocytotic activity in guinea-pig basophils following experimentally produced basophilia. DESAGA *et al.* (1971), who carried out a similar experiment on humans, failed to confirm RINGOEN's results. They found no evidence of phagocytosis in the freshly emigrated basophils in skin biopsy specimens studied light- and electron-microscopically. In an effort to establish the normal range of variation of human basophil granules, we examined both semi-thin and ultra-thin sections of over 600 blood basophils. We found no evidence for the incorporation of foreign bodies in these cells (PARWARESCH *et al.*, 1976). Results reported by other authors seem to be in good agreement with these findings (SHIBATA *et al.*, 1966).

SAMPSON and ARCHER (1967) made phase-contrast optical studies of blood basophils in leukocyte concentrates and reported that on glass blood basophils started to develop an ameboid motility after a time lapse of 5 min.

The time lapse was reduced when polystrene coated slides were used. After incubation of basophils from blood group 0 with suspended erythrocytes from group A in an anti-A serum, the blood basophils were observed to move toward the corresponding lyzed erythrocytes. Upon the addition of fresh immune sera, active phagocytosis of the lyzed erythrocytes through the group 0 blood basophils was observed. The phagocytic activity increased after the addition of antiserum-treated erythrocytes that had been stored at 0° C for 30 min. CHARCOT-LEYDEN crystals were sometimes observed in the degenerating blood basophils. The incubation of blood basophils with zymosan also led to the incorporation of zymosan particles.

FORKNER (1900), SABIN (1923), PHILIPSBORN (1930), and HEDENIUS (1940) were among the first to systematically investigate vital and/or supravital stained blood basophils.

Among the dyes used, the purely basic dyes have proved effective due to their great affinity for blood basophil polyanions. The best results are obtained with dilute toluidine-blue solutions. Under proper conditions toluidine blue gives a metachromatic coloration of basophil granules, enabling them to be distinguished from other leukocytes. For the supravital staining of basophil granules, thionine, methylene blue, Nile blue sulfate, brilliant cresyl blue, and neutral red have been used in addition to toluidine-blue (HAMMAR, 1912; SABIN, 1923). Thionine and brilliant cresyl blue give similar results to toluidine blue. Nile blue sulfate stains the cytoplasm more intensely than the other dyes.

Neutral red, usually in conjunction with Janus green, has often been used in supravital staining of blood basophils (SIMPSON, 1921 a, b, c; 1922 a, b; SABIN, 1923; 1932; MASUGI, 1926; TOMPKINS, 1932; 1955; GABL, 1960 and others). The basophils turn a strong yellow-orange. A preferential accumulation of the dye occurs in the basophil granules. The blood basophils are then easily distinguished from the other types of granulocytes (SHIBATA *et al.*, 1966).

Methylene blue proved unsuitable as a supravital stain for basophils, and toluidine blue is best used in very dilute form. HEDENIUS (1940) used a 3.8% sodium citrate solution which contained 0.02% toluidine blue. MISSMAHL (1964) recommended a 0.5% solution to be mixed with citrate blood in the ratio 2 : 10. The concentration of the dye has a decisive influence on the results. Concentrations below 0.02% give too weak a stain, while too high a concentration results in over-staining and will obscure the metachromasia. The incubation temperature is also critical. A much longer exposure time is needed at room temperature. Unduly long incubation leads to autolytic alterations. With a 0.02% toluidine blue solution at room temperature, 45 min incubation would be needed to achieve results equal to those obtained after 30 min at 37° C. When toluidine blue is correctly applied in supravital staining, the erythrocytes remain unstained. The leukocytes generally, turn bluish and the cytoplasm almost always takes on a faint bluish colour; the nuclei can hardly be distinguished. The basophil granules stain strongly red to violet and look like coarse lumps of cytoplasm. If the slide is heated to 60° C the metachromasia disappears, appearing again upon cooling. The results achieved by light microscopy to a large extent confirm those revealed by phase-contrast microscopic investigations. The kinematic documentation of basophil behavior has afforded a good insight into the kinetics of their granule discharge.

With polarization optics, blood basophils are non-refractive (MAXIMOW, 1929; MICHELS, 1938; ACKERMAN and BELLIOS, 1955; SELYE, 1965). Establishing an elliptical compensation, they show a slight degree of anisotropy in an unstained form with a gear variance of 1 μ (MISSMAHL, 1964 a, b, c). By addition of a supravital stain it is possible to strengthen the weak anisotropy in basophil granules. This is throught to result from the parallel deposition of dye micelles on the granule matrix. The blood basophils will then glow red to green between intersecting poles (MISSMAHL, 1965 a, b). The granules of neutrophils and eosinophils behave isotropically and are therefore easily differentiated from the basophil granules (MISSMAHL, 1965 a, b). The circular arrangement of parallel dye micelles and the occurrence of negative polar crossings signify, according to MISSMAHL, that the basophil granules are composed of numerous stratified, ellipsoidic layers in a concentric arrangement.

IV. Electron-Optical Morphology

Few electron-optical studies have been conducted on blood basophils and most of them concern animal blood basophils (GREY and BEISELE, 1955; PEASE, 1955; 1956; OSAKO, 1959; POLLICARD *et al.*, 1959; WINQUIST, 1963; WETZEL *et al.*, 1967; SPIECER *et al.*, 1968). As in light-microscopic studies of blood basophils, the fixatives commonly used in ultrastructural studies (osmic acid etc.) do not ensure satisfactory preservation of these cells and their granules (ZUCKER-FRANKLIN, 1967; MIURA *et al.*, 1968).

KAUTZ and DE MARSH (1953) carried out the first electron-microscopic examinations of normal human blood basophils. They used a 10% gelatin solution in order to process the leukocyte layers (buffy coat) together. A 0.25% osmic acid solution of pH 7.35 was used as the fixative and only a few basophils could be observed. The basophils displayed an indented nucleus and meager, electron-dense, homogeneous granules up to 1 μ in diameter surrounded by a thin membrane. Mitochondria and abundant osmophilic spherical structures, interpreted as lipid enclosures, were also encountered. BRAUNSTEINER and PAKESH (1957) used a 1% osmic acid solution and identified the basophil granules as rounded, electron-dense, homogeneous structures without any definite membrane. The techniques so far mentioned have not given satisfactory results. A far better method is that of ZUCKER-FRANKLIN (1967), who used a 3% glutaraldehyde solution in a phosphate buffer of pH 7.4. The addition of 1% acrolein with subsequent fixing in 2% osmic acid solution resulted in a far better preservation of the basophil granules. For the electron-microscopic investigation ultrathin sections were contrasted with either uranyl acetate (WATSON, 1958) or lead hydroxide (MILLONIG, 1961). In such preparations the basophil granulocytes appear as polymorphonuclear cells with a coarse nuclear chromatin which seems to be connected with the nuclear membrane pores. The granules are irregularly dispersed and present considerable variations in size, number, and shape. An electron-dense lamellary structure consisting of several concentric membranes has been observed within the granules. These structures have been referred to as myelin figures or KURLOFF bodies. WATANABE *et al.* (1967) showed many intermediate stages between intact granules and myelin figures.

Even though the fixatives hitherto used in ultrastructural studies of blood basophils cannot be considered optimal, many new results have been brought out by submicroscopic studies of these cells. Electron microscopy has proved highly valuable in detecting the ultrastructural alterations caused by functional activities. Furthermore, neoplastic aberrations of blood basophils which eluded clarification by light microscopy are now better understood on the basis of submicroscopic information.

We studied over 600 basophils in blood samples of 10 healthy donors (PARWARESCH *et al.,* 1976). Preliminary studies were undertaken to investigate the influence of various fixatives on the general morphology and preservation of basophil granules. The best results were achieved with the solutions suggested by ZUCKER-FRANKLIN (1967), i.e. 3% glutaraldehyde and 1% acrolein in a 0.1 M sodium cacodylate buffer of pH 7.3. This solution renders fairly satisfactory conservation of basophil granules along with good general structural preservation (Table 2).

A survey of our results concerning the normal electron-optical morphology of human basophils is given below.

Table 2. Effect of different fixatives on general morphology and preservation of basophil granules as seen in the electron microscope

Fixative	General Cell Morphology	Preservation of Granules
1 – Glutaraldehyde (5%) in 0.1 M-sodium cacodylate buffer (pH 7.3)	+ + + +	+ +
2 – Glutaraldehyde-formalaldehyde (KARNOVSKY, 1965)	+ + +	+
3 – Glutaraldehyde (5%) and calcium acetate (2%) in 0.1 M sodium cacodylate buffer (pH 7.3)	+ +	+ +
4 – Glutaraldehyde (5%) and N-cetylpyridinium chloride (0.2%) in 0.1 M sodium cacodylate buffer (pH 7.3)	+	+
5 – Glutaraldehyde (5%) and 5-aminoacridine (2%) in 0.1 M sodium cacodylate buffer (pH 7.3)	+	+ +
6 – Glutaraldehyde and acrolein (1%) in 0.1 M sodium cacodylate buffer (pH 7.3) (ZUCKER-FRANKLIN, 1967)	+ + +	+ + +

To determine granule size, 500 sectional planes of granules with the same final magnification were measured and the diameters interpolated. With the aid of a mathematical procedure, the distribution curve of the interpolated diameters was compared with that of the "true" diameters calculated on the basis of the following integral formula (BACH, 1959):

$$g(r)=2r\int_{r}^{\infty}\frac{f(R)d(R)}{\sqrt{R^2-r^2}}+\delta f(r).$$

The size distribution curves of the granules were obtained from the measured distribution curves of the sectional planes of the granules observed in electron micrographs.

g(r) is the dispersion of the radii of the circular sections, f(r) is the dispersion of the sphere radii, and δ the thickness of the section. f(R) is the dispersion function of the distribution of the sphere radii, as defined by the values of its function at n equidistant values 1, . . . n of the sphere radii R.

This equation was worked out on a computer by BRÖCKER (1971). During the computations the function f(R) proved extremely sensitive to very small variations in g(R). The variation of frequency in particular granule sections can thus be of only qualitative interest, if this computation is extended to take in curves that delimit the span of the error g(R) (BRÖCKER, 1971).

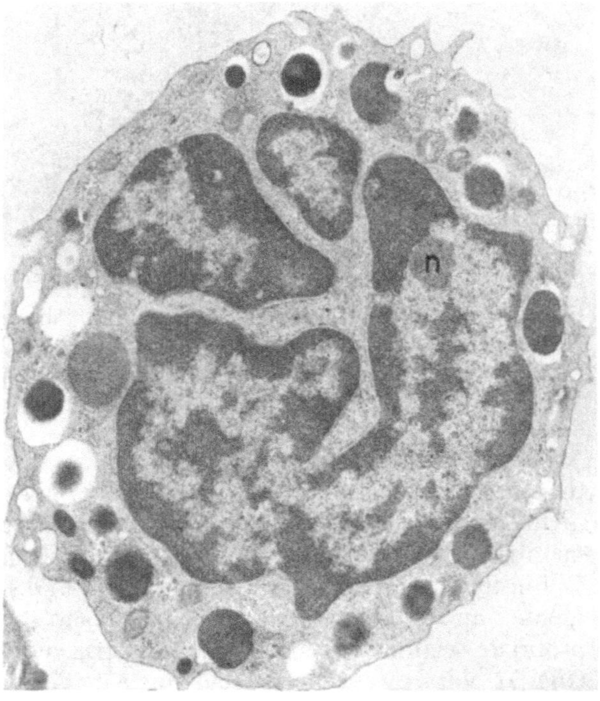

Fig. 3. The extremely rare incidence of a nucleolus (*n*) in the nucleus of a normal basophil from the peripheral blood; ×13,100

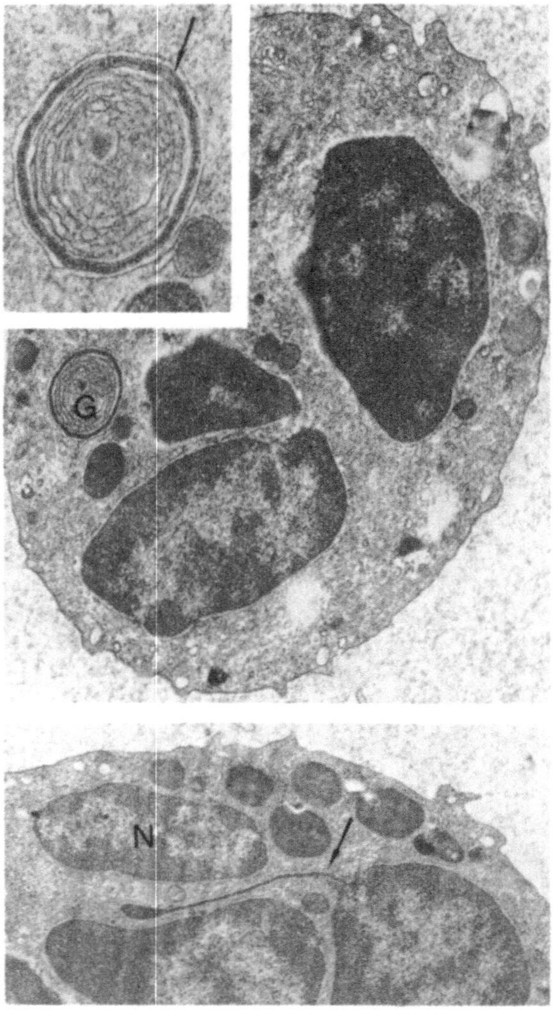

a

b

Fig. 4 a and b. (a) Peripheral blood basophil. Above: Tubular prolongation of nucleus (arrow) surrounding the Golgi complex (*G*); ×27,300. (b) Membrane-like prolongation of nucleus (arrow) between two unaltered nuclear segments (*N*); ×13,100

Ultrastructure of basophil nucleus. Because of its irregular segmentation, the nucleus of the blood basophil is generally cut into 1 to 4 different segments (Fig. 3) with medium chromatin-dense zones along the inner nuclear membrane. Coarse, lumpy aggregations of chromatin are irregularly strewn within the karyoplasm. The euchromatin looks coarsely granulated or filamented and in the nuclear pores reaches to the nuclear membrane. In appropriate sections one small electron-opaque nucleolus is occasionally seen (Fig. 3). Very rarely there occur nuclear indentations or "nuclear pockets" (Fig. 4); these form on the furthermost regions of the nuclear segment. They show small nuclear striations marked off by a proper nuclear membrane

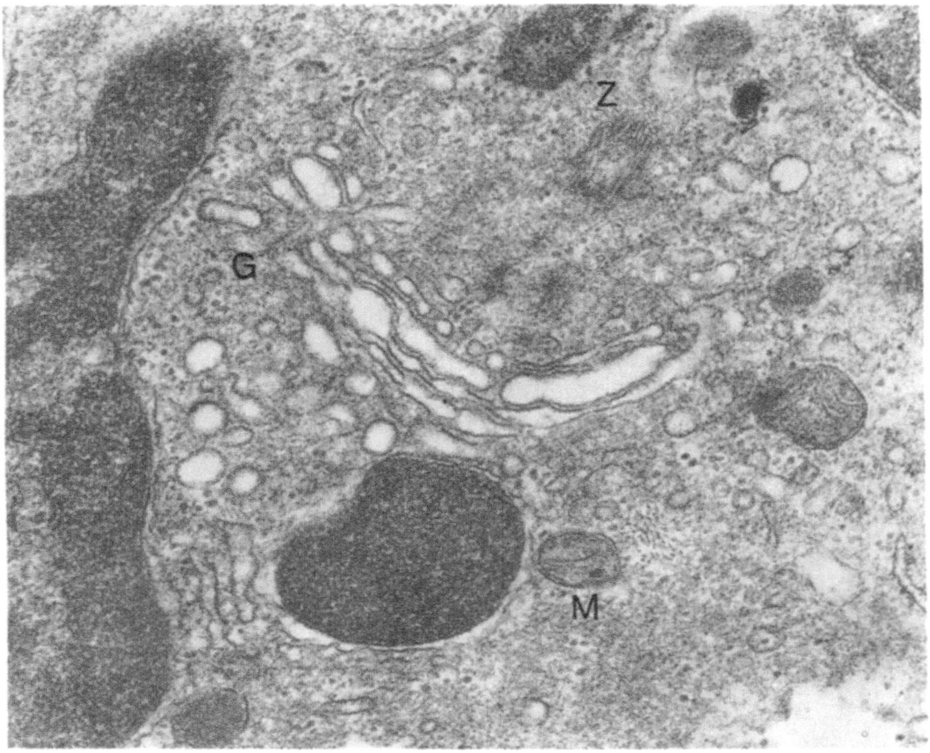

Fig. 5. Golgi complex of a blood basophil. Obliquely cut tubulovesicular structures (*G*) concentrically arranged around the centriole (*Z*). Mitochondria (*M*); ×55,700

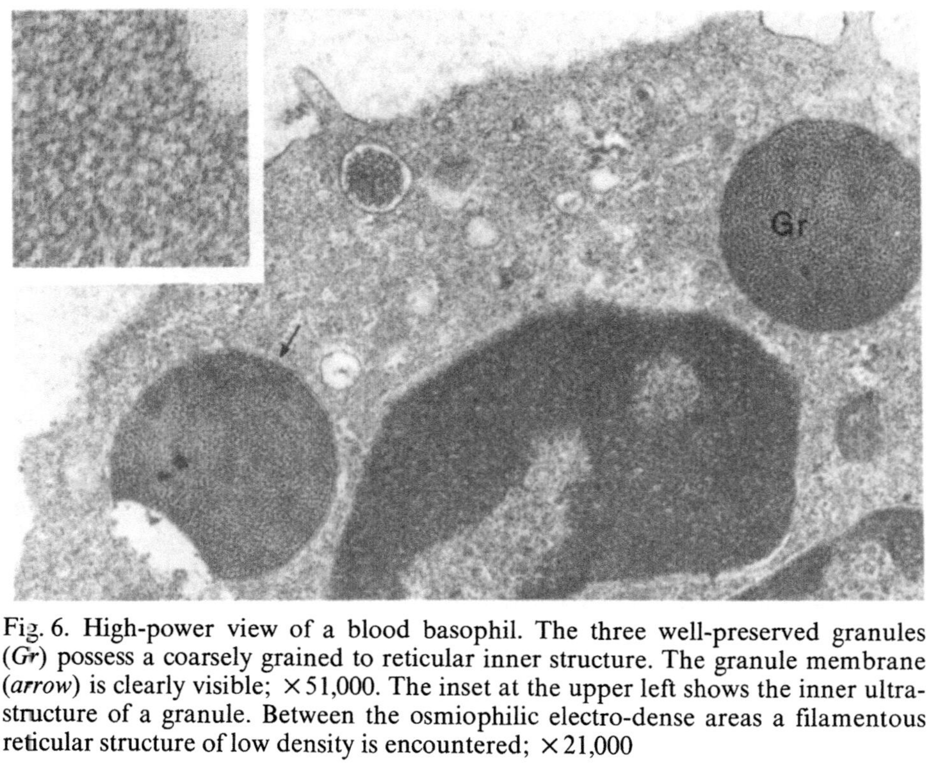

Fig. 6. High-power view of a blood basophil. The three well-preserved granules (*Gr*) possess a coarsely grained to reticular inner structure. The granule membrane (*arrow*) is clearly visible; ×51,000. The inset at the upper left shows the inner ultrastructure of a granule. Between the osmiophilic electro-dense areas a filamentous reticular structure of low density is encountered; ×21,000

and often surrounding large areas of cytoplasm. A cytoplasmatic area surrounded by nuclear pockets can include partly or completely cytoplasmic organelles. We observed filamental inclusions and Golgi vesicles, both of which were surrounded by nuclear pockets. Among 600 electron-optically observed blood basophils, only five exhibited nuclear pockets. The causes and the exact mechanisms of formation of nuclear pockets are still unclear. Since they are much more common in cases of leukemia, they may represent a degenerative phenomenon or damage to the nuclear membrane.

Ultrastructure of basophil cytoplasm. In well-preserved basophils the groundplasm appears fine-grained and is of moderate electron density. Smooth endoplasmic reticulum occurs sometimes in basophils, and can be

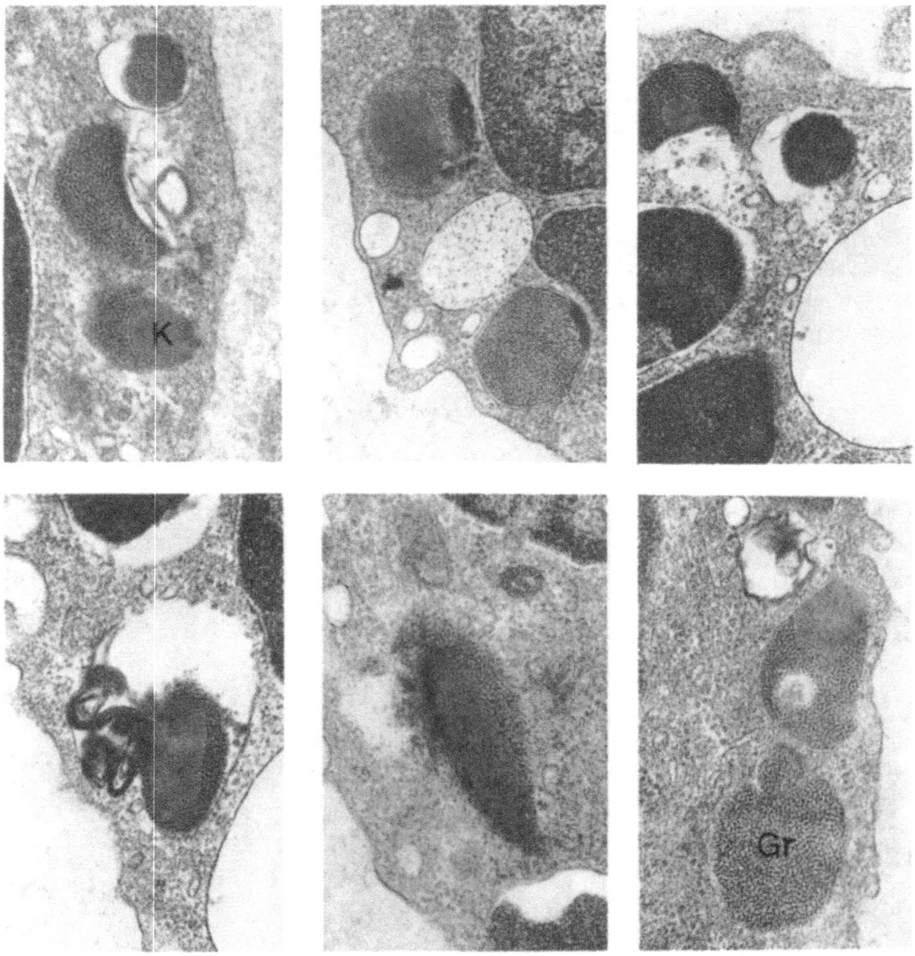

Fig. 7. Spectrum of ultrastructural variation of basophil granules. The granules (*Gr*) are well preserved and often show a concentric arrangement of their grainy intragranular structures. Most of the granules show a homogeneous, crystalline central zone (*K*); ×21,800

dilated to show a cisternlike form. Upon examination of a large number of blood basophils, it is often possible to find short ergastoplasm tubes. The Golgi field is well developed in some cells (Fig. 5); it consists of tubular or vesicular structures in polar arrangement around the centriole. Electron-dense spherules are seen in some vesicles. Mitochondria are a regular feature of the basophil cytoplasm. In well-preserved specimens mitochondria of the meager type are present. Long mitochondria with clearly identifiable cristae occur very seldom. Single ribosomes are regularly observed, usually strewn about within the cytoplasm. The so-called tonofilaments, or bundles of fine fibrils of moderate density, which occur in other granulocytes, are seldom observed in blood basophil cytoplasm. Glycogen appears as rounded, compact grains of considerable electron density in basophil cytoplasm.

The cell membrane is usually smooth and possesses only a few single, coarse offshoots. Pinocytotic vesicles occur in many basophils, and empty vacuoles about 0.2 μ in diameter can sometimes be seen close to the inner surface of the cell membrane. They can be clearly distinguished from the empty vacuoles caused by dissolved basophil granules. It has not been possible to determine whether these longish vacuoles represent collapsed pinocytotic blisters or other structures.

Ultrastructure of basophil granules. Specific granules in blood basophil cytoplasm show up as very characteristic structures when electron-optically

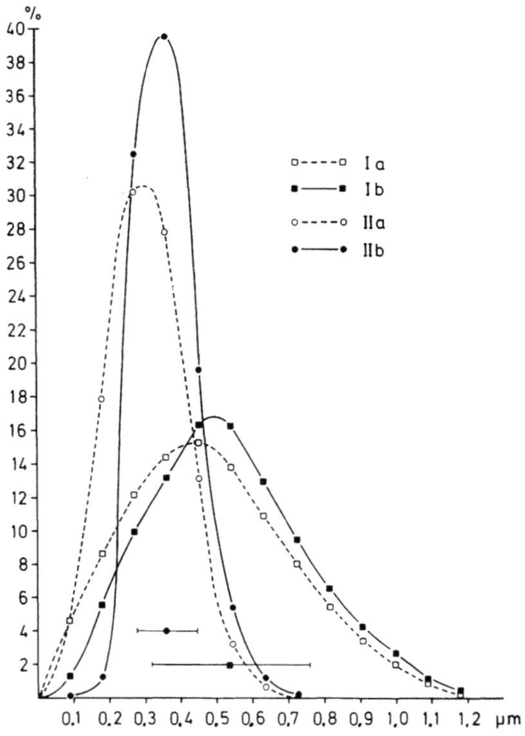

Fig. 8. Graph showing the electron optically obtained diameters of the granules of normal blood basophils (*I a*) and the correspondingly computed "true" granule size (*I b*). Note the average size ($\bar{X}$ = 0.54 μm) and the considerable variation (s = ±21). Compare the same data (*II a* and *b*) for the granules of leukemic blood basophils (0.35 ± 0.08 μm). Ordinate: Number of granules as %. Abscissa: Granule size in μm

observed. They are quite electron-dense when in a good state of preservation, usually round or slightly oval, sometimes with an obvious indentation and strewn unevenly throughout the cytoplasm. They possess a plainly recognizable unit membrane. Though granules within one cell may present varying degrees of density, the variation is about the same in all cells of the same blood samples. The specific granules possess a similar and typical inner structure of grainy appearance (Figs. 6 and 7), measuring about 100 to

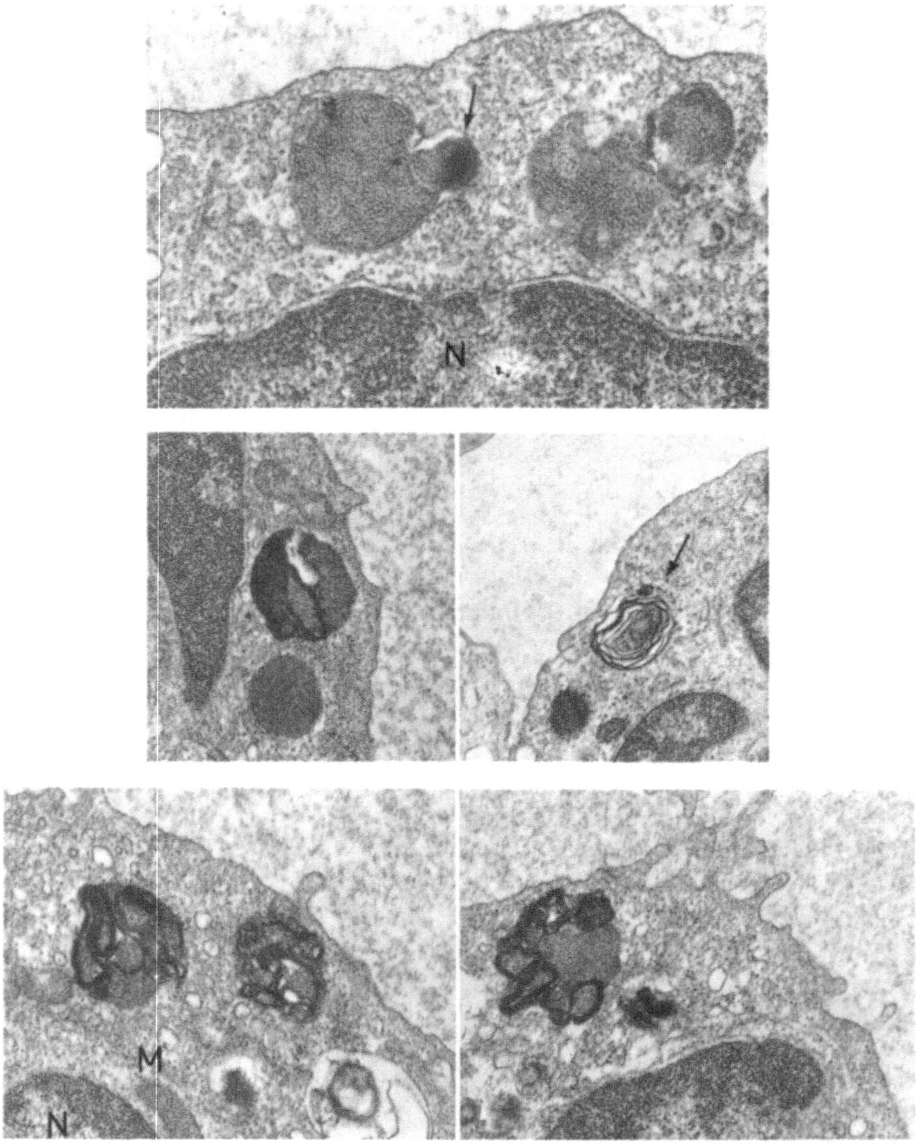

Fig. 9. So-called myeline figures (*arrows*) arising singly or in multiples from the specific basophil granules. Nucleus (*N*), mitochondria (*M*); ×24,600

150 Å. These particles are arranged concentrically and are irregularly dispersed toward the granule center. The space between these particles has a somewhat lower optical density. Computations made from sample measurements of the granule section surfaces, assuming the actual granule volume to represent a sphere, gave an average diameter of 0.54 μ with a standard deviation of ± 0.21 μ (Fig. 8).

The state of preservation of the granules varies considerably according to the fixative used. Besides well-defined granules with grainy, electron-dense structures, there are also loosely-structured basophil granules with a fine reticular content of minor optical density within their membraneous border. Homogeneous polygonal crystalloid formations of medium density are observed in the center of some well-preserved granules (Fig. 7). Forty percent of all normal basophils display one or two membrane whorls within or attached to obviously well-preserved granules (Fig. 9).

It is possible that the use of glutaraldehyde as fixative alters the phospholipids, giving rise, to formation of such membraneous precipitates. They can be solitary or multiple. Some granules contain several myelin figures, giving the basophil granule a multicentric appearance. Membrane whorls have also been found in cells rich in membranes or phospholipids without any glutaraldehyde treatment. The exact mechanism of their formation is unclear. They are unlikely to be mere artifacts, especially since they occur in many basophils in great numbers. Poorly fixed basophils show a complete loss of intragranular structures.

References

Ackerman, G. A., Bellios, N. C.: A study of the morphology of the living cells of blood and bone marrow in vital films with the phase-contrast microscope. I. Normal blood and bone marrow. Blood **10,** 3 – 16 (1955).

Ackerman, G. A.: Cytochemical properties of the blood basophilic granulocytes. Ann. N. Y. Acad. Sci. **103,** 376 – 393 (1963).

Albritton, E. C.: Standard Values in Blood. London: Saunders Co. 1953.

Angeli, G., Tedeschi, G., Cavazzuti, F.: Il tasso dei basofili del sangue periferico nel soggetto normale, valutato con un nuovo metodo di conta diretta. Progr. med. (Napoli) **10,** 742 – 756 (1954).

Arase, S.: On the fundamental and clinical studies with respect to the number of circulating basophils and eosinophils. Iryo **23,** 306 – 317 (1969).

Arneth, F.: Die qualitative Blutlehre. Leipzig: Klinkhardt (1920 a).

Arneth, F.: Über das Mastzellenblutbild. Berlin: Klin. Wschr. **57,** 109 (1920 b).

Bach, G.: Über die Größenverteilung von Kugelschnitten in durchsichtigen Schnitten endlicher Dicke, S. 1 – 33, Bd. 57. Gießen: Mitt. Math. Seminar 1959.

Bersani, R. B.: The blood basophil in urticaria and other dermatoses. University of Zürich 1959.

Bessis, M.: Living Blood Cells and Their Ultrastructure. Springer-Verlag: Berlin-Heidelberg-New York 1973.

Boseila, A. W. A.: Influence of cortisone on the basophil granulocytes and the total white cell count in rabbit blood. Acta endocr. (Copenhagen) **29,** 253 – 256 (1958 a).

Boseila, A. W. A.: Influence of corticotrophin on the circulating basophils in the rabbit. Acta endocr. (Copenhagen) **29,** 355 – 360 (1958 b).

BOSEILA, A. W. A.: The normal count of basophil leucocytes in human blood. Acta med. scand. **163**, 525 – 529 (1959 a).

BOSEILA, A. W. A.: Variation in the blood-basophil count induced by sexual stimulation in the rabbit. Acta endocr. (Copenhagen) **30**, 477 – 480 (1959 b).

BOSEILA, A. W. A.: Normal count and physiological variability of rabbit blood basophils. Experientia (Basel) **15**, 149 – 150 (1959 c).

BOSEILA, A. W. A.: Hormonal influence on blood and tissue basophilic granulocytes. Ann. N. Y. Acad. Sci. **103**, 394 – 408 (1963 a).

BOSEILA, A. W. A.: Discussion on Boseila's paper. Ann. N. Y. Acad. Sci. **103**, 408 – 420 (1963 b).

BOSEILA, A. W. A., MOLTKE, E.: Influence of L-thyroxine on the circulating basophil leukocytes in rabbit. Acta endocr. (Copenhagen) **29**, 273 – 278 (1958).

BOSEILA, A. W. A., UHRBRAND, H.: Basophil-eosinophil relationship in human blood. Studies on the effect of ACTH. Acta endocr. (Copenhagen) **28**, 49 – 53 (1958).

BRAUNSTEINER, H., PAKESH, F.: Elektronenmikroskopische Untersuchungen der Granula menschlicher Leukocyten. Acta haemat. (Basel) **17**, 136 – 142 (1957).

BRAUNSTEINER, H., THUMB, N.: Quantitative Veränderungen der Blutbasophilen und ihre klinische Bedeutung. Acta haemat. (Basel) **20**, 339 – 349 (1958 a).

BRAUNSTEINER, H., THUMB, N.: Über quantitative Veränderungen der basophilen Leukocyten und ihre Stoffwechselbedeutung. Wien. Z. inn. Med. **39**, 285 – 288 (1958 b).

BRAUNSTEINER, H., SAILER, S., SANDHOFER, F.: The relationship between level of triglycerides in plasma and number of basophils in blood. Metabolism **14**, 1071 – 1075 (1965).

BRÖCKER, E.-B.: Die Lipidtropfen in der Nebennierenrinde der weiblichen Maus und Beziehungen ihrer Größenverteilungen zum Cyclus. Z. Zellforsch. **113**, 188 – 202 (1971).

CAMERADA, P., LEO, P.: Il tasso dei leucociti basofili nel sangue circolante di soggetti normali. Rass. med. sarda. **57**, 45 – 51 (1955 a).

CAMERADA, P., LEO, P.: Modificationi indotte dalla tiroxina sul tasso ematico dei leucociti basofili. Rass. med. sarda. **57**, 163 – 169 (1955 b).

CAVAZZUTI, F., TEDESCHI, G., ANGELI, G.: Rapporti tra funzionalità tiroidea e leucociti basofili. Min. Med. **50**, 2352 – 2358 (1959).

CHARTON, F.: Das weiße Blutbild nach Operationen. Dissertation, Kiel 1969.

CODE, C. F.: Eosinophils, basophils and platelets as histamine carriers. In: Ciba Found. Symp. Histamine. C. E. W. WOLSTENHOLME and C. M. O'CONNOR (eds.), London: Churchill 1956.

CODE, C. F., MITCHELL, R. G.: Histamine, eosinophils and basophils in the blood. J. Physiol. (Lond.) **136**, 449 – 468 (1957).

CODE, C. F., MITCHELL, R. G., KENNEDY, J. C.: The effect of cortisone on the number of circulating basophils and eosinophils: Is there a relationship between these cells? Proc. Mayo Clin. **29**, 200 – 204 (1954).

COOPER, J. K., CRUICKSHANK, C. N. D.: Improved method for direct counting of basophil leucocytes. J. clin. Path. **19**, 402 – 403 (1966).

CUNNINGHAM, R. S., TOMPKIN, E. H.: The supravital staining of normal human blood cells. Folia haemat. (Lpz.) **42**, 257 – 270 (1930).

DESAGA, J. F., PARWARESCH, M. R., MÜLLER-HERMELINK, H. K.: Die cytochemische Identifikation der Mastzellvorstufen bei der Ratte. Z. Zellforsch. **121**, 292 – 300 (1971).

DUNÉR, H., PERNOW, B.: Histamine and leucocytes in blood during muscular work in man. Scand. J. clin. Lab. Invest. **10,** 394 – 396 (1958).

EHRLICH, P.: Über die spezifischen Granulationen des Blutes. Arch. Anat. Physiol., Phys. Abt. **3,** 571 – 579 (1879).

FERRATA, A., GOLINELLI, A.: Sui globuli bianchi con granulazione basofili. Fol. clin. chim. Micros. Bologna 3, **2,** fasc. 5 (1910).

FORKNER, C. E.: Blood and bone marrow cells of the domestic fowl. 1900. Cited in: J. exp. Med. **50,** 121 – 141 (1929).

FOSSATI, C.: The basophil cells of the blood in tuberculosis. Acta med. scand. **138,** 457 – 462 (1950).

FREDRICK, R. E., MOLONEY, W. C.: The basophilic granulocytes. Blood **14,** 571 – 583 (1959).

FRICK, G.: Zur Absolutzählung der basophilen Leukozyten. Dtsch. Gesundh.-Wes. **21,** 1548 – 1550 (1966).

FRICK, G., FRICK, U.: Zur Rolle der basophilen Leukocyten und Mastzellen in Fibrinolyse und Allergie. I. Wirkung von Fibrinolytika und Antifibrinolytika auf den Degranulierungsgrad von basophilen Leukocyten. Folia haemat. (Basel) **86,** 389 – 403 (1966 a).

FRICK, G., FRICK, U.: Zur Rolle der basophilen Leukocyten und Mastzellen in Fibrinolyse und Allergie. II. Wirkung eines Antihistaminikums und einer allergischen Sofortreaktion auf Zahl und Degranulierung basophiler Leukocyten. Folia haemat. (Basel) **87,** 178 – 189 (1966 b).

FRICK, G., KONRAD, H.: Sofortreaktionen im peripheren Blutbild nach Glukokortikoiden, Adrenalin, ACTH und Pyrogenen. Folia haemat. (Basel) **81,** 377 – 405 (1963).

FRICK, G., KONRAD, H.: Basophile und Heparin in der Sofortreaktion nach Glukosteroiden. Folia haemat. (Basel) **82,** 369 – 381 (1964).

GABL, F.: Supravitalfärbung. In: Handbuch der gesamten Haematologie. Bd. II, 1. München, Berlin: Urban & Schwarzenberg 1960.

GILBERT, H. S., ORNSTEIN, L.: Basophil counting with a new staining method using alcian blue. Blood. **46,** 279 – 286 (1975).

GOMORI, G.: Aldehyde-fuchsin: A new stain for elastic tissue. Amer. J. clin. Path. **20,** 665 – 666 (1950).

GRABENER, E.: Die Glukokortikoid-Basopenie. Blut **12,** 219 – 225 (1966).

GRABENER, E.: Funktionsanalytische Untersuchungen an Blutbasophilen. Kiel: Habilitationsschrift 1969.

GRAF, W., SVENSSON, R.: Experimental investigations on local changes in the white blood cell picture following perforating injury to blood vessels. J. Path. Bact. **62,** 419 – 427 (1950).

GREY, C. E., BIESELE, J. J.: Thin-section electron microscopy of circulating white blood cells. Rev. Hémat. **10,** 283 – 299 (1955).

HAMERSTON, O., ELVEBACK, L., HALBERG, F., GULLY, K. J.: Correlation of absolute basophil-eosinophil counts in blood from institutionalized human subjects. J. appl. Physiol. **9,** 205 – 207 (1956).

HAMMAR, J. A.: Lipoidbildung in den weißen Blutkörperchen. Kngl. Svenska Vetenskapsakademiens Handlingar 1912.

HARMS, H.: Über Schwankungen der relativen Basophilen-Zahl im peripheren Kaninchenblut, unter verschiedenartigen Entnahme- und Färbebedingungen, sowie nach Colchicinbehandlung. Folia haemat. (Lpz.) **72,** 129 – 135 (1954).

HEDENIUS, P.: Über wahre Metachromasie der weißen Blutkörperchen. Acta med. scand. (Suppl. 109) 3 – 60 (1940).

HELLY, K.: In: H. NOTHNAGEL: Spezielle Pathologie und Therapie, Bd. VIII, 1. und 2., pp. 1 – 205. Die haemapoetischen Organe in ihren Beziehungen zur Pathologie des Blutes. Wien: Hölder 1906.

HOLMGREN, H.: Funktion und Chemie der Ehrlichschen Mastzellen. Verh. anat. Ges. (Jena) **83**, 31 – 37 (1937).

INAGAKI, S.: The relationship between the level of circulating basophil leukocytes and thyroid function. Acta endocrin. (Copenhagen) **26**, 477 – 488 (1957).

JAMES, G. W., WRIGHT, D. U., WILKERSON, V., SHELLENBERG, K.: Observations on the absolute basophil count in health and disease. Clin. Res. Proc. **3**, 31 (1955).

JOLLY, J.: Action des rayons ultraviolets sur les mouvements améboïdes des leucocytes. C. R. Soc. Biol. **99**, 1554 – 1556 (1928).

JUHLIN, L.: Basophil and eosinophil leukocytes in various internal disorders. Acta med. scand. **174**, 249 – 255 (1963).

KARVONEN, M. J., KUNNAS, M.: Factor analysis of haematological changes in heavy manual work. Acta physiol. scand. **29**, 220 – 231 (1953).

KAUTZ, J., DE MARSH, Q. B.: An electron-microscope study of sectioned cells of peripheral blood and bone marrow. Blood **9**, 24 – 38 (1953).

KEHNSCHERPER, M., BLAU, H.: Das postprandiale Verhalten von Blutbasophilen und veresterten Serumfettsäuren im Kindesalter. Klin. Wschr. **44**, 847 – 848 (1966).

KELEMAN, E., BIKICH, G.: Insufficiency of acute response of basophil and eosinophil leucocytes and of blood histamine after the administration of ACTH and cortisone in untreated myelocytic leukaemia. Acta haemat. (Basel) **15**, 202 – 206 (1956).

KIMURA, I., MORITANI, Y., NISHIZAKI, Y., TANIZAKI, Y.: Clinical significance of basophil leukocytes in bronchial asthma. Acta Med. Okayama **22**, 203 – 208 (1968).

KOVACS, G. S. VON: A simple direct method for absolute basophil and eosinophil counts from the same blood sample. Folia haemat. (Frankfurt) **5**, 166 – 175 (1961).

LABENDZINSKI, F.: Recherches quantitatives sur les basophiles du sang périférique au moyen de la goutte épaisse. Sang **27**, 432 – 437 (1956).

LABENDZINSKI, F., BROZOZOWSKA, W.: Wplyw nicktorych lekow ua poziom bazofilow krwi (Influence of certain drugs on the basophil level in the blood). Arch. Med. Wewnet Rzneg. **27**, 463 – 471 (1957).

LENNERT, K.: Zur Praxis der pathologisch-anatomischen Knochenmarksuntersuchung. Frankf. Z. Path. **63**, 267 – 299 (1952).

LENNERT, K.: Lymphknoten. Diagnostik in Schnitt und Ausstrich. In: Handbuch der speziellen pathologischen Anatomie, Bd. I/3 A. Berlin-Göttingen-Heidelberg: Springer 1961.

LENNERT, K., PARWARESCH, M. R.: Die Reaktion der basophilen Granulocyten auf eine postprandiale Hyperlipaemie. Schweiz. med. Wschr. **33**, 1410 – 1414 (1970).

LENNERT, K., SCHUBERT, J. F. C.: Zur Cytochemie der Blut- und Gewebsmastzellen. Verh. dtsch. Ges. inn. Med. **66**, 1061 – 1065 (1960).

LINDAHL, U.: Comment on the use of cetylpyridinium chloride in the isolation of connective tissue proteoglycan. Biochem. J. **113**, 569 – 570 (1969).

MASUGI, M.: Über die Beziehungen zwischen Monocyten und Histiocyten. Beitr. path. Anat. **76**, 396 – 443 (1926).

MAXIMOW, A.: Über entzündliche Bindegewebsneubildung beim Axolote. Beitr. path. Anat. **39**, 333 – 336 (1906).

MAXIMOW, A.: Über die Histogenese der entzündlichen Reaktion. Nachprüfung der v. Möllendorffschen Trypanblauversuche. Beitr. path. Anat. **82,** 1 – 26 (1929).

MENEGHINI, C. L., LEVI, L.: Cutaneous reactivity in relation to histamine-liberating substances. G. ital. Derm. **100,** 255 – 262 (1959 a).

MENEGHINI, C. L., LEVI, L.: Histaminemia and circulating mast cells in some allergic dermatoses. G. ital. Derm. **100,** 449 – 460 (1959 b).

MICHAELIS, L.: Über Mastzellen. Münch. med. Wschr. **49,** 225 – 226 (1902).

MICHELS, N. A.: The mast cells. In: Downey's Handbook of Hematology, Vol. 1, p. 326 – 350. New York: P. B. Hoeber 1938.

MILLONIG, G.: A modified procedure for lead staining of thin sections. J. biophys. biochem. Cytol. **11,** 736 – 739 (1961).

MISSMAHL, H. P.: Metachromasie durch gerichtete Zusammenlagerung von Farbstoffteilchen, erläutert am optischen Verhalten des Toluidinblau. Histochemie **3,** 396 – 412 (1964 a).

MISSMAHL, H. P.: Doppelbrechung im Protoplasma der Leukocyten des peripheren Blutes. 1. Tag. Südwestdtsch. Ges. inn. Med. (1964 b).

MISSMAHL, H. P.: Nachweis von doppelbrechenden Strukturen im Protoplasma der Leukocyten des peripheren Blutes nach Supravitalfärbung mit Toluidinblau beim Menschen. Klin. Wschr. **42,** 750 – 751 (1964 c).

MISSMAHL, H. P.: Doppelbrechung in Leukocyten des peripheren menschlichen Blutes nach Supravitalfärbung mit Toluidinblau. Blut **XII,** 149 – 158 (1965 a).

MISSMAHL, H. P.: Der feinstrukturelle Aufbau der Granula basophiler Leukocyten des menschlichen Blutes. Blut **XII,** 159 – 163 (1965 b).

MIURA, A. B., SHIBATA, A., ONODERA, S., SUZUKI, A., SAKAMOTO, S., SUZUKI, CH.: The ultrastructure of basophile leukocytes in human chronic myelogenous leukaemia. Tohoku J. exp. Med. **96,** 87 – 95 (1968).

MOORE, J. E., JAMES, G. W.: A simple direct method for absolute basophil leucocyte count. Proc. Soc. exp. Biol. (N. Y.). **82,** 601 – 603 (1953).

MORELLE, L.: Sur le comportement des leucocytes basophiles en certains chocs experimentaux. C. R. Soc. Biol. (Paris) **107,** 904 – 905 (1931).

NAEGELI, O.: Blutkrankheiten und Blutdiagnostik, 2. Edn. Berlin: Julius Springer 1920.

NOMURA, Z.: (Japan.) 1928. Cited by INAGAKI: The relationship between the level of circulating basophil leukocytes and thyroid function. Acta endocr. (Copenhagen) **26,** 477 – 488 (1957).

OSADA, Y.: Parallel changes in the numbers of circulating eosinophils and basophils induced by ACTH administration. Bull. Inst. pub. Health **4,** 12 – 18 (1954).

OSADA, Y.: Diurnal rhythms in the numbers of circulating basophils and eosinophils in healthy adults. Bull. Inst. pub. Health **5,** 5 – 9 (1956).

OSAKO, R.: An electron microscopic observation on the specific granules of eosinophil leukocytes of vertebrates. Acta haemat. jap. **22,** 134 – 150 (1959).

PADAWER, J., GORDON, F.: Hormonal influences upon the mast cells of peritoneal fluid. Anat. Rec. **118,** 402 (1954).

PARWARESCH, M. R., LENNERT, K.: Löslichkeit und Fixierungsmöglichkeiten der Blutbasophilen-Granula des Menschen. Z. Zellforsch. **83,** 279 – 287 (1967).

PARWARESCH, M. R.: Eine neue Anreicherung der Blutleukocyten, besonders der Blutbasophilen. Blut **XVII,** 260 – 265 (1968).

PARWARESCH, M. R., MÜLLER-HERMELINK, H. K., TESSMANN, H.: Elektronenoptische Untersuchung der Blutbasophilen bei alimentärer Hyperlipaemie. In preparation (1976).

PEASE, D. C.: Marrow cells seen with the electron microscope after ultra-thin sectioning. Rev. Hémat. **10,** 300 – 313 (1955).

PEASE, D. C.: An electron microscopic study of red bone marrow. Blood **XI** (6), 501 – 526 (1956).

PETROVA, T. R.: On the reaction of basophil and eosinophil leukocytes to hormones and heparin. Probl. endokr. Gormonoter. **12,** 53 – 57 (1966).

PHILIPSBORN, E. VON: Die amöboide Beweglichkeit der Leukocyten. Folia haemat. (Lpz.) **43,** 142 – 191 (1930).

PIETTE, M., PIETTE, C.: Etude critique des méthodes de numération directe des granulocytes basophiles dans le sang humain: Proposition d'une technique. Ann. Biol. clin. **20,** 197 – 205 (1962).

POLICARD, A., COLLET, A., PRÉGERMAIN, S.: Les cellules basophiles et éosinophiles du sang et des tissues chez le rat. Etude au microscope électronique. Rev. Hémat. **14,** 278 – 293 (1959).

POTUZHEK, O. VON, THUMB, N. T., BRAITENBERG, H., BRAUNSTEINER, H.: Quantitative Veränderungen der Blutbasophilen durch Schwangerschaft, Zyklus und Sexualhormone. Wien. klin. Wschr. **71,** 595 – 598 (1959).

RIND, H.: Atlas der Phasenkontrastmikroskopie. Berlin: Akademie-Verlag 1958.

RINGOEN, A. H.: The mast leucocytes in the adult guinea pig under experimental conditions. Amer. J. Anat. **31,** 319 – 337 (1923).

RORSMAN, H.: Basophil leucocytes and urticaria. Acta derm.-venereol. (Stockh.) **37,** 121 – 128 (1957).

RORSMAN, H.: Normal variation in the count of circulating basophil leucocytes in man. Acta allerg. (Kbh.) **XVII,** 49 – 65 (1962).

RORSMAN, H., ROSENGREN, R.: Basophil leucocytes and blood histamine in urticaria. Acta derm.-venereol. (Stockh.) **38,** 377 – 393 (1958).

SABIN, F. R.: Studies of living human blood cells. Bull. Johns Hopk. Hosp. **34,** 277 – 288 (1923).

SABIN, F. R.: Cellular studies in tuberculosis. Amer. Rev. Tuberc. **25,** 153 – 171 (1932).

SAMPSON, D., ARCHER, G. T.: Release of histamine from human basophils. Blood **29,** 722 – 736 (1967).

SCOTT, J. E.: Aliphatic ammonium salts in the assay of acidic polysaccharides from tissues. Meth. biochem. Anal. **8,** 145 – 197 (1960).

SELYE, H.: The mast cells. Washington: Butterworth & Co. 1965.

SHELLEY, W. B., PARNES, H. M.: The absolute basophil count. J. amer. med. Ass. **192,** 108 – 110 (1965).

SHIBATA, A., TAKASE, S., OYODERA, S., MIURA, A. B., SUZUKI, A., SAKAMOTO, S., OIKAWA, A., SATO, T.: Cytological studies on basophil leukocytes. Acta haem. jap. **29,** 879 – 889 (1966).

SIMPSON, M. E.: On the reaction of the living blood cells to dyes. Anat. Rec. **21,** 82 (1921 a).

SIMPSON, M. E.: Vital staining of human blood with special reference to the separation of the monocytes. Univ. Calif. Publ. Anat. **1,** 1 – 9 (1921 b).

SIMPSON, M. E.: The experimental production of circulating of endothelial macrophages and the relation of these cells to the monocytes. Univ. Calif. Publ. Anat. **1,** 11 – 19 (1921 c).

SIMPSON, M. E.: Vital staining of human mammalian blood with special reference to the separation of monocytes. Anat. Rec. **23,** 37 (1922 a).

SIMPSON, M. E.: The experimental production of macrophages in the circulating blood. J. med. Res. **43,** 77 – 144 (1922 b).

SPICER, S. S., HORN, R. G., WETZEL, B. K.: Ultrastructural and cytochemical characteristics of leukocytes in various stages of development. Biochem. Pharmacol. Suppl. 143 – 157 (1968).

SUNDBERG, M., WASASTJERNA, C.: Occurrence of basophilic granulocytes in blood. Finska Läk.-Sällsk. Handl. **96**, 208 – 215 (1953).

TATAI, K., OSADA, Y.: The adrenocortical stimulating effect of adrenochrome derivatives as administered to healthy young males. J. med. Progr. Jap. **32**, 441 – 448 (1957).

TEDESCHI, G., CAVAZZUTI, F.: Variazioni quantitative dei basofilie ematici indotte dalle somministrazione di alcuni ormoni. Boll. Soc. med.-chir. Modena **59**, 1 – 4 (1959).

TEDESCHI, G., CAVAZZUTI, F., ANGELI, G.: Variazioni quantitative dei granulociti basofili del sangue periferico in diverse condizione patologiche. Min. Med. **50**, 1535 – 1541 (1959).

THONNARD-NEUMANN, E.: Basophile Leukocyten und Ovarialfunktion. Ärztl. Forsch. **8**, 443 – 451 (1954).

THONNARD-NEUMANN, E.: Basophile Leukocyten und Steroidhormone. Med. Welt **27/28**, 1087 – 1090 (1958).

THONNARD-NEUMANN, E.: The influence of hormones on the basophilic leukocytes. Acta haemat. (Basel) **25**, 261 – 270 (1961).

THONNARD-NEUMANN, E., TAYLOR, W. L., NOSAU, M.: Changes over time in blood basophil counts of x-irradiated rabbits. Blut **19**, 537 – 544 (1969).

THUMB, N., POTUZHEK, O., BRAITENBERG, H., BRAUNSTEINER, H.: Hochgradige Verminderung der Blutbasophilen während der Schwangerschaft. Wien. Z. inn. Med. **40**, 129 (1959).

TOKUÉ, K.: The blood mast cell and its oxidase and peroxidase reaction. Tohoku J. exp. Med. **12**, 459 – 464 (1929).

TOMPKINS, E. H.: Clinical applications of supravital staining. J. lab. clin. Med. **17**, 921 – 931 (1932).

TOMPKINS, E. H.: The monocyte. Ann. N. Y. Acad. Sci. **59**, 732 – 745 (1955).

TURIN, M.: Blutveränderungen unter dem Einfluß der Schilddrüse und Schilddrüsensubstanz. Dtsch. Z. Chir. **107**, 343 – 366 (1910).

UNDRITZ, E.: Die nicht zur Blutkörperchenbildung gehörenden Zellen intravitaler Knochenmarkspunktate nebst Auszählungsschema für Myelogramme. Schweiz. med. Wschr. **2**, 333 – 337 (1946).

WATANABE, J., DONAHUE, S., HOGGATT, N.: Method for electron-microscopic studies of circulating human leukocytes and observations on their fine structure. J. ultrastruct. Res. **20**, 366 – 382 (1967).

WATSON, M. L.: Staining of tissue sections for electron microscopy with heavy metals. J. biophys. biochem. Cytol. **46**, 475 – 478 (1958).

WEIDENREICH, F.: Studien über das Blut und die blutbildenden und -zerstörenden Organe. III. Bau und morphologische Stellung der Blutlymphdrüsen. Arch. mikr. Anat. **65**, 1 – 77 (1905).

WEIDENREICH, F.: Alexander Maximow, 1874 – 1928. Anat. Anz. **67**, 360 – 368 (1929).

WESTERHOFF, H.: Untersuchungen der Blutbasophilen bei verschiedenen Arthropathien unter besonderer Berücksichtigung der Gicht. Dissertation. Münster 1966.

WESTPHAL, E.: Über Mastzellen. In: Farbenanalytische Untersuchungen zur Histologie und Klinik des Blutes, Part 1, pp. 17 – 41. Ed. P. EHRLICH. Berlin: A. Hirschwald 1891.

WETZEL, B. K., HORN, R. G., SPICER, S. S.: Fine structural studies on the development of heterophil, eosinophil and basophil granulocytes in rabbit. Lab. Invest. **16**, 349 – 382 (1967).
WINQVIST, G.: Electron microscopy of the basophilic granulocyte. Ann. N. Y. Acad. Sci. **103**, 352 – 375 (1963).
WOLF-JÜRGENSEN, P.: Leukocytes: Eosinophils, basophils, biochemistry. Series haematologica **I**, 45 – 68 (1968).
YANAGIHARA, K.: The parallel changes of circulating eosinophils and basophils in the rabbit with insulin administration. Bull. Inst. publ. Health Jap. **7**, 14 – 19 (1958).
ZACHARIAE, F., ASBOE-HANSEN, G., BOSEILA, A. W. A.: Studies on the mechanism of ovulation. Migration of basophil leucocytes from blood to genital organs at ovulation in the rabbit. Acta endocr. (Copenhagen) **28**, 547 – 552 (1958).
ZUCKER-FRANKLIN, D.: Electron microscopic study of human basophils. Blood **29**, 878 – 890 (1967).

V. Cytochemistry of Blood Basophils

Few cells in the human body possess such a multifaceted and complex biochemical make-up as the blood basophil and the closely related tissue mast cell.

Tissue mast cells are more readily available for chemical analysis than are blood basophils. They can be cultured in quantities sufficient for biochemical analysis, whereas blood basophils occur in very limited numbers and do not withstand preparatory operations. This is probably the reason why indirect techniques of cytochemistry have been so extensively applied to the basophils.

In the following section we consider the topochemistry of a group of substances whose occurrence in blood basophils has been definitely ascertained, or at least shown to be highly probable by direct methods. The functional significance of these substances is discussed in detail in Chapter C.

The carbohydrates in blood basophils consist of simple polysaccharides, primarily glycogen, which is localized in the intergranular cytoplasm and is dependent upon the current cell metabolism. Blood basophils are further distinguished by a high content of highly sulfated and highly polymerized acid glucomucans. These are found in extraordinarily high concentrations in the specific basophil granules.

Furthermore, blood basophils are said to contain polyribonucleotides. It remains unclear whether this class of substances can enrich in a special way, or whether they are merely components of the ribosomal RNA attached to the occasionally observable rough endoplasmic reticulum.

The enzymes contained in blood basophils include both hydrolases and oxidoreductases. The presence of the majority of the hydrolases can readily be demonstrated by means of the different esterase reactions, but their function still remains unclear. However, they do shed light on cytogenesis, as well as being a valuable diagnostic aid, and should therefore be specially considered from this point of view.

Finally, we discuss the significance of histamine, the decarboxylation product of the amino acid histidine, which occurs in the specific basophil granules. The presence of histamine in tissue mast cells has been confirmed by fluorescent histochemical methods, but this has not proved possible for human blood basophils.

1. Lipids

A battery of chemical and physical techniques is available for the detection and identification of lipids and related substances, yet reliable conclusions can only be reached through a combination of various methods. Among the numerous extraction procedures, the technique reported by Baker (1946) has been the most extensively used in hematology. In addition, nonpolar dyes have been applied for the visualization of tissue lipids. The Sudan colorants, particularly Sudan red and Sudan black B, are of special importance here (Lennert and Weitzel, 1952 a, b; Lennert, 1955).

Sudan black B exhibits a wider staining spectrum than the usual nonpolar stains. After prior extraction of neutral fats this dye selectively stains many tissue phospholipids. Sudan black B-positive structures occur in human leukocytes (Shehan, 1939) and are not removed by subsequent treatment with organic solvents. The so-called sudanophilia of human leukocytes is observed exclusively in eosinophils, neutrophils, and monocytes, which also give a positive peroxidase reaction (Undritz, 1961; Hayhoe and Quaglino, 1964; Merker, 1968). As exogenous peroxidase was found to block sudanophilia of human leukocytes, Schäfer and Fischer (1970) concluded that the so-called stable sudanophilia of leukocytes depends upon their peroxidase content. According to these authors, Sudan black B, both spontaneously as well as in combination with phenols, undergoes an oxidative coupling in the presence of myeloperoxidase, thereby serving as a substrate for the myeloperoxidase which occurs constantly in eosinophils and neutrophils and occasionally in monocytes and basophils. Bailif and Kinbrough (1947) and Storti and Perugini (1949 a; 1951) could find no sudanophilia in human monocytes and basophils, whereas Rheingold and Wislocki (1948) established the presence of lipids in the specific granules of blood basophils by adding phenol to a slightly alkaline medium. The controversy that centered around the sudanophilia of blood basophils was reopened in 1953 by Hayhoe and systematically investigated. He was unable to establish the presence of sudanophilic structures in blood basophils. In contrast, Bloom and Wislocki (1950), using a modification of Baker's method, observed numerous fat-positive granules in blood basophils. After subsequent pyridine extraction the reaction product completely disappeared. The hematin-positive pyridine-extractable structures were claimed to be phospholipids. Corini *et al.* (1955) maintained that 8 to 28% of normal blood basophils contain Sudan black B-positive structures, whereas the percentage of Sudan-positive blood basophils is definetely higher in cases of myeloid leukemias and amounts to over 50% of the total basophil population; in the so-called basophil leukemias, practically all of the blood basophils contain Sudan black B-positive structures. Similar results have also been obtained by LENNERT and SCHUBERT (1960) and SHIBATA *et al.* (1966). Taking into consideration the results of SCHÄFER and FISCHER (1970), it is possible to reduce the whole controversy to a common denominator, i.e. myeloperoxidase can be visualized by phenol-containing Sudan black B solutions. Normal blood basophils contain some weak and irregular peroxidase activity. In myeloproliferative diseases a much larger percentage of blood basophils give a positive reaction, producing coarsely granular precipitates. Sudanophil structures are identical with the peroxidase-containing basophil granules and so are also covered by the peroxidase reaction. The clear cytotopographic agreement of both reactions bound preferentially to specific granules, and the fact that sudanophilia can only be demonstrated in fresh slides provide further evidence to support the above view.

The structures that can be observed with the hematin-pyridine technique are not bound to any specific granules. They occur mostly between the specific granules and are far smaller. Some of these structures may represent mitochondria, which become visible through treatment by BAKER's technique. The size and arrangement of these particles correspond to the distribution pattern of the mitochondria identified by phase-contrast microscopy. It is already known that lipids appear in noticeable quantities in purified, mitochondrial fractions. The ratio of lipids to protein in mitochondrial fractions is 1 : 0.4 and therefore lies beyond the histochemically attainable borderline. It is a matter of structural lipids which consist of up to 90% of phospholipids (phosphatidyl choline and phosphatidyl ethanolamine, etc.), all of which yield a positive hematin-pyridine reaction. To sum up: structures in blood basophils which contain peroxidase can be identified with the usual phenol-containing Sudan black B solutions. In contrast, the hematin-pyridine technique stains the extra-granular structural lipids, which in all probability correspond to the mitochondria.

2. Glycogen

The glycogen content of human basophils has been repeatedly disputed. SMITH (1949) and WISLOCKI *et al.* (1949) were able to detect glycogen in blood basophils by means of diastase digestion and subsequent PAS staining. This finding was supported by GIBB and STOWELL (1949). PIETTE and PIETTE (1956) could only partially confirm these results. They pointed out that approximately 40% of blood basophils are PAS-negative.

Many contradictory opinions exist concerning the localization of the PAS-positive and diastase-labile structures in blood basophils. Compact particles about 250 to 300 Å in diameter, localized in groups in intergranular space as detected by electron microscope (BIAVA, 1963; REVEL, 1964; ZUCKER-FRANKLIN, 1968), were believed to be glycogen. WATANABE *et al.* (1967) also concluded on the basis of their ultrastructural investigations that the intergranular particles appearing in blood basophils must be glycogen.

The results of ASTALDI *et al.* (1952) contradict these findings; after diastase treatment they could find no difference in the intensity of the PAS reaction in blood basophils, although the intensity of the PAS reaction decreased in the neutrophil granulocytes. An irregular weak PAS reaction in human basophils was encountered by ACKERMAN (1963). The findings of SMITH (1949), ACKERMAN (1963), and HAYHOE (1963) support the view that the specific granules do indeed contain PAS-positive material, but that this material is diastase-resistant. PAS-positive deposits in the intergranular space have been found to be regularly lysed by diastase treatment (INAGAKI, 1968). The PAS positivity and the glycogen content of blood basophils have been thoroughly dealt with in a report by KAUNG (1969), who clearly showed that the specific granules of blood basophils always give a PAS-negative reaction. A weak positive reaction was observed in the intergranular space but disappeared when treated with saliva diastase. These results were further substantiated by findings from semithin sections and subsequently ultrathin sections for electron microscopy.

The inconsistent reports regarding glycogen in blood basophils are mostly due to the fact that the glycogen content depends upon the momentary metabolic condition of the cell and is therefore subject to great fluctuations. Many of the studies reported do not really make clear whether the authors believe the site of glycogen storage to be the specific granules or the intergranular cytoplasm. Metachromatic basophil granules definitely do not contain glycogen. The PAS-positive reaction occasionally observed in specific granules is essentially due to the presence of acidic mucopolysaccharides and phospholipids. The glycogen-induced PAS positivity of the intergranular cytoplasm is relatively weak and the fact that it disappears after diastase treatment can easily be overlooked. In addition, the specific granules dissolve when treated with aqueous solutions, making exact cytotopographic orientation almost impossible.

In our experience glycogen regularly occurs in blood basophils. The amount and its distribution within the cytoplasm varies according to the metabolic state of the cell. Under normal circumstances, glycogen is present in limited quantities; it is fine-grained and evenly distributed throughout the cytoplasm of the blood basophils. It can be detected in the intergranular spaces by electron microscope or light microscope on the basis of its weak, diastase-labile PAS-positivity.

A localized accumulation of glycogen in blood basophils (coarsely granular precipitates positive to the PAS reaction) indicates a severe disturbance of the cellular metabolism with impaired glycogen catabolism. This finding in blood basophils is elevated in myeloproliferative diseases and is a valuable criterion for cell atypia.

3. Acid Mucopolysaccharides (Glycosamino-Glycans)

EHRLICH believed the granules of tissue mast cells and blood basophils to consist of proteins. PAPPENHEIM (1906) and his students (STAEMMLER, 1921; HAUSER, 1937) pointed out the similarities in the staining of the metachromatic granules and mucin. VAN HERWERDEN (1919) attempted to produce evidence of the nucleic acid character of the granules. STAEMMLER (1921) suggested that the metachromatic staining property of the granules was an indication of their acidic content. NAGAYO (1928) emphasized the histochemical similarity of these cells to cartilage and stated that there must be a close chemical relationship between these granules and cartilage. On the basis of their histochemical investigations with dyes like carmine and iodine as well as with the MILLONS and BIURET reactions, WERMEL and SASSUCHIN (1927) took the view that the metachromatic material in these structures represents glycoprotein.

BERGSTRÖM (1930; 1935), JORPES (1935), LISON (1935; 1936) and JORPES and BERGSTRÖM (1936; 1937) showed that a dilute heparin solution with a dilute basic dye – for example a 0.001% toluidine-blue solution – induced a clear metachromatic shift. In 1937, HOLMGREN and WILANDER were able to prove that the metachromatically reacting contents of tissue mast cell granules were identical with the substance described by HOWELL and HOLT (1918), namely, heparin. Later, numerous other authors confirmed these results (WISLOCKI and DEMPSEY, 1946; WISLOCKI *et al.*, 1947; RHEINGOLD and WISLOCKI, 1948, ASTALDI *et al.*, 1954). The acid-mucopolysaccharide nature of the metachromatic granules was further substantiated partly on the basis of chemical analyses and partly by cytochemical methods such as colloidal iron, the PAS-reaction, and basic stains (SMITH, 1949; WISLOCKI *et al.*, 1949; LAVES and THOMA, 1950; BEHRENS and TAUBERT, 1952; LAVES, 1952; ASTALDI, 1953; ASTALDI *et al.*, 1953; MARTIN and ROKA, 1953; BOIVIN and ROBINEAUX, 1957; AMANN and MARTIN, 1961; BRAUNSTEINER, 1962; ACKERMAN, 1963).

Many valuable cytochemical methods exist today for the selective staining of glycosaminoglycans, but only a minority of them can be applied to human basophils. A brief survey of some of these methods is provided.

a) Bismarck Brown

Bismarck brown was one of the first dyes employed in histochemistry. In a solution containing 0.5% dye in a mixture of hydrochloric acid and alcohol the basophil granules appear as dirty yellow structures (HARDIE and WESBROOK, 1895; LEACH, 1947; LILLIE, 1954; SPATZ, 1960). As a basic diazo stain, Bismarck brown was also widely used in the portrayal of nuclear chromatin (LILLIE, 1954). The mode of reaction appears to be a true salt bonding. Bismarck brown offers no significant advantages over other dyes.

b) Colloidal Iron

Glycosaminoglycans can be visualized with colloidal ferric hydroxide. Basophil granules can also be stained by this technique (ASTALDI *et al.*, 1953). The mechanism is an elective bonding of ferric hydroxide (Fe^{+++}) to the strongly dissociated acidic groups at low pH (WOLMAN, 1956; MOWRY, 1957; CASSELMAN, 1959). The absorbed iron can then easily be visualized by the prussian blue reaction ($K_4Fe(CN)6 \cdot 3\ H_2O$). The glycosaminoglycans show up as luminous blue (HALE, 1946). This method is far too susceptible and very sensitive to pH fluctuations.

c) Phthalocyanine Stains

Adequate coloration of glycosaminoglycans is readily provided by the phthalocyanine stains (Alcian blue 8 GS, Alcian blue 8 GX, Alcian green 2 GX, Alcian green 3 BX, Astra blue), first described by STEEDMAN (1950). Further modifications were reported by VIALLI (1951), LISON (1953), MOWRY (1956 a, b), PIOCH (1957) and LANDING and WILSON (1959).

The exact structural formulae and the mode of action of this group of stains have not yet been fully explained. Both a salt-linkage and a hydrogen bond or a coordinative accumulation of the copper nucleus of the dye have been discussed. The affinity for different acidic groups depends on the H-ion concentration of the solution being limited to uronic acid at pH 2 and confined to sulfuric groups at pH 1 (SPICER, 1960; LEV and SPICER, 1964).

The coloration is a luminous blue or light green and widely insensitive to acidic and alkaline decolorants.

Aqueous solutions of these dyes are not satisfactory (LINDNER, 1961), whereas 0.1% dye in 0.6 to 0.7 n HCL (pH 0.2), as recommended by BLOOM and KELLY (1960), gives excellent results.

It is possible to enhance the specific affinity of Alcian blue for the different tissular acidic groups by adding electrolytes (HCl, NaCl, KCl, and $MgCl_2$) in various molarities (QUINTARELLI *et al.*, 1964 a, b; SCOTT *et al.*, 1964; QUINTARELLI and DELOVO, 1965; SCOTT and DORLING, 1965). The histochemical exploitation of this phenomenon, called critical electrolyte concentration, provides a selective demonstration of carboxyl groups at a 0.2 M $MgCl_2$ concentration and of sulfate groups at molarities above 0.8.

By gradually increasing the salt molarity, the nonsulfated glycosaminoglycans can be differentiated from those which are sulfated. It is further possible to differentiate the sulfated glycosaminoglycans according to degree of sulfation. Investigations using critical electrolyte concentrations of Alcian blue yielded results which were fairly comparable with those obtained from the so-called pH series on the basis of basic dyes.

For a simultaneous portrayal of both blood basophils and tissue mast cells in bone marrow smears INAGAKI (1969) developed a staining technique employing Astra blue, a stain introduced into histochemistry by GEDIGK (1956), PIOCH (1957), and FASSKE (1957). Astra blue is a hemin-like phthalocyanine compound with a copper nucleus. It is obtainable as an acetate (Astra blue FM, Chroma 10110). BLOOM and KELLY (1959; 1960) applied this dye to the mast cells. With INAGAKI's technique blood basophils in fresh smears are distinguishable as blue-green, optically dense structures. Older smears are unsuitable for this technique because almost all granulocytes, especially eosinophils, take up the same color.

d) Aldehyde Fuchsin

Among the group of triarylphenylmethane dyes, aldehyde fuchsin possesses a remarkable affinity for sulfate ions (GOMORI, 1950; MELI and DAVIES,

1953; SCOTT and CLAYTON, 1953; BANGLE, 1954; RABENOVITCH *et al.,* 1954; SPICER and MEYER, 1960; ABUL HAY and RINEHART, 1962). The chemical mechanism of this reaction is not yet fully understood. It is probably explained by the acidic depolymerization of paraldehyde and a subsequent reaction of acetaldehyde with the free perarosaniline amino group (CONN and BANGLE, 1954; ELFTMAN, 1959; ORTMAN *et al.,* 1966). The acid structures then show a luminous purple to violet color (Fig. 16). However, since other structures, such as cells rich in cystine, the thyroid colloid, or the elastic fibers are also well colored, the selectivity of this stain is limited. According to SCOTT and CLAYTON (1953), prior acid oxidation should be avoided when a selective staining of the sulfated components is desired.

Aldehyde fuchsin, though not suitable for routine work on blood basophils, has proved indispensable for certain studies. In our investigations we used chloroform-extracted aldehyde fuchsin for autoradiographic studies of blood basophils. Compared to numerous other stains, aldehyde fuchsin displayed in these studies considerable advantages, such as particular stability to organic solvents, pH fluctuations, and shifts in ionic strength. A further advantage of aldehyde fuchsin is that it produces neither a positive nor a negative chemographism. Following GOMORI (1950), we used a 0.5% dye solution in 70% ethanol to which 1% (v/v) paraldehyde and 1% concentrated hydrochloric acid were added. The selectivity of the staining solution seems to depend upon the predominance of azomethine over pararosaniline. In old solutions, however, the staining components with blockaded amino groups predominate. This is supported by the fact that solutions over 1 week old become light blue in colour. They display the same spectral photometric characteristic as methyl violet 2B and crystal violet. Aldehyde fuchsin stain is not suitable for successive enzyme-cytochemical studies. Naphthol AS-D chloroacetate esterase, to cite one instance, is normally highly resistant, but when used in combination with aldehyde fuchsin it was found to be completely inactivated.

e) The PAS-Reaction

Numerous modifications of the PAS-reaction are used for the histochemical portrayal of polysaccharides (MCMANUS, 1946; 1949; HOTCHKISS, 1948). The chemical mechanism of this reaction has been thoroughly investigated. A number of very different compounds show a positive reaction. Among simple polysaccharides (homoglycans), glycogen, starch, and cellulose give a positive reaction; among the heteroglycans, sialoglycan, and among the glycoproteins, most epithelial mucins as well as chorionic gonadotrophin, the hypophyseal gonadotrophins (FSH and LH), thyroglobulin, and blood-group substance A all give a PAS-positive reaction. Further positive reactions occur with gangliosides, cerebrosides and sphingomyelins. Not all acidic glycosaminoglycans show a positive reaction; free hyaluronic acid is PAS-negative. In contrast, sulfated hyaluronic acid and many chondroitin sulfates are said to be PAS-positive. According to JORPES *et al.* (1948) and GOMORI (1953), low-sulfated heparinates are PAS-positive, whereas the highly sulfated heparin chains are PAS-negative.

Mast cells and blood basophils have often been investigated for their PAS reaction (GIBB and STOWELL, 1949; SMITH, 1949; WISLOCKI *et al.*, 1949; LEBLOND, 1950; LILLIE, 1950; ASTALDI *et al.*, 1953; RILEY, 1953; HALE, 1957; LONGLEY, 1958; BOSEILA and UHRBRAND, 1958; LENNERT and SCHUBERT, 1960; LENNERT, 1962; ACKERMAN, 1963; HAYHOE, 1963; DUNN and SPICER, 1968; INAGAKI, 1968; KAUNG, 1969).

Regarding the PAS positivity of basophils, the reaction of the specific granules and that of the intergranular cytoplasmatic space have to be considered separately. Like the other kinds of granulocytes, blood basophils contain glycogen in amounts depending upon their functional condition. Glycogen yields a positive PAS-reaction; it is localized exclusively in the intergranular spaces and can be eliminated by diastase treatment. ACKERMAN (1963) established that blood basophils contain both diastase-labile and diastase-stable PAS-positive granules. Only diastase-resistant, PAS-positive granules can be considered specific. Opposing this, ASTALDI and STROSSELLI (1963) maintained that leukemic blood basophils treated with either saliva or taka diastase show no decrease in PAS intensity, in contrast to the neutrophils. The positive PAS-reaction was ascribed to the presence of polysaccharides because, after treatment of the blood smears with a M/20 Na_2SO_2 solution (blockading of the aldehyde groups according to LILLIE, 1954), the PAS reaction turns negative. The reversible decrease in PAS intensity following acetylation for 45 min was regarded as indicative of 1,2 glycol groups. Furthermore, ASTALDI and STROSSELLI (1963) considered a proportion of the PAS-positive substances in the basophil granules to be lipids.

The intensity of the PAS reaction in blood basophils is said to decline radically after treatment with lipid solvents such as pyridine or methanol. Long-term acetylation, after which the basophil granules become irreversibly PAS-negative, is also considered by LILLIE (1954) and ASTALDI and STROSSELLI (1963) as evidence for the presence of PAS-positive lipids.

Recent results by INAGAKI (1968), DUNN and SPICER (1968) and KAUNG (1969) seem to have brought the debate about the PAS reaction in blood basophils to a close. INAGAKI (1968) was able to show that the solubility of basophil granules in water was the limiting factor in determining the PAS positivity of the specific granules, which proved to be always PAS-negative. PAS-positive structures were more or less diffusely distributed and limited to the intergranular space. KAUNG (1969), who investigated blood basophils both light- and electron-microscopically, reported similar findings. Good conformity was found between the sites of PAS activity in semithin sections and the distribution of glycogen particles in the corresponding ultrathin sections.

To summarize: For assessment of the PAS-reaction on basophil, special fixing steps to preserve the water-soluble granules are necessary. The diastase-labile PAS positivity is always confined to the extragranular space. Both the saliva amylase investigations and electron-microscopic findings support the premise that the PAS-positive structures in blood basophils represent glycogen. The glycosaminoglycans of the specific granules are PAS-negative. This is in good agreement with the cytochemical classification of polysaccharides established by Spicer *et al.* (1965). According to this classification, the group S mucopolysaccharide A (10.0, $MgCl_2$), which also contains keratin sulfate and heparin, is PAS-negative.

f) Thiazine Dyes

This group of dyes has acquired special importance for the cytochemical portrayal of glycosaminoglycans. They enjoy particularly widespread use in connection with panoptic stains (Giemsa, Pappenheim, Leishman, Wright, etc.). The thiazine dyes are basic substances which have a strong affinity for acidic organic compounds. They are chemically derived from thionine. The site of the positive charge of the common chromophore component was specified differently for different molecular forms. Thionine occurs in two mesomers as 1,2(ortho)chinoid and 1,4(para)chinoid, where either the sulfur or nitrogen atom can be positively charged. According to Harms (1965), the chinoid in para form possesses a far stronger color intensity due to its greater oscillation distance.

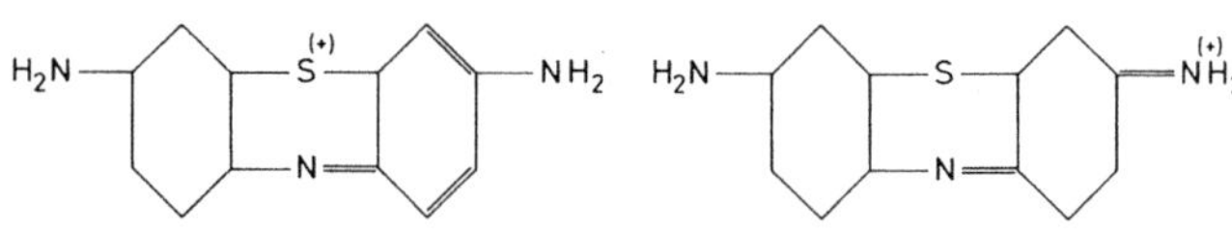

1,2 (ortho) chinoid 1,4 (para) chinoid

In addition to thionine, methylene blue (tetramethylthionine), azure B (trimethylthionine), azure A (dimethylthionine), azure C (monomethylthionine), and especially toluidine blue 0 (C-methylated azure A) are all used in the histochemistry of glycosaminoglycans. According to Wilander's investigations, toluidine blue 0, under appropriate conditions combines stoichiometrically with heparin (Wilander, 1937). Since then quite a number of staining techniques with toluidine blue have been developed. Its solubility in various alcohols amounts to approximately 0.5%. In water and in aqueous media, higher concentrations can be achieved. Acidic structures – basophil granules, for example – show a red to light violet metachromasia when stained with toluidine blue. The cytoplasm is only vaguely demonstrated. The nuclei become visible with alcohol solutions within a range of light to dark blue, depending upon concentration and duration of staining. In aqueous dye solutions the nuclear color depends upon the hydrogen-ion concentration, being blue-violet at pH above 4 and turning light blue with decreasing pH.

g) Metachromasia

During his studies with aniline dyes, in particular with monophenyl rose aniline, Ehrlich (1877) discovered the mast cells, due to their peculiar tinctorial properties. He observed this property in cartilage as well and named it metachromasia. Metachromasia is the shift in color of the stained structures from the original color of the dye employed. The principal mechanisms underlying metachromasia have now been largely clarified. It is also possible to make deductions concerning the chemical nature of the structures exhibiting the phenomenon of metachromasia. For instance, the glycosaminoglycans and polynucleotides are the only components affected when dilute basic (cationic) dyes of the thiazine group are employed. Basophil granulocytes, like tissue mast cells, contain large amounts of glycosaminoglycans, which is why they react metachromatically.

Table 3. Shilfts in absorption maxima of basic dyes implying metachromasia (KELLY, 1956)

Dyes	Absorption maxima (nm) Orthochromasia	Metachromasia
Toluidine blue	630	480 – 540
Azure A	620	480 – 530
Methylene blue	665	570
Cresyl blue	625	530
Crystal violet	590	510
Basic fuchsin	543	510
Thionine	597	557

Metachromasia is due mainly to a shift in the absorption maximum of an organic dye induced by certain substances (chromotropes). The absorption maximum of the dye shifts to shorter wavelengths, so that the absorption maximum of the molar extinction coefficent diminishes. Except for a few anionic stains which have not yet been sufficiently investigated, only basic dyes have been used in histochemistry. For a true, stable metachromasia (survey by LISON, 1935) the basic stains of the thiazine group have proven especially suitable. Table 3 (taken from KELLY, 1956) lists the absorption maxima of toluidine blue, azure A, methylene blue, cresyl blue, crystal violet, basic fuchsin, and thionine in both the ortho- and metachromatic states.

The metachromasia of toluidine blue has been well investigated. Chemically, toluidine blue is a 2-amino-7-dimethylamino-3-methyl-diphenylacetonium chloride, a C-methylated azure A. It is very similar in color to methylene blue. Toluidine blue is superior to other dyes in its metachromatic characteristics because of its tendency to association and the well-separated absorption maxima of the stain dimers and polymers, with their clearly differentiated color tones. Very dilute toluidine-blue solutions show an absorption maximum of 630 nm (alpha bands of the monomer). Any increase in stain concentration induces a tendency toward micellar aggregation. Already at a concentration of 2.9×10^{-5} M (0.87 mg%), a hypsochromic shift to 590 nm (beta bands of the dimer) occurs. Further increases in concentration produce absorption maxima at even shorter wavelengths of 540 and

520 nm (gamma and μ bands of the higher molecular aggregates). Along with this hyposochromic shift, a clearly visible change occurs in the reflected light fractions (blue-violet-red) (MICHAELIS, 1947; KUHN, 1949; SCHUBERT and LEVINE, 1955; SCHUBERT and HAMERMANN, 1956).

The metachromasia of a chromotropic substrate can be influenced by various factors. Those of significant importance are:

1. Chemical composition of the solvents used (LISON, 1936; KELLY, 1956).
2. Temperature (KELLY, 1936; BANK *et al.*, 1939; BAKER, 1958).
3. Concentration of the reaction partner (MICHAELIS, 1947; KELLY, 1956; BAKER, 1958).
4. Duration of coloring time (KRAMER and WINDRUM, 1955).
5. Degree of purity of the stain (KELLY, 1935; BANK *et al.*, 1939).
6. Hydrogen-ion concentration at which the staining is performed (PISCHINGER, 1926).

Lowering the temperature favors the hypsochromic shift and gives rise to metachromasia. Sedimentation of the dye by adding solutions of salts such as ammonium sulfate effects a similar shift in the absorption maxima by changing the aggregation rates. The metachromasia of a chromotropic substance is further influenced by the solvent, especially by its dielectric constant. One is reminded here of the disappearance of metachromasia in aqueous heparin or chondroitin sulfate solutions after addition of dioxane or similar substances. Dioxane, acetone, and long-chained alcohols radically lower the dielectric constant of water. The bathmochromic effect of temperature in alcoholic staining solutions is based on a similar principle. At low temperature the dielectric constant of alcohol (DK 26) is 2 or 3 times greater and is near the dielectric constant of water (EILUND and PERSSON, 1949).

Metachromatic tissular structures have certain features in common. All chromotropes bear dissociable, negatively charged groups of varying ion strengths. There are the acid hydroxyl groups of the aromatic carbohydrate bonds, carboxyl groups, and the stronger inorganic anionic groups such as phosphates and sulfates. The surface density of the negative charges has a further bearing on the appearance of metachromasia. The denser the surface charge of the anion to be stained, the greater will be the intensity of metachromatic staining (SYLVEN, 1954). A maximum distance of 5 Å between the sites of the anionic groups is considered to be the borderline value for formation of metachromasia. The size of the chromotropic molecule is also of importance for metachromatic behavior (LISON, 1935). Small molecules like ethylene sulfate ($C_2H_5HSO_4$) do not offer the conditions necessary for micellar aggregation of the cations. However, very small quantities of dextran sulfate, an anionic polyelectrolyte of sufficient molecular size, show high metachromatic activity. The development of metachromasia hence depends upon a local accumulation of the dye which, by inducing polymerization of micellar aggregates of the dye molecules, gives rise to a color change.

Metachromasia can be repressed (KELLY, 1955) by salts or even proteins (SINGER, 1954). This effect is largely pH-dependent and is especially pronounced in strong cationic additions. The proteins compete with the ionized dye molecules for the substrate valencies so that the inhibiting effect vanishes after adjustment of the isoelectric points of the added proteins. The competition of the cations for the anionic substrate groups and their sensitivity to pH fluctuations stimulated investigations into the nature of the chromotropic groups. LANDSMEER (1951) assumed that the acid groups of the metachromatic material (tissue mast cells and blood basophil granules, for example) could be occupied by either cationic metal ions or cationic dye ions. Therefore it must be possible to ascertain a definite concentration of metal ions above which further bonding of metal or dye (staining) could no longer occur because the negative charges were already saturated by the metal ions available in excess. Thus, depending on the chromotropic groups, typical relationships arise from which revealing conclusions about the nature of the acidic groups can be drawn.

Further information can be obtained from the pH values that favor the dissociation of the respective acidic groups. WITTIAN's concept of the physicochemical nature of the staining reaction as a heteropolar linkage rests on the observation that the state of dissociation of the reactants determines the degree of coloration to a great extent. If the dissociation of the chromotropes is pH-dependent, then the staining reaction must similarly depend upon the H-ion concentration of the dye solution. Various authors (MATTHEWS, 1898; PISCHINGER, 1926; MOMMSEN, 1927; SCHWARTZ and KARSTEN, 1927; LEVINE, 1940) have systematically investigated the influence of H-ion concentration upon the color reaction with reference to the IE point of the amphoteric biological material. Considering the inhomogeneous character of the tissue substrate, it is more exact to speak of an isoelectric range. What has in fact to be considered is the conversion range on the pH scale in which the acidophilia of the tissue structures makes room for basophilia. It thus becomes clear that the amount of stain absorbed (and therefore the color intensity) will be greater with increasing difference in pH between the isoelectric range of the tissue to be stained and that of the dye solution. The dissociation ranges of the tissular acidic groups have different pH values. VICKERSTAFF (1954), using model substrates, was able to assess the approximate dissociation ranges at various pH values of dye solutions. With substrates of IE value 5, the ratio $-COOH : -COO^{(-)}$ up to pH 2.0 was 100 : 0. With increasing pH, the dissociation increased in the following order: at pH 4.4 the dissociation ratio was 50 : 50; at pH 5.0 it was 20 : 80, and at pH values over 7.0, almost complete ionization was achieved with a ratio of 0 : 100. VICKERSTAFF did not consider stronger acidic groups, such as phosphoric acid and sulfo groups. In contrast, BAKER (1958) ascertained 100% dissociation of the $-COOH$ groups only at pH 11. Similar investigations are available for the phosphate and sulfo groups.

Under the conditions prevailing in hematology, a dissociation ratio suitable for such staining reactions is reached at pH 6.0 for the phosphate groups (MICHAELIS, 1947; WEISSMAN *et al.,* 1952; BERGERON and SINGER,

1958). The corresponding dissociation situation for even stronger acid groups, such as the sulfo groups, lies at significantly lower pH levels. An increase in the H-ion concentration of the staining solution represses first the dissociation of the carboxyl groups, then of the phosphate groups, and finally, at rather low pH, of the sulfo groups. In other words, the use of cationic dyes in acidic solutions permits elective staining of strongly acidic structures within the histological material. The capacity of tissue structures to bind basic stains with increasing acidity is gradually released until only the strongest acidic components – those containing organic acid groups, for instance, sulfated glycosaminoglycans – remain stainable by the cationic dye (PARWARESCH and LENNERT, 1969). This is the basic mechanism underlying the use of the so-called pH scales in the histochemistry of mast cells and blood basophils.

The Toluidine-Blue pH Scale. The selective tingibility of tissular amphoters at characteristic pH levels reveals information about the IE range of the tissular structures. Thus, conclusions can be drawn about their acidity, and in the case of sulfated glycosaminoglycans, about their polymerization and sulfate content. Toluidine blue is the dye most widely used in this context, but other dyes have been applied in the same manner (DEMPSEY and SINGER, 1946; SCHÜMMELFEDER and STOCK, 1956; SZIRMAI and BALASZ, 1958).

The toluidine blue pH scale worked out by LENNERT and SCHUBERT (1959) has proved useful in the cytochemical assessment of tissue mast cells and blood basophils, particularly with respect to their maturity, functional alterations, and neoplastic anomalies. We applied the procedure suggested by LENNERT and SCHUBERT (1960) as modified by LENNERT and BACH (1961). Air-dried smears of leukocyte concentrates were fixed and treated with dilute toluidine-blue solutions in 0.1 M buffers at pH ranging from 2.8 to 5.8 in 0.2 steps. The slides were then differentiated in the same buffer and dehydrated in isopropyl alcohol. The basophils were destained between each pH step by transferring the slides to buffer solutions of higher pH values.

After each staining the number of basophils with metachromatic granules was counted and expressed as a percentage of the highest value observed. These values yield a characteristic curve on plotting against the pH intervals. The toluidine-blue pH series can also be used to determine the isoelectric range of the glycosaminoglycans that occur in cartilage, vessel wall, and connective tissue. The results can then be compared with those obtained from the critical electrolyte concentrations.

With the toluidine blue pH series the blood basophils consistently display a typical tinctorial pattern. Under normal conditions the great majority of blood basophils appear metachromatically in the pH range 2.8 to 3.8. With decreasing H-ion concentration of the dye solution, the total number of metachromatically stained basophils decreases markedly. Although some blood basophils are stainable at apparently irregular pH intervals, others under identical conditions do not appear at all. The same was found to be true of the granules of single basophils; some remained stained at different pH levels, for example 2.8, 3.0 and 3.2, presenting an identical distribution of metachromasia, whereas the same cell at higher pH levels displayed an

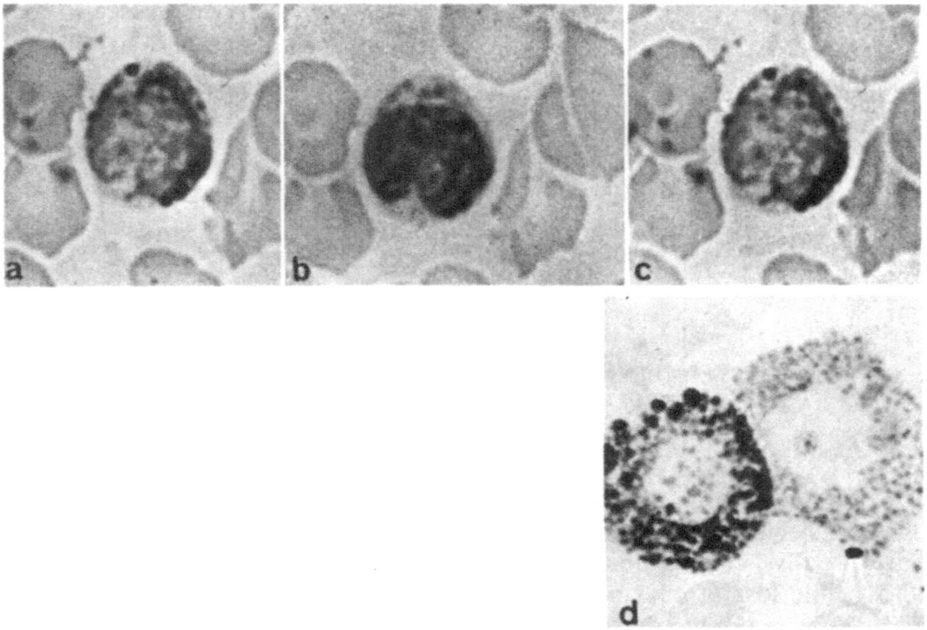

Fig. 10 a – d. Selective staining of the metachromatic structures in blood basophils and tissue mast cells with dilute toluidine-blue solutions at various pH levels. Above: The same blood basophil (a) at pH 2.8, (b) at pH 3.8 and (c) at pH 4.8. Below: Difference in the tinctorial property of tissue mast cells (d) at pH 4.6. Only the upper one of the two tissue mast cells is stained. × 1,400

entirely different granule pattern (Fig. 10). The total number of blood basophil counted at all pH levels includes a relatively large number of cells that are repeatedly considered.

With experience, it is possible to obtain a certain pH range which covers most or all of the blood basophils. This range offers the maximum metachromatic staining for a given cell population; for normal human basophils of the peripheral blood this range is 2.8 to 3.8 (Parwaresch and Lennert, 1969), as is well shown by the location of the calculated median of the relevant toluidine-blue pH curves.

Figure 11 presents the typical toluidine-blue pH curve obtained from 20 healthy fasting subjects. All items represent mean values. As a reference point for statistical comparisons, the mean value of the curve median with its standard deviation is computed. The curve median ($\tilde{x}$) reflects, in quantitative terms, the maximum metachromatic tingibility of the basophils. It thus affords an insight into the acidic capacity, e.g. glycosaminoglycan content, of the basophil population in question. A shift to the right of the curve median will reflect a significant decrease in the basophil content of anionic groups which can be the result of insufficient sulfation or reduced polymerization. Both conditions occur in immature basophil populations like that of normal bone marrow. Similar curve patterns are also encountered in neoplastic basophil populations in connection with myeloproliferative diseases.

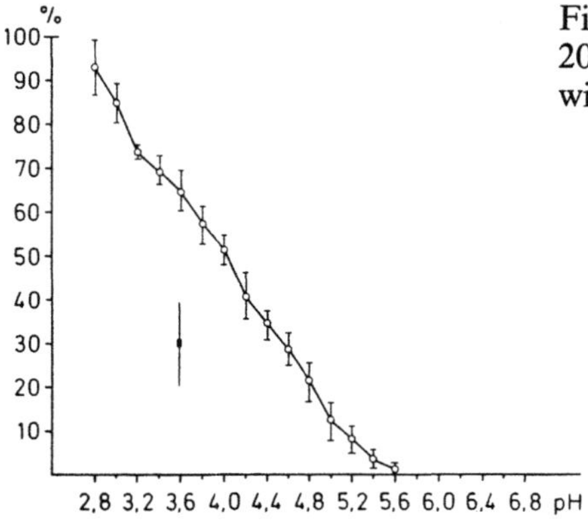

Fig. 11. Toluidine-blue pH curve obtained from 20 healthy subjects. Mean of curve medians with small standard deviation at pH 3.6

4. Enzymes

Because of the rarity of blood basophils, no direct biochemical assay of the enzymes occurring in them has yet proved possible. Cytochemical methods have usually been applied in spite of the water solubility of basophil granules. Some loss of enzyme activity almost always occurred when reliable fixatives were used to preserve the structure of the granules.

Hydrolases, despite their low substrate specificity (MERKER, 1968) are important in hematologic diagnoses because they are relatively more stable than oxidoreductases. Their physiological significance, however, is not well understood (ZURWEHME *et al.*, 1970). While adequate functional information is available on the mitochondrial and lysosomal enzymes of the energy-delivering metabolism, they are very susceptible to inactivation by preparative measures.

a) Oxidoreductases

Oxidative enzymes can be cytochemically displayed in blood basophils by means of tetrazolium salts, in particular nitro-BT (a ditetrazolium salt) and MTT (a triazolyl-substituted monotetrazolium compound) (PEARSE, 1957; 1958; SCARPELLI *et al.*, 1958; PEARSE *et al.*, 1960; PEARSE and HESS, 1961). In the meantime, a number of reports on the activity of oxidoreductase in blood basophils has appeared (KOPPEL and OLWIN, 1954; MARTIN *et al.*, 1955; NACHLASS *et al.*, 1957; 1958 a, b; DE SOUZA and KOTHARE, 1959; QUAGLINO and HAYHOE, 1960).

Reliable fixatives, though indispensable for structural preservation, always cause a great loss in enzyme activity. We must allow for the fact that unfixed cells possess higher enzyme activities. Despite the many refinements in techniques, the cytochemical methods for studying oxidases, diaphorases and dehydrogenases are still unsatisfactory for routine work (NOVIKOFF and MASEK, 1953; NOVIKOFF *et al.*, 1960; QUAGLINO and HAYHOE, 1960; ECKSTEIN and LINDNER, 1961; WALKER and SELIGMAN, 1961; MORRISON and KRONHEIM, 1962). The ready solubility of basophil granules greatly complicates matters (BALOGH and COHEN, 1961; FISCHER, 1963).

In a microprocedure a minimum of incubation solution between cover glass and slide permits direct phase-contrast microscopic observation of the cells in the course of the enzyme reaction. BALOGH and COHEN (1961) used a tetrazolium salt: 2,2-di-(p-nitrophenyl)-5,5-diphenyl-3,3(3,3-demithoxy-4,4-biphenylene)-ditetrazolium chloride. The results were reported to be satisfactory with respect to both enzyme activity and structure preservation.

In principle, all cells of the granulocytic system show a marked decrease in dehydrogenase activity in the course of maturation. Compared with monocytes and lymphocytes, the granulocytes react somewhat more weakly. The eosinophils and especially the blood basophils show lower enzyme activities than the neutrophils. DPNH and TPNH diaphorases, as well as succinate, lactate, malate, glutamate, beta-hydroxybutyric acid, glucose-6-phosphate and 6-phosphogluconate dehydrogenases are all detectable in blood basophils; a distinct activity of isocitric acid dehydrogenase is also encountered. Diphosphopyridine nucleotide (NADH) or triphosphopyridine nucleotide (NADPH) is usually employed as hydrogen acceptor in such experiments. The highest level of activity was encountered for NADH diaphorase and lactate diaphorase. Compared with the eosinophils, the activity produced by lactate dehydrogenase was higher in blood basophils and that of glucose-6-phosphate dehydrogenase significantly lower. Traces of succinate dehydrogenase can be detected in blood basophils. Malate, glutamate and isocitrate dehydrogenase activity is also slight. The enzyme that oxidizes gluconolactone to gluconic acid (gluconolactone-6-phosphate dehydrogenase) has also been detected in human blood basophils. Furthermore, according to BECK and VALENTIN (1953) and BECK (1958), human blood basophils contain glucose-oxidizing enzymes in addition to the glycolytic enzymes. In blood basophils the catabolic pathways of the intermediate carbohydrate metabolism appear to set off, not just the glycolytic chain and the citric-acid cycle, but also direct oxidation and decarboxylation of glucose (C1 oxidation of glucose). The presence of gluconolactone-6-phosphate-dehydrogenase in human blood basophils points in this direction.

Recent studies confirm earlier information on the dehydrogenase activity in blood basophils. After careful prefixation in 40% cold acetone for 30 sec, ACKERMAN (1963) detected a weak but definite activity in human blood basophils of the succinic, lactic, maleic acid and glucose-6-phosphate-dehydrogenases, as well as DPNH and TPNH diaphorases. SHIBATA *et al.* (1966) reported results completely in agreement. Of the various enzymes of the tricarbonic-acid cycle and lactic acid and glucose-6-phosphate dehydrogenases, he described beta-hydroxybutyric acid dehydrogenase as being of low activity in the blood basophils.

Disregarding diffusion artifacts, dehydrogenase and diaphorase activity appears to be confined to the intergranular cytoplasm. The specific granules do not contain these enzymes. Table 4 lists the activity of diaphorases and dehydrogenases for the various myeloid leukocytes as reported by BALOGH and COHEN (1961). Diaphorases and dehydrogenases display a somewhat weaker activity in blood basophils than in neutrophil granulocytes, and lymphocytes and monocytes possess a higher enzyme content than neutrophils, eosinophils, and basophils. The activity of choline dehydrogenase appears in varying levels in monocytes and reaches high levels in eosinophils. Blood basophils always react weakly. Of the cytochromoxidases, $NADH_2$-cytochrome-c-diaphorase and $NADPH_2$-cytochrome-c-diaphorase have been detected in blood basophils. Both types of oxidases promote a weak reaction. The NADI reaction indicating cytochromoxidase activity was recorded with greater intensity in blood basophils when studied with the modification of INAGAKI (1964). 3,4-dihydroxyphenylalanine (DOPA) is readily oxidized by the cytochromoxidases. In fixed specimens the reaction is confined to the myeloid cells. Human basophils without exception give a positive reaction (INAGAKI, 1965 a).

Besides the positive DOPA and NADI reactions, the myeloid cells including monocytes oxidize other phenols and diamines into chinoid compounds (GOMORI, 1953; MERKER, 1968). Blood basophils have also been

Table 4. Activity of dehydrogenases (DH) involved in biologic oxidative processes in normal human monocytes, neutrophils, eosinophils and blood basophils

Enzymes	Monocytes	Neutrophils	Eosinophils	Basophils
Succinate-DH	++	+	+	+
Glutamate-DH	++	+	+	+
Glycerin-1-phosphate-DH	++	+	+	+
Lactate-DH (NAD)	++	++	+	+
Malate-DH (NAD)	++	++	+	+
-glycerophosophate-DH (NAD)	+	++	+	+
Glucose-6-phosphate-DH (NADP)	+++	++	+	+
-hydroxybutyrate-DH (NAD)	+	++	++	+
Choline-DH	Ø / +++	++	++++	+
Isocitrate-DH (NADP)	++	+	+	+
Dihydroorotic acid-DH	+ / ++	+ / ++	+	+
$NADH_2$-cytochrome-c-diaphorase	+++	++	+	+
$NADPH_2$-cytochrome-c-diaphorase	++	++	+	+
Oxidase (phenoloxidase, diaminooxidase, peroxidase):				
NAD-reaction	+	+	+	+
DOPA-reaction	+	+	+	+
Adrenalineoxidation	+	+	+	+
Myeloperoxidase (SATO, GRAHAM, LEDER)	Ø / +	++++	++++	Ø / +

found to react positively: in concentrated adrenaline solutions they take on a strong yellow-brown color at strongly alkaline pH (INAGAKI, 1965 b). The relatively stable oxidative activity of myeloid cells in the NADI, dihydroxyphenylanaline, and adrenaline reactions has been attributed to a phenol-oxidizing property of the incubation solution. Since such oxidative reactions also take place with fixed preparations, it is debatable whether this is, in fact, due to peroxide decomposition (DEANE *et al.*, 1960).

To sum up: blood basophils possess most of the key enzymes for energy-delivering metabolic processes. The enzyme activities correspond to those of the eosinophil and neutrophil granulocytes but the reactions of blood basophils are much less intense than those of lymphocytes and monocytes.

Dihydroorotic Acid Dehydrogenase. Dihydroorotic acid dehydrogenase was first cytochemically detected by SMITH and BAKER (1959) and PEARSE and HESS (1961). They confirmed that all blood cells, with the exception of erythrocytes, posses a more or less strong enzyme activity.

Among the dehydrogenases, dihydroorotic acid dehydrogenase deserves attention as it provides an insight into the proliferation tendency of the cells. Orotic acid results from the biosynthesis of the pyrimidine ring in connection with nucleotide synthesis. Uridine-5-phosphate arises from the reaction of orotic acid and phosphoribosyl-pyrophosphate under separation of 2-phosphoric acid residues (from ribose C1) and subsequent decarboxylation. Thus the orotic acid represents the biochemical origin of pyrimidine nucleosides. The orotic acid dehydrogenase oxidizes the dihydroorotic acid to orotic acid. Riboflavin monophosphate and flavin adenine dinucleotide are considered as coenzymes (LIEBERMANN and KORNBERG, 1954; FRIEDMANN and WENNESLAND, 1958; SMITH and BAKER, 1959).

The activity of dihydroorotic acid dehydrogenase in the blood cells of both healthy and diseased children was investigated by NARTSISSOV (1965). A high enzyme activity was observed in cases of reactive leukocytosis, acute leukemias, and aplastic anemias.

CASTOLDI *et al.* (1968) subjected this enzyme to a systematic cytochemical investigation. They studied the influence of fixatives, storage, variations in pH, incubation time, and reduction indicators upon its activity. The enzyme was up to 90% inhibited by the application of p-chloromercuric-benzoate in a concentration of 10^{-3} M. The reaction intensity in the eosinophils and basophils was weak, but in some of the neutrophils the activity was somewhat higher. Lymphocytes and monocytes reacted much more strongly. Here, too, enzyme activity tends to decrease in the course of cell maturation. High enzyme activity was observed in myeloproliferative diseases and in chronic lymphatic leukemia, the highest activity being observed in cases of acute leukemia.

Myeloperoxidase. The peroxidase reaction was implemented in hematology in order to separate the myeloid cells from the nonmyeloid blood and bone marrow cells. Since then, numerous modifications have been developed. The peroxidase content of blood basophils is the subject of continuing debate. Positive peroxidase reaction has been found in normal human blood basophils by several authors (SCHULZE, 1909; DUNN, 1910; KREIBICH,

1910; PAPPENHEIM and NAKANO, 1912). NAEGELI (1919) maintained that human blood basophils can be separated from tissue mast cells by virtue of their peroxidase activity.

These results stand in opposition to those of other authors who could not detect any significant peroxidase activity in normal human basophils (GRAHAM, 1920; HIRSCHFELD, 1924; MICHELS, 1938). TOKUE (1929) explicitly stressed that human blood basophils are generally peroxidase-negative and can thus be distinguished from peroxidase-positive guinea-pig basophils. According to his results, 90% of human blood basophils show a negative reaction, 5% a very weak and 5% a weak peroxidase reaction. These results caused him to contradict EHRLICH's postulate on the myelogenous origin of human blood basophils. BRAUNSTEINER and ZUCKER-FRANKLIN (1957) stated that blood basophils are generally peroxidase-negative and that only a few of them demonstrate a weak activity.

LENNERT and SCHUBERT (1961) using a more sensitive technique could detect some peroxidase activity in blood basophils. UNDRITZ (1961) believed blood basophils to be peroxidase-positive and stated that, even after 5 years, old blood smears still displayed some activity. However, in his systematic investigations of the cytochemistry of blood basophils ACKERMAN (1963) could not detect any peroxidase in blood basophils, neither with the GRAHAM method nor with that of SATO. SHIBATA *et al.* (1966) obtained a definite positive peroxidase reaction in blood basophils but, as is often the case in the literature, their investigations were conducted upon leukemic basophils. In the meantime, further methods for the cytochemical detection of myeloperoxidase in basophil granulocytes have been developed (INAGAKI, 1963; SCHUBERT and MARTIN, 1968 a, b). SCHAEFER and FISCHER (1968) developed a new technique for peroxidase delineation in blood smears and paraffin-embedded material using 3-amino-9-ethylcarbazole as hydrogen donor. They did not report upon the state of preservation of the blood basophils, but they did mention that, basically, basophil granulocytes, like monocytes, react positively in some cases, depending upon species.

We attempted to visualize this enzyme light- and electron-microscopically in normal and leukemic blood basophils by applying the different methods hitherto used. We found blood basophils to contain a very small amount of myeloperoxidase. The activity within the cells fluctuates considerably. Some single blood basophils demonstrate a peroxidase-positive reaction with very careful procedures to preserve their soluble granules. The majority of normal blood basophils, however, reveal a negative reaction. Simultaneous demonstration of granule metachromasia and peroxidase reaction could only be achieved in a few basophils.

The occurrence of peroxidase in normal human basophils is best shown by a successive demonstration of metachromasia and enzyme activity in one and the same basophil (Fig. 12.)

Table 5 surveys the myeloperoxidase activity of normal blood and bone-marrow cells.

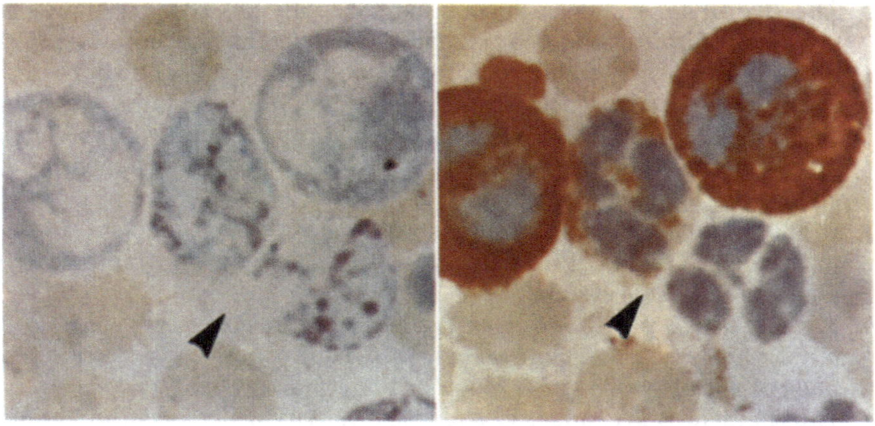

Fig. 12. Buffy coat smear with two basophils (arrow) and two neutrophils, subjected to the myeloperoxidase reaction (right) following supravital staining with toluidine blue (left). ×1,800

Table 5. Myeloperoxidase activity in normal human blood and bone-marrow leukocytes. All other cells react negatively

Maturation Stages Cell Lines	Promyelo- cytes	Myelo- cytes	Metamyelo- cytes	Band- forms[a]	Seg- mented
Neutrophils	++++	+++	+++	+++	+++
Eosinophils	++++	+++	+++	+++	+++
Basophils	++++	+++	+	±	±
		Promono- cytes	Monocytes	Monocytogenic Cells	
Monocytes	++++	++	±	–	

[a] Blood-Marrow Border

b) Hydrolases

With the evidence of the presence of hydrolytic enzymes in blood cells, a new phase in hematology began. This was not so much because of the promise of new insights into certain metabolic processes of blood cells but rather because these enzyme reactions brought a new cytochemical tool for the morphogenetic investigation of the hematopoietic system. Genetically related cell series could be easily distinguished by their content of certain enzymes or by a specific enzyme pattern. New criteria for routine hematology were provided by these reactions, enabling more precise classification of blood dyscrasia. Several features of the hydrolytic enzymes make them of special value in the recognition and differentiation of blood cells, their cytogenetic relationships, and their neoplastic atypias.

1. The hydrolytic enzymes, in comparison with the oxidoreductases, are markedly more resistant to fixatives. The relevant reactions can be carried out using fairly well-fixed cells in good structural condition.
2. The intensity of the reaction product and its cytotopographic distribution are subject to relatively strict rules and appear quite independent of the metabolic state of the cell at any given time. These reactions yield good reproducible typical results.
3. A good many hydrolyses demonstrate a strict cytogenetic specificity – a phenomenon that is of fundamental significance for morphological analysis of hemopoetic system.
4. Some hydrolases in the course of cellular maturation show typical quantitative and qualitative changes which permit conclusions concerning the stage of maturity of a given blood or bone-marrow cell.
5. The characteristic changes in hydrolase activity which occur in neoplastic and reactive blood disorders permit a clearcut differential diagnosis.

The weak substrate specifity of the hydrolases used in hematology can give rise to nonspecific reactions. A good example of this is the naphthol-AS-D chloroacetate-esterase positivity of the actually negative bone-marrow reticulum cells, which occurs due to insufficient inactivation (fixing!) of other esterases. Such technical shortcomings easily lead to mistaken interpretations. In the following section we go more closly into those hydrolases of interest for blood basophils.

Leucine Aminopeptidase. Leucine aminopeptidase in human blood and bone-marrow cells has been only sporadically investigated.

ACKERMANN (1961; 1963), using different fixatives, attempted to detect alanine and leucine-beta-naphthyl-formamide hydrolyzing aminopeptidase in blood basophils. He failed to detect even N-benzyl-D-beta-naphthyl-amid-hydrochloride hydrolyzing aminopeptidase, which is very similar to trypsin and often appears in tissue mast cells, in normal human blood basophils.

SCHUBERT and KATZENMEYER (1963) investigated blood smears from 220 patients and 50 healthy persons by the technique of ACKERMANN (1961). A positive reaction could be detected in 31% of the polymorphonuclear neutrophils and in some eosinophils. Due to poor fixation, some of the basophil granules were dissolved and the remainder revealed no enzyme activity. On the other hand, the bone-marrow tissue mast cells displayed a moderate reaction. In a later report, SCHUBERT and MARTIN (1968) described normal human blood basophils as being weakly enzyme-positive. Mature neoplastic basophils also display a positive reaction. Immature leukemic blood basophils, however, proved to be enzyme-negative.

Sulfatase. Sulfatase activity has only occasionally been studied in blood cells (RUTHENBURG *et al.*, 1952; AUSTIN and BISCHEL, 1961), and most authors do not cover blood basophils at all. AUSTIN and BISCHEL (1961) studied 5 patients with an extremely high blood basophil count and pointed out that their technique would not clearly distinguish blood basophils from neutrophil granulocytes. They stated, however, that blood basophils were also sulfatase-positive, since they behave similarly to neutrophils.

Phosphatase. The phosphatase activity of human leukocytes has been dealt with in a considerable body of publications (TAKAMATSU, 1938; 1939; GOMORI, 1939; 1941 a, b; KABAT and FURTH, 1941; reviews by PEARSE, 1960; KAPLOW, 1968; MERKER, 1968). The phosphomonoesterases, especially those with an activity optimum in the alkaline region (pH 9.2 to 9.4) have received special attention in routine hematology because of their diagnostic value in differentiating the chronic myeloid leukemias from cases of reactive leukocytosis. In the former, mostly low activities or negative reactions are found, while the latter usually give high enzyme activities. In cases of myelofibrosis with myeloid metaplasia and in the beginning phase of polycytemia vera a considerable enhancement in the activity of polymorphonuclear neutrophils to the alkaline phosphatase is found. These divergences from the normal state have been shown to be helpful in arriving at certain hematological diagnoses, although a diagnosis cannot be made on the basis of such a finding alone, since no strict reglarity could be established in the behavior of the leukocyte alkaline phosphatase activity.

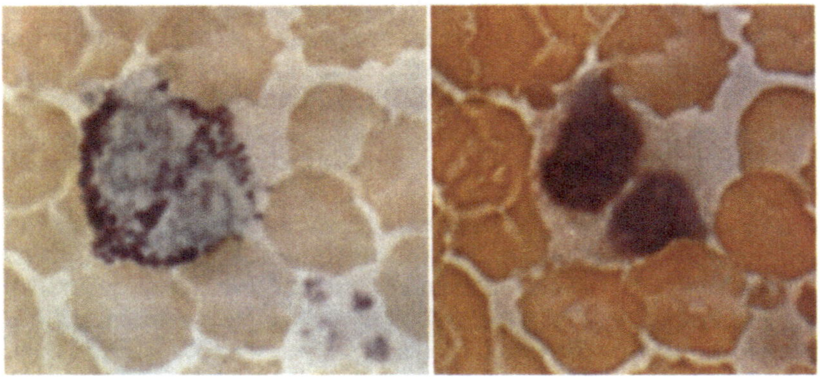

Fig. 13. Successive application of toluidine-blue (left) and alkaline phosphatase reaction to normal blood. Basophils give a negative enzyme reaction; × 1,800

Normal human basophils give a constant negative reaction to the alkaline phosphatase (GOMORI, 1952; WILTSHAW and MOLONEY, 1955; LENNERT and SCHUBERT, 1960; MERKER, 1963). This is shown in Fig. 13 by successive toluidine-blue staining and enzyme reaction in one and the same cell. A survey of the activities of normal blood and bone-marrow cells to the alkaline phosphatase reaction is provided in Table 6.

Contradictory results have been reported as regards the acid phosphatase activity of basophils. A positive reaction was found by LENNERT and SCHUBERT (1960) and LENNERT (1961). ACKERMAN (1963) and MERKER (1963), however, could not confirm these results. In our experience, normal human basophils present an intense acid phosphatase activity as detected by the successive demonstration of metachromasia and enzyme reaction

Table 6. Alkaline phosophatase activity in blood and bone marrow cells

Polymorphonuclear neutrophils	+ + (variable)
Capillary endothelium	+ + + +
Fibroblasts	+ + (variable)

(Fig. 14). The reaction pattern of basophils and other blood and bone-marrow cells is fairly constant and for some cells highly specific.

Nonspecific Esterases. Among the nonspecific esterases the naphthol AS-(D) acetate esterase and the alpha-naphthyl acetate esterase have successfully been employed in hematology (LEDER, 1967). Both reactions give a more or less selective portrayal of monocytes. Human blood basophils have been reported to react positively to both techniques (LENNERT and SCHUBERT, 1960), although the reaction intensity is considerably weaker than that of monocytes (LÖFFLER, 1961; 1962; QUAGLINO *et al.*, 1962; BAKALOS *et al.*, 1963; LEDER and NICOLAS, 1963; MERKER, 1964). A similar reaction was found in leukemic basophils (SHIBATA *et al.*, 1966). A survey of the reactivity of different granulocytic cells to the nonspecific esterase is given in Table 7.

Naphthol AS-D Chloroacetate Esterase (LEDER's esterase). Neutrophil granulocytes split naphthol-substituted chloroacyl (GOMORI, 1953; BURSTONE, 1957). The replacement as coupling agent of fast garnet GBS by pararosaniline (LEDER, 1964) opened up a new approach to the understanding of cytogenetic relationships in the hematopoietic system because

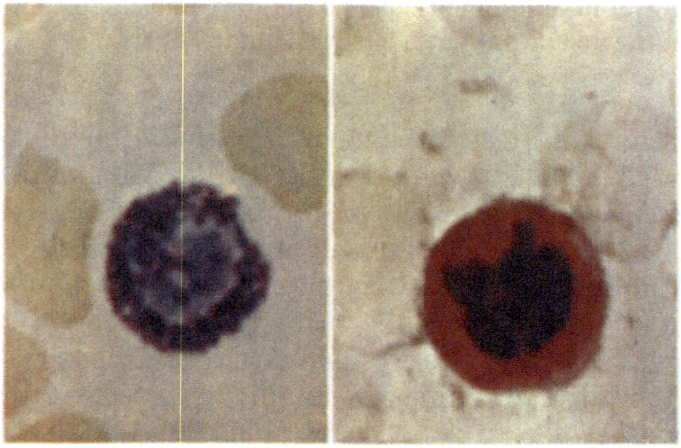

Fig. 14. Normal blood smear. Left: A blood basophil stained with toluidine blue. Right: The same cell stained for the acid phosphatase reaction. Note the diffuse strong positivity of the enzyme reaction; × 1,800

Table 7. Reactivity of myelogenous cell lines to the nonspecific esterase

Cell lines	Maturation Stages: Promyelo-cytes	Myelo-cytes	Metamyelo-cytes	Band-forms	Seg-mented
Neutrophils	–	+	–	–	–
Eosinophils	–	–	–	–	–
Basophils	–	–	–	±	+
Monocytes	–	+	++	+++	

the reaction could be carried out in the commonly processed paraffin-embedded sections (LEDER, 1964) even after extensive exposure to alcohols, and formaldehyde.

LEDER's esterase is basically seen as a distinctive mark of promyelocytes. Being chiefly bound to the so-called primary granules, it serves as a strictly specific and regular tracer of a genetically fixed property of the myelogenous system. Human blood basophils in the mature stage of segmented nuclear forms regularly react negatively to LEDER's esterase (MOLONEY *et al.*, 1960; LAMBERS and BAUER-SIC 1963; LEDER, 1964). In the usual technique, basophils lose their specific granules and can hardly be distinguished, which may explain why some authors believed them to react positively (MERKER, 1963). Reports to the contrary stimulated further investigations in this field, which definitely proved the naphthol AS-D chloroacetate negativity of mature basophils (LANGNER and STEIGLEDER, 1966). Using toluidine blue, we stained over 1200 blood basophils from 15 healthy subjects and 5 cases of reactive leukocytosis. The smears were then destained and LEDER's esterase reaction was implemented. We found no single instance of positively reacting mature normal basophils (PARWARESCH *et al.*, 1970; 1971), which seems to justy the statement that normal mature basophils never react positively to the LEDER's esterase, even in cases of accelerated emergence. This is shown in Fig. 15, where a basophil displaying typical toluidine-blue metachromasia is subjected to the enzyme reaction.

The constant behavior of hematopoietic cells as regards their reactivity to LEDER's esterase is summarized in Table 8. It will be noted that, in contrast to normal polymorphonuclear basophils, their progenitors always display considerable activity to LEDER's esterase, and neoplastic basophils in cases of myeloproliferative diseases partly do so. This question will be dealt with in later chapters.

Histidine Decarboxylase. The origin of the histamine in basophils has been much debated. The view that histamine is produced by certain strains of intestinal microflora resorbed and accumulated in blood basophils seemed to find support in the evidence of histidine decarboxylase activity

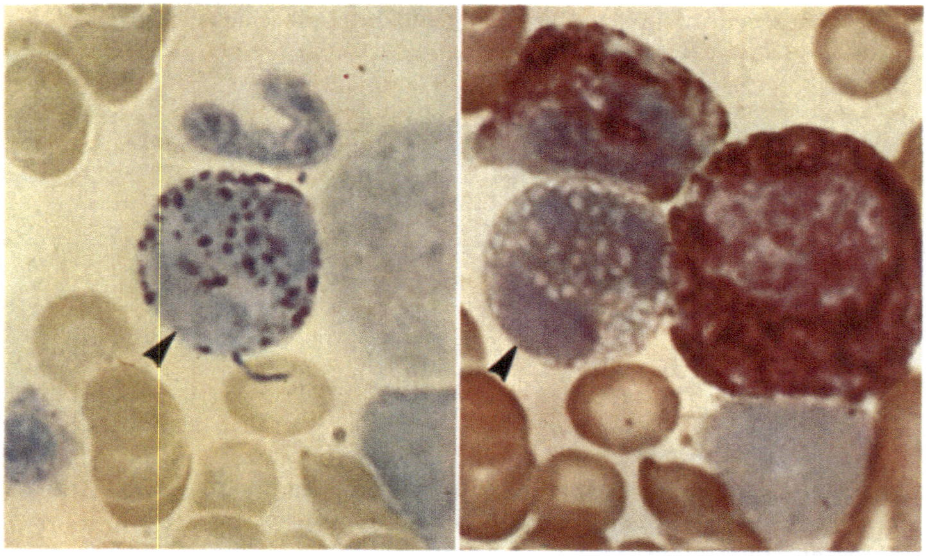

Fig. 15. Normal marrow smear. Left: Polymorphonuclear basophil stained with toluidine blue at pH 2.8 (*arrow*). Right: The same cell treated for the naphthol AS-D chloroacetate esterase reaction and haemalum counter stained. ×1,800

in these bacteria (WOLSTENHOLME and O'CONNOR, 1956; RILEY, 1959). Later, however, histidine decarboxylase activity could also be demonstrated in leukocyte concentrates rich in blood basophils. HARTMANN *et al.* (1960), using L-histidine-2(ring)-^{14}C as substrate and pyridoxal-5-phosphate as coenzyme, presented unequivocal evidence of histamine production, even under sterile conditions that precluded possible bacterial decarboxylase activity. According to SCHAYER (1960; 1963), histidine decarboxylase is an adaptive enzyme which under certain circumstances reaches high activities, while pyridoxal-5-phosphate is the natural coenzyme. Tissue mast cells, which contain considerable amounts of histamine, have been shown to contain pyridoxal-5-phosphate in their intergranular cytoplasm (BENDITT, 1968).

Table 8. Reactivity of granulocytic system to LEDER's esterase. With the exception of tissue mast cells, all other cells give a negative reaction

	Maturation Stages				
Cell lines	Promyelocytes	Myelocytes	Metamyelocytes	Band-forms	Segmented
Neutrophils	++++	+++	+++	++	++
Eosinopils	+	–	–	–	–
Basophils	++++	+++	++	+	–
Monocytes	++++	+++	++		±

5. Biogenic Amines (Histamine)

Due to their high amine content, tissue mast cells and blood basophils have often been assumed to be part of a transmitter system serving the adaptive reactions of the organism in response to injurious stimuli. Quantitative and qualitative changes in blood basophils have been reported in connection with stress, acute inflammation, shock, and hyperergic reactions. A great deal of interest has been focused on the release of histamine by basophils shedding their specific granules into the surrounding medium.

There is still no satisfactory method for the cytochemical demonstration of biogenic amines in basophils, although quite a number of extremely sensitive techniques have been developed for the visualization of biogenic amines in tissue mast cells. It is only a matter of time before there a method that can be used on blood basophils becomes available.

The occurrence of histamine in tissue mast cells, first proposed by CAZAL (1942), was experimentally verified 10 years later by RILEY and WEST (1952, 1953 a, b, 1955 a, b). Of the biogenic amines, only histamine appears in human tissue mast cells, whereas 5-hydroxytryptamine is also claimed to occur in rodent mast cells (review by RILEY, 1959; SELYE, 1965; BOOZ, 1967).

CODE and MACDONALD (1937) extracted histamine from leukocyte concentrates of various species. In 1952, GRAHAM *et al.*, succeeded in detecting histamine in human blood basophils. They established that blood basophils contain 50 times as much histamine as any other blood cell. Later results were in full agreement with these findings (VALENTINE *et al.*, 1955; CODE and MITCHELL, 1957; SAMPSON and ARCHER, 1967). The biochemical evidence of the presence of histamine and other biogenic amines in tissue mast cells, blood basophils, and especially nerve cells stressed the need to make these substances accessible to cytochemical methods. The discovery by CARLSON *et al.* (1961) and FALK (1962) that the condensation of biogenic amines with formaldehyde (EHRLEN, 1948; HESS and UDENFRIEND, 1959) under special conditions confers a strong fluorescence on cytoplasm of tissue mast cells paved the way for the development of highly sensitive cytochemical methods for the demonstration of dopamine (CORRODI and HILLARP, 1964; CORRODI *et al.*, 1964), noradrenaline (FALK and TORP, 1962; ANGELAKOS and KING, 1965; COUPLAND, 1965; RITZEN, 1966; EL-BADWI and SCHENK, 1967), adrenaline (COUPLAND, 1965), hydroxytryptamine (COUPLAND, 1965; CORRODI and JONSSON, 1965; FUXE and JONSSON, 1967; RITZEN, 1967), 3,4-dehydrophenyl-alanine (CORRODI and JONSSON, 1966), and 5-hydroxytryptophan (RITZEN and HAMMARSTRÖM, 1965). The cytotopographic localization of monoamine-containing structures has been of great help in studies on the metabolism, synthesis, accumulation, and liberation of the biogenic amines (DAHLSTRÖM and FUXE, 1964; 1965; MALMFORS, 1965; NORBERG, 1965; ANDEN *et al.*, 1966). In 1959 SCHAUER and WERLE attempted to visualize histamine precipitated as REINECKE salt through treatment with diazotized sulfanilic acid. The method had to be given up due to insensitivity and artifacts. The fluorescence produced by formalin vapor (LAGUNOFF *et al.*, 1961) was believed to be specific for histamine. Later studies have shown, however, that the formaldehyde fluorescence has no connection with the histamine content (LISON, 1966; CORRODI and JONSSON, 1967; SHELLEY *et al.*, 1968). The decisive step forward in the cytochemical visualization of histamine was taken by JUHLIN and SHELLEY (1966). They converted the fluorometric method of SHORE *et al.* (1959) into a cytochemical technique. The method consisted of a condensation of o-phthalaldehyde with histamine in a strongly alkaline medium. In acidic pH regions the condensation product displays under monochrome light (3500 Å) a strongly yellowish fluorescence with an absorption maximum at 5400 Å. For cytochemical uses, a 1% o-phthalaldehyde solution in ethylene benzol is suitable. The preparation is incubated for 4 min in a damp chamber at room temperature, then immediately covered with tetrahydrofurfurol (JUHLIN and SHELLEY, 1966; SHELLEY and JUHLIN, 1966; EHINGER and THUNBERG, 1967; JUHLIN, 1967 a and b; SHELLEY *et al.*, 1968; ENERBÄCK, 1969). SHELLEY *et al.* (1968) tested large numbers of compounds for their fluoreophoric properties, using o-phthalaldehyde in ethylene benzol. Among the many amines tested, DL-beta 3,4-dihydroxyphenylalanine (DOPA) showed a green fluorescence, adrenaline a bluish green, glutathion in reduced from a luminous blue, noradrenaline an orange-blue, procaine HCl a yellowish brown, and taurine a weak ocher color. In the control tests, only L-histidine dihydrochloride displayed a weak yellow fluorescence. This guaranteed the specificity of the method for histamine. As the lowest limit for detectable histamine concentration, the authors recommended a dilution ratio of $1 : 10^4$ (less than 0.1 μg free base), which, however, applies only to their own histochemical models. SHORE *et al.* (1959) were able to detect by means of the spectral fluorometric method concentrations as low as 0.005 μg/ml. According to our calculations and those in the literature, the tissue mast cells contain 7 to 50×10^{-6} μg histamine as the equivalent of free base in a cell (RILEY, 1953; GRAHAM *et al.*, 1955; PATON, 1957). Blood basophils, which contain only $2.5 \pm 0.6 \times 10^{-6}$ μg histamine per cell (SAMPSON and ARCHER, 1967), could not so far be handled with the same technique. Our attempts to produce an o-phthaldehyde fluorescence in variously fixed blood basophils also failed.

The fact that basophil granules are readily soluble in water is one more technical difficulty, added to all the others. The only attribute of most fixatives is their ability to preserve the glycosaminoglycans in the basophil granules. The solubility of histamine has received little consideration.

6. Trace Elements (Zinc, Copper)

WOLFF (1956), using leukocyte concentrates from human blood, ascertained a zinc content of 22.5 μg/10^9 cells, which is more than that found in erythrocytes. Earlier reports from WEITZEL and FRETZDORFF (1953; 1956) and WEITZEL (1956) established that zinc is usually found combined with histamine, or with histamine and heparin (KERP and STEINHÄUSER, 1961).

The zinc content of blood basophils was investigated by AMANN and WOLFF (1955; 1956). Using the dithizone reaction, AMANN (1963) and RASKOVIC and GEREBTZOFF (1963) reported that zinc was detectable in neutrophils, as well as in eosinophils and basophils. According to SZIMIGIELSKI and LITWIN (1965), zinc appears first in metamyelocytes and the amount increases as the cell matures. Thus, the polymorphonuclear granulocytes, including the mature basophils, yield the highest content. The leukocyte zinc content is said to vary in typical ways in different diseases (FREDERICKS *et al.*, 1960; 1964).

The total leukocyte zinc content does not correlate with the blood basophil count, for example, in cases of basophilia. SMITH *et al.* (1969) were able to develop a special fluorescent microscopic method for the cytochemical demonstration of zinc, derived from a modification of the zinc detection technique of MAHANAND and HOUCK (1968). According to this technique, blood smears were incubated for 15 min in a mixture of 0.1 ml of 3% 8-hydroxyquinoline in absolute ethanol and 25 ml MICHAELIS universal buffer at pH 8. The fluorescent optical investigation was done with a mercury lamp at 395 nm. In this technique, which is preferred to other methods because it is much less susceptible to artifacts, the blood basophil granules give clearly positive results.

Tissue mast cell granules and eosinophil granulocytes have been investigated for their copper content by various cytochemical methods (OKAMOTO, 1942; AMANN and WOLFF, 1956). AMANN later (1963) questioned his own original findings, which showed a positive reaction in basophil granules (1961). Further investigations have thrown doubt on whether copper really does occur in blood basophils.

7. Amino Acids

Some amino acids, among them arginine, histidine, tyrosine, cystine, and tryptophane, have been reported to be detectable in human basophils (ACKERMANN, 1964). It has not yet been determined whether there is a relationship between these amino acids and the crystalline structures occasionally observed in basophil granules.

References

ABUL HAJ, S. K., RINEHART, J. F.: 1962. Cited in ACKERMAN, G. A.: Cytochemical properties of the blood basophilic granulocyte. Ann. N. Y. Acad. Sci. **103,** 376 – 393 (1963). Ed. PADAWER, J.

ACKERMAN, G. A.: Histochemistry of the centrioles and centrosomes of the leukemic cells from human myeloblastic leukemia. J. biophys. biochem. Cytol. **11,** 717 – 719 (1961).

ACKERMAN, G. A.: Histochemical demonstration of aminopeptidase activity in the cells of the blood and bone marrow from various hematological disorders. Nature (Lond.) **197,** 189 – 190 (1963).

ACKERMAN, G. A.: Leukopoiesis in health and disease. Ann. N. Y. Acad. Sci. **113,** 537 – 565 (1964). Ed. H. R. BIERMAN.

AMANN, R.: Zur Physiologie und Biochemie der Mastzellen. Arch. klin. exp. Derm. **213**, 565 – 572 (1961).

AMANN, R.: Histochemischer Schwermetallnachweis in Blut- und Gewebsmastzellen. In: Zyto- und Histochemie in der Haematologie, Ed. H. MERKER. Berlin-Göttingen-Heidelberg; Springer 1963.

AMANN, R., MARTIN, H.: Blutmastzellen und Heparin. Acta haemat. (Basel) **25**, 209 – 219 (1961).

AMANN, R., WOLFF, H. R.: 1955, 5. Kongreß Europ. Ges. Haematol. Cited in: H. R. WOLFF, D. RINGLEB und R. AMANN: Histochemische Untersuchungen über das Inselzink; histophotometrische Messungen. Z. ges. exp. Med. **126**, 390 – 416 (1955).

AMANN, R., WOLFF, H. R.: Schwermetalle in Leukocyten. Z. ges. exp. Med. **127**, 281 – 292 (1956).

ANDEN, N. R., CORRODI, H., DAHLSTRÖM, A., FUXE, K., HÖKFELT, T.: Effects of tyrosine hydroxylase inhibition on the intra-neutronal amine levels of the central monoamine neurons. Life Sci. **5**, 561 – 568 (1966).

ANGELAKOS, E. T., KING, M. P.: A new histochemical method for the specific demonstration of catecholamine-containing structures. Fed. Proc. **24**, 389 (1965).

ASTALDI, G.: La fosfatasi nelle cellule eritopoietiche. Haematologica **37**, 599 – 626 (1953).

ASTALDI, G., BERNADELLI, E., RONDANELLI, G.: Richerche sul contenuto in glicogeno delle cellule del sangue e del midollo osseo. Folia haemat. (Lpz.) **36**, 749 – 771 (1952).

ASTALDI, G., RONDANELLI, E. G., BERNADELLI, E.: Recherches cytochimiques sur la moelle osseuse et le sang d'une leucémie à basocytes. Rev. Hémat. **8**, 105 – 118 (1953).

ASTALDI, G., RONDANELLI, E. G., BERNADELLI E.: Ricerche istochimiche sul contenuto dei granuli delle mastcellule del midollo osseo umano. Haematologica **38**, 967 – 991 (1954).

ASTALDI, G., STROSSELLI, E.: Cytochemie der Leukocytengranulation bei seltenen Blutkrankheiten. In: Zyto-Histochemie in der Hämatologie. Berlin-Göttingen-Heidelberg: Springer 1963.

AUSTIN, J. H., BISCHEL, M.: A histochemical method for sulfatase activity in hemic cells and organ imprints. Blood **17**, 216 – 224 (1961).

BAILLIF, R. N., KINBROUGH, C.: Studies on leucocyte granules after staining with Sudan black B and MAY-GRÜNWALD-Giemsa. J. Lab. clin. Med. **32**, 155 – 166 (1947).

BAKALOS, D., PETROPOULOS, P.: The non-specific esterase activity of the monocyte. A further contribution to the myeloid origin of moncytes. Blut **9**, 7 – 20 (1963).

BAKER, J. R.: The histochemical recongnition of lipine. Quart. J. micr. Sci. **87**, 441 – 470 (1946).

BAKER, J. R.: Principles of Biological Microtechnique, pp. 19 – 44, 89 – 138, 149 – 150. New York: John Wiley and Sons Inc. 1958.

BALOGH, K. Jr., COHEN, B.: Histochemical demonstration of diaphorases and dehydrogenases in normal human leucocytes and platelets. Blood **17**, 491 – 496 (1961).

BANGLE, R., Jr.: Gomori's paraldehyde-fuchsin stain. I. Physico-chemical and staining properties of the dye. J. Histochem. Cytochem. **2**, 291 – 299 (1954).

BANK, O., BUNGENBERG DE JONG, H. G.: Untersuchungen über Metachromasie. Protoplasma **32**, 489 – 516 (1939).

BECK, W. S.: Occurrence and control of the phospho-gluconate oxidation pathway in normal and leukemic leukocytes. J. biol. Chem. **232,** 271 – 285 (1958).

BECK, W. S., VALENTINE, W. N.: Carbohydrate metabolism of leukocytes. Cancer Res. **13,** 309 – 317 (1953).

BEHRENS, M., TAUBERT, M.: Der Nachweis von Heparin in den basophilen Leukocyten. Klin. Wschr. **30,** 76 – 78 (1952).

BENDITT, E. P.: 5-Hydroxytryptamine and 5-hydroxytryptophan decarboxylase in rat mast cells. 5-hydroxytryptamine, p. 32. New York: Pergamon Press 1968.

BERGERON, J. A., SINGER, M.: Metachromasia: An experimental and theoretical reevaluation. J. biophys. biochem. Cytol. **4,** 433 – 457 (1958).

BERGSTRÖM, S.: 1930. Cited in: S. BERGSTRÖM: Über die Wirkungsgruppe des Heparins. Naturwissenschaften **23,** 706 (1935).

BERGSTRÖM, S.: Über die Wirkungsgruppe des Heparins. Naturwissenschaften **23,** 706 (1935).

BIAVA, C.: Identification and structural forms of human particulate glycogen. Lab. Invest. **12,** 1179 – 1197 (1963).

BLOOM, M. L., WISLOCKI, G. B.: The localization of lipids in human blood and bone marrow cells. Blood **5,** 79 – 88 (1950).

BLOOM, G., KELLY, J. W.: The copper phthalocyanine dye "Astrablau" and its staining properties, especially the staining of mast cells. Histochemie **2,** 48 – 57 (1960).

BOIVIN, P., ROBINEAUX, R.: Cytochimie des leukocytes. (Cytochemistry of leukocytes). Rev. franç. clin. Biol. **2,** 495 – 516 (1957).

BOOZ, K. H.: Der histochemische Nachweis des Tryptophans, 5-Hydroxytryptamins und der Monoaminoxydase in den Mastzellen der Ratte. Verh. anat. Ges. (Jena) **62,** 547 – 556 (1967).

BOSEILA, A. W. A., UHRBRAND, H.: see page 22.

BRAUNSTEINER, H.: In: BRAUNSTEINER und ZUCKER-FRANKLIN. New York: Grune & Stratton, 1962.

BRAUNSTEINER, H., ZUCKER-FRANKLIN, D.: Mast cells and basophil leukocytes. In: The Physiology and Pathology of Leukocytes, pp. 46 – 62. Ed. H. BRAUNSTEINER and D. ZUCKER-FRANKLIN New York: Grune & Stratton 1957.

BURSTONE, M. S.: Esterase activity of developing bones and teeth. AMA Arch. Path. **63,** 164 – 167 (1957).

CARLSSON, A., FALCK, B., HILLARP, N.-Å., THIEME, G., TORP, A.: A new histochemical method for visualization of tissue catecholamines. Med. Exp. **4,** 123 – 125 (1961).

CASSELMAN, W. G. B.: Histochemical Technique, pp. 48 – 51, 55 – 56, 91 – 109, 134 – 135. New York: John Wiley and Sons, Inc. 1959.

CASTOLDI, G. L., YAM, L. T., MITUS, W. J.: Cytochemical demonstration of dihydroorotic dehydrogenase in blood and bone marrow cells. Acta haemat. (Basel) **39,** 203 – 213 (1968).

CAZAL, P.: Un nouvel aspect de la médicine tissulaire: les réticulopathies, et le systéme reticulo-histiocytaire. Paris: Vigot 1942.

CODE, C. F., MACDONALD: The histamine-like activity of blood. Lancet **1937 II,** 730 – 738.

CODE, C. F., MITCHELL, R. G.: see page 22.

CONN, E., BANGLE, R.: 1954. Cited in: R. C. CURRAN and J. S. KENNEDY: The distribution of the sulfated mucopoly-saccharides in the mouse. J. Path. Bact. **70,** 449 – 457 (1955).

CORRODI, H., HILLARP, N.-Å.: Fluorescenzmethoden zur histochemischen Sichtbarmachung von Monoaminen. 2. Identifizierung des fluorescierenden Produktes aus Dopamin und Formaldehyd. Helv. chim. Acta. **47,** 911 – 918 (1964).

CORRODI, H., HILLARP, N.-Å., JONSSON, G.: Fluorescence methods for the histochemical demonstration of monoamines. 3. Sodium borohydride reduction of the fluorescent compounds as a specificity test. J. Histochem. Cytochem. **15,** 582 – 586 (1964).

CORRODI, H., JONSSON, G.: Fluorescence methods for the histochemical demonstration of monoamines. 4. Histochemical differentiation between dopamine and noradrenaline in models. J. Histochem. Cytochem. **13,** 484 – 487 (1965 a).

CORRODI, H., JONSSON, G.: Fluorescenzmethoden zur histochemischen Sichtbarmachung von Monoaminen. 5. Identifizierung des fluorescierenden Produktes aus Modellversuchen mit 5-Methoxytryptamin und Formaldehyd. Acta Histochem. (Jena) **22,** 247 – 258 (1965 b).

CORRODI, H., JONSSON, G.: Fluorescenzmethoden zur histochemischen Sichtbarmachung von Monoaminen. 6. Identifizierung der fluorescierenden Produkte aus m-Hydroxyphenylaethylaminen und Formaldehyd. Helv. chim. Acta **49,** 798 – 806 (1966).

CORRODI, H., JONSSON, G.: The formaldehyde fluorescence method for the histochemical demonstration of biogenic amines. A review on the methodology. J. Histochem. Cytochem. **15,** 65 – 78 (1967).

COUPLAND, R. E.: The Natural History of the Chromaffin Cell. London: Longmans Green 1965.

DAHLSTRÖM, A., FUXE, K.: A method for the demonstration of monoamine-containing nerve fibers in the central nervous system. Acta physiol. scand. **60,** 293 – 294 (1964).

DAHLSTRÖM, A., FUXE, K.: Evidence for the existence of monoamine neurons in the central nervous system. II. Experimentally induced changes in the intraneuronal amine levels of bulbospinal neuron systems. Acta physiol. scand. **64,** Suppl. 247, 1 – 36 (1965).

DEANE, H. W., BARRNETT, R. J., SELIGMAN, A. M.: Histochemische Methoden zum Nachweis der Enzymaktivität. In: W. GRAUMANN und K. NEUMANN (Hrsg.): Handbuch der Histochemie, Bd. VII/1. Stuttgart: Gustav Fischer 1960.

DEMPSEY, E. W., SINGER, M.: Observations on the chemical cytology of the thyroid gland at different functional stages. Endocrinology **38,** 270 – 295 (1946).

DE SOUZA, E. J., KOTHARE, S. N.: A method for the cytochemical demonstration of succinic dehydrogenase in human leucocytes. J. Histochem. Cytochem. **7,** 77 – 79 (1959).

DUNN, J. S.: The oxydase reaction in myeloid tissues. J. Path. Bact. (Cambridge) **15,** 20 – 30 (1910/1911).

DUNN, W. B., SPICER, S. S.: Sulfated mucosubstances and basic proteins in human granulocytes. Hematology **1,** 671 (1968).

ECKSTEIN, M., LINDNER, J.: Cytochemie der Mastzellen. Verh. 8. Kongr. Europ. Ges. Haematol., III, 41 – 94. Wien 1961.

EHINGER, B., THUNBERG, R.: Induction of fluorescence in histamine-containing cells. Exp. Cell Res. **47,** 116 – 122 (1967).

EHRLEN, J.: Fluorimetric determination of adrenalin. Farm. Rev. (Stockh.) 1948.

EHRLICH, P.: Beiträge zur Kenntnis der Anilinfärbungen und ihrer Verwendung in der mikroskopischen Technik. Arch. mikr. Anat. **13,** 263 – 277 (1877).

EILUND, R., PERSSON, B. H.: The influence of polar solvents on the metachromatic reaction in vitro. Experientia (Basel) **5,** 210 – 211 (1949).

El-Badawi, A., Schenk, E. A.: Histochemical methods for separate consecutive and simultaneous demonstration of acetylcholinesterase and norepinephrine in cryostat sections. J. Histochem. Cytochem. **15,** 580 – 587 (1967).

Elftman, H.: A Schiff reagent of calibrated sensitivity. J. Histochem. Cytochem. **7,** 93 – 97 (1959 a).

Elftman, H.: Combined aldehyde-fuchsin and periodic acid-Schiff staining of the pituitary. Stain Technol. **34,** 77 – 80 (1959 b).

Enerbäck, L.: Detection of histamine in mast cells by o-phthalaldehyde reaction after liquid fixation. J. Histochem. Cytochem. **17,** 757 – 759 (1969).

Falck, B.: Observations on the possibilities of the cellular localization of monoamines by a fluorescence method. Acta physiol. scand., Suppl. **197,** 1 – 25 (1962).

Falck, B., Torp, A.: New evidence for the localization of noradrenaline in the adrenergic nerve terminales. Med. Exp. **6,** 169 – 172 (1962).

Fasske, E.: Zur Darstellung der sauren Mucopolysaccharide im Bereich der Zwischensubstanz mesenchymaler Gewebe. Zbl. allg. Path. path. Anat. **97,** 174 – 179 (1957).

Fischer, R.: Probleme der Enzymhistochemie beim Nachweis oxydativer Fermente an Blutzellen. In: Cyto- und Histochemie in der Haematologie. 9. Freiburger Symposion. Hrsg. H. Merker: Berlin-Göttingen-Heidelberg: Springer 1963.

Fredericks, R. E., Tanaka, K. R., Valentine, W. N.: Zinc in human blood cells: normal values and abnormalities associated with liver disease. J. clin. Invest. **39,** 1651 – 1656 (1960).

Fredericks, R. E., Tanaka, K. R., Valentine, W. N.: Variations of human blood cell zinc in disease. J. clin. Invest. **43,** 304 – 315 (1964).

Friedmann, H. C., Vennesland, B.: Purification and properties of dihydroorotic dehydrogenase. J. biol. Chem. **233,** 1398 – 1406 (1958).

Fuxe, K., Jonsson, G.: A modification of the histochemical fluorescence method for the improved localization of 5-hydroxytryptamine. Histochemie **11,** 161 – 166 (1967).

Gedigk, P.: Über neue Färbeverfahren für Mucopolysaccharide und Phospholipide. Zbl. allg. Path. path. Anat. **95,** 486 (1956).

Gibb, R. P., Stowell, R. E.: Glycogen in human blood cells. Blood **4,** 569 – 579 (1949).

Gomori, G.: Microtechnical demonstration of phosophatase I. Histochemische Untersuchungsmethodik der Phosphatase und deren Verteilung in verschiedenen Organen und Geweben. Trans. Soc. Path. Jap. **29,** 492 – 498 (1939).

Gomori, G.: Distribution of phospatase in normal organs and tissues. J. cell comp. Physiol. **17,** 71 – 83 (1941).

Gomori, G.: Distribution of acid phosphatase in the tissue under normal and under pathologic conditions. Arch. Path. **32,** 189 – 199 (1941).

Gomori, G.: see page 23.

Gomori, G.: Microscopic histochemistry, principles and practice. Chicago: University of Chicago Press, 1952.

Gomori, G.: Oxydase reaction of myeloid elements. H. Histochem. Cytochem. **1,** 486 – 492 (1953).

Gomori, G.: Chloroacylesters as histochemical substrate J. Histochem. Cytochem. **1,** 469 – 470 (1953).

Graham, G. S.: The hemic basophil. J. exp. Med. **31,** 209 – 231 (1920).

Graham, H. T., Wheelwright, F., Parish, H. H., Jr., Marks, A. R., Lowry, O. H.: Distribution of histamine among blood elements. Fed. Proc. **11,** 350 (1952).

GRAHAM, H. T., LOWRY, O. H., WHEELWRIGHT, F., LENZ, M. A., PARISH, H. H., Jr.: Distribution of histamine among leukocytes and platelets. Blood **10,** 467 – 481 (1955).

HALE, C. W.: Histochemical demonstration of acid polysaccharides in animal tissues. Nature (Lond.) **157,** 802 (1946).

HALE, C. W.: The histochemistry of polysaccharides. In: International Review of Cytology. Bourne, G. H. and J. F. Danielli (eds)., Vol. 6, pp. 193 – 263. New York: Academic Press Inc. 1957.

HARDIE, W. B., WESBROOK, F. F.: The wandering cells of the alimentary canals. J. Physiol. (Lond.) **18,** 490 – 524 (1895).

HARMS, H.: Handbuch der Farbstoffe für die Mikroskopie. Kamp-Lintfort: Staufen-Verlag 1965.

HARTMANN, W. J., CLARK, W. G., CYR, S. D.: Histine decarboxylase activity of basophils from chronic myelogenous leukemic patients. Origin of blood histamine. Proc. Soc. exp. Biol. **107,** 123 – 125 (1960).

HAUSER, H.: Über Bau und Funktion der Wiederkäuerparotis. Z. mikro.-anat. Forsch. **41,** 177 – 228 (1937).

HAYHOE, F. G. J.: The cytochemical demonstration of lipids in blood and bonemarrow cells. J. Path. Bact. **65,** 413 – 421 (1953).

HAYHOE, F. G. J.: In: Whitby & Britton: Disorders of the Blood. London: Churchill 1963.

HAYHOE, F. G. J., QUAGLINO, D.: Autoradiographic investigations of RNA and DNA metabolism of human leukocytes cultured with phytohaemagglutinin; uridine-5-3H als a specific precursor of RNA. Nature (Lond.): **205,** 151 – 154 (1964).

HERWERDEN, M. A.: Über das Voluntin und seine chemische Zusammensetzung. Fol. microbiol. **5,** 18 – 30 (1919).

HESS, S. M., UDENFRIEND, S.: A fluorometric procedure for the measurement of tryptamine in tissues. J. Pharmacol. exp. Ther. **127,** 175 – 177 (1959).

HIRSHFELD, H.: Erfahrungen mit der Oxydase- und Peroxydasereaktion. Med. Klin. **20,** 249 – 250 (1924).

HOLMGREN, H., WILLANDER, O.: Beitrag zur Kenntnis der Chemie und Funktion der Ehrlichschen Mastzellen. Z. mikr.-anat. Forsch. **42,** 242 – 278 (1937).

HOTCHKISS, R. D. A.: A microchemical reaction resulting in the staining of polysaccharide structures in fixed tissue preparations. Arch. Biochem. **16,** 131 – 141 (1948).

HOWELL, G. H., HOLT, E.: Two new factors in blood coagulation: heparin and proantithrombin. Amer. J. Physiol. **47,** 328 – 345 (1918).

INAGAKI, S.: Cytochemical reactions of basophil leucocytes. I. Peroxidase staining. Acta haemat. jap. **26,** 544 – 548 (1963).

INAGAKI, S.: Cytochemical reactions of basophil leucocytes. II. NADI staining. Acta haemat. jap. **27,** 431 – 435 (1964).

INAGAKI, S.: Cytochemical reactions of basophil leucocytes. III. DOPA staining. Acta haemat. jap. **28,** 125 – 129 (1965 a).

INAGAKI, S.: Cytochemical reactions of basophil leucocytes. IV. Adrenaline staining. Acta haemat. jap. **28,** 618 – 622 (1965 b).

INAGAKI, S.: Cytochemical reactions of basophil leucocytes. VII. Periodic acid-Schiff (PAS) reaction. Acta haemat. jap. **31,** 169 – 174 (1968).

INAGAKI, S.: Cytochemical reactions of basophil leucocytes. VIII. Astra blue staining. Acta haemat. jap. **32,** 148 – 153 (1969).

JORPES, E.: The chemistry of heparin. Biochem. J. **29,** 1817 (1935).

JORPES, J. E., WERNER, B., ABERG, B.: The fuchsin-sulfurous acid test after periodate oxidation of heparin and allied polysaccharides. J. biol. Chem. **176,** 277 – 282 (1948).

JUHLIN, L.: Localization and content of histamine in normal and diseased skin. Acta derm.-venereol. (Stockh.) **47,** 383 – 391 (1967 a).

JUHLIN, L.: Determination of histamine in small biopsies and histological sections. Acta physiol. scand. **71,** 30 – 36 (1967 b).

JUHLIN, L., SHELLEY, W. B.: Detection of histamine by a new fluorescent o-phthalaldehyde stain. J. Histochem. Cytochem. **14,** 525 – 528 (1966).

KABAT, E. A., FURTH, J.: A histochemical study of the distribution of alkaline phosphatase in various normal and neoplastic tissue. Amer. J. Path. **17,** 303 – 318 (1941).

KAPLOW, L. S.: Leukocyte alkaline phosphatase cytochemistry: applications and methods. Ann. N. Y. Acad. Sci. **155,** 911 – 947 (1968).

KAUNG, D. T.: Periodic acid-Schiff reaction in human basophilic leucocytes. Acta haemat. (Basel) **42,** 269 – 274 (1969).

KELLY, G. F.: 1935. Cited in: G. F. KELLY: Eosinophilia. Amer. J. Dis. Child. **49,** 403 – 407 (1936).

KELLY, G. F.: Eosinophilia. Amer. J. Dis. Child. **49,** 403 – 407 (1936).

KELLY, J. W.: Suppression of metachromasia by basic proteins. Arch. Biochem. Biophys. **55,** 130 – 137 (1955).

KELLY, J. W.: The metachromatic reaction, Protoplasma **2,** 1 – 98 (1956).

KERP, L., STEINHÄUSER, G.: Über einen tertiären Heparin-Metall-Histamin-Komplex. Klin. Wschr. **39,** 762 – 764 (1961).

KOPPEL, J. L., OLWIN, J. H.: Dehydrogenase activities of human platelets. Proc. Soc. exp. Biol. (N. Y.) **86,** 641 – 645 (1954).

KRAMER, H., WINDRUM, G. M.: The metachromatic staining reaction. J. Histochem. Cytochem. **3,** 227 – 237 (1955).

KREIBICH, C.: Leukocytendarstellung in Gewebe durch Adrenalin. Wien. klin. Wschr. **41,** 701 – 702 (1910).

KUHN, H.: A quantum-mechanical theory of light absorption of organic dyes and similar compounds. J. chem. Phys. **17,** 1198 – 1212 (1949).

LAGUNOFF, A., PHILLIPS, M., BENDITT, E. P.: The histochemical demonstration of histamine in mast cells. J. Histochem. Cytochem. **9,** 534 – 541 (1961).

LAMBERS, K., BAUER-SICK, P.: Hydrolytische Enzyme in der klinischen Diagnostik. In: Zyto- und Histochemie der Haematologie. Ed. H. MERKER. 9. Freiburger Symposion. Berlin-Göttingen-Heidelberg: Springer 1963.

LANDING, B. H., WILSON, H. E.: Effects of inorganic oxides, sulfides, chlorides, and acid chlorides on metachromasia and other staining properties. Stain Technol. **34,** 273 – 277 (1959).

LANDSMEER, J. M. F.: Some colloid chemical aspects of metachromasia. Influence of pH and salts on metachromatic phenomena evoked by toluidine blue in animal tissue. Acta physiol. pharmacol. neerl. **2,** 112 – 128 (1951).

LANGNER, R., STEIGLEDER, G. K.: Läßt sich eine Naphthol-AS-D-Chloracetat-Esterase Aktivität in den basophilen Granulocyten des Blutes nachweisen? Klin. Wschr. **44,** 900 – 901 (1966).

LAVES, W.: Über die Anwendung von Enzymen in der Haematologie und die physiologische Bedeutung der Nukleasen für die periphere Leukocyten-Steuerung. Acta haemat (Basel) **8,** 1 – 28 (1952).

LAVES, W., THOMA, K.: Histoenzymatische Untersuchungen an den Mastzellen des Blutes. Klin. Wschr. **28,** 95 – 96 (1950).

LEACH, E. H.: Bismarck brown as a stain for mucoproteins. Stain Technol. **22**, 73 – 76 (1947).

LEBLOND, C. P.: Distribution of periodic acid reactive carbohydrates in the adult rat. Amer. J. Anat. **86**, 1 – 50 (1950).

LEDER, L.-D., NICOLAS, R.: Fermentcytochemische Untersuchungen zur Genese der Makrophagen an Hautfensterpräparaten. Frankfurt. Z. Path. **73**, 228 – 244 (1963).

LEDER, L.-D.: Über die selektive fermentcytochemische Darstellung von neutrophilen myeloischen Zellen und Gewebsmastzellen im Paraffinschnitt. Klin. Wschr. **42**, 553 (1964).

LEDER, L.-D.: Die fermentcytochemische Erkennung normaler und neoplastischer Erythropoiesezellen im Schnitt und Ausstrich. Blut **15**, 289 – 293 (1967).

LENNERT, K.: Zur Kenntnis der Mastzellenleukämie. Verh. dtsch. Ges. Path. **39**, 257 – 259 (1955).

LENNERT, K.: In: Handbuch der speziellen pathologischen Anatomie und Histologie, Vol I/3, p. 106 Lymphknoten. Berlin-Göttingen-Heidelberg: Springer 1961.

LENNERT, K.: Zur pathologischen Anatomie der „Mastocytosen" mit einigen Bemerkungen zur Cytochemie der Mastzellen. Arch. klin. exp. Derm. **213**, 606 – 624 (1961).

LENNERT, K.: Zur pathologischen Anatomie von Urticaria pigmentosa und Mastzellenretikulose. Klin. Wschr. **40**, 61 –67 (1962).

LENNERT, K.: Bildung und Differenzierung der Blutzellen, insbesondere der Lymphocyten, pp. 163 – 213 50. Tg. Verh. dtsch. Ges. Path. Heidelberg 1966. Stuttgart: Gustav Fischer Verlag 1966.

LENNERT, K., SCHUBERT, J. F. C.: Untersuchungen über die sauren Mucopolysaccharide der Gewebsmastzellen im menschlichen Knochenmark. Frankfurt. Z. Path. **69**, 579 – 590 (1959).

LENNERT, K., LENNERT, K., SCHUBERT, J. F. C.: Zur Histochemie der Gewebsmastzelle im menschlichen Lymphknoten. Frankfurt. Z. Path. **69**, 591 – 595 (1959).

LENNERT, K., SCHUBERT, J. F. C.: see page 24.

LENNERT, K., WEITZEL, G.: Morphologie und Histochemie der Bürzeldrüse von Enten. Z. mikr.-anat. Forsch. **58**, 208 – 229 (1952 a).

LENNERT, K., WEITZEL, G.: Zur Spezifität der histologischen Fettfärbungsmethoden. Z. wiss. Mikr. **61**, 20 – 29 (1952 b).

LENNERT, K., BACH, G.: Eine verfeinerte Technik der Toluidinblau-pH-Reihe zur Mastzellendarstellung. Klin. Wschr. **39**, 1026 – 1027 (1961).

LENNERT, K., SCHUBERT, J. F. C.: Cytochemischer Nachweis von Esteraseaktivität in den „Kugelhäufchen" (MOESCHLIN) der Megaloblasten. Klin. Wschr. **39**, 1027 – 1028 (1961).

LEV, R., SPICER, S. S.: Specific staining of sulphate groups with alcian blue at low pH. J. Histochem. Cytochem. **12**, 309 (1964).

LEVINE, N. D.: The determination of apparent isoelectric points of cell structures by staining at controlled reactions. Stain Technol. **15**, 91 – 112 (1940).

LIEBERMAN, I., KORNBERG, A.: Enzymatic synthesis and breakdown of a pyrimidine, orotic acid. II. Dihydroorotic acid, ureidosuccinic acid and 5-carboxymethylhydantoin. J. biol. Chem. **207**, 911 – 924 (1954).

LILLIE, R. D.: Further exploration of the HIO_4-Schiff reaction with remarks on its significance, Anat. Rec. **108**, 239 – 253 (1950).

LILLIE, R. D.: Argentaffin and Schiff reactions after periodic acid oxidation and aldehyde blocking reactions. J. Histochem. Cytochem. **2**, 127 – 136 (1954).

LILLIE, R. D.: Histopathological Technic and Practical Histochemistry, pp. 31 – 48 and 175. New York: The Blakiston Co. 1954.

LINDNER, J.: In: K. LENNERT und J. LINDNER: Cytochemie der Mastzellen, III, pp. 41 – 94, 1962. Congr. europ. Soc. Haemat. Vienna 1961.

LISON, L.: Etudes sur la métachromasie. Colorants métachromatiques et substances chromatropes. Arch. Biol. (Lièges) **46,** 1 – 70 (1935).

LISON, L.: Histochimie animale: méthodes et problèmes, pp. 227 – 228, 231, 236 –242. Paris: Gauthier-Villars 1936.

LISON, L.: Hystochemie. Paris: Gauthier Villars 1953.

LISON, L.: Histochimie des mastocytes. In: Histamine and Antihistamines, p. 136 M. ROCHA E SILVA (ed.). New York: Springer 1966.

LÖFFLER, H.: Cytochemischer Nachweis von unspezifischer Esterase in Erythroblasten, pp. 475 – 478. 8. Kongr. d. Europ. Ges. f. Haematologie. Wien 1961.

LÖFFLER, H.: Cytochemischer Nachweis von unspezifischen Esterasen und Blutzellen, III, pp. 32 – 34 Proc. 8th Congr. europ. Soc. Hemat. Vienna 1962.

LONGLEY, J. B.: Methylation and the periodic acid-Schiff reaction of mast cells (abstract). J. Histochem. Cytochem. **6,** 399 (1958).

MAHANAND, D., HOUCK, J. C.: Fluorometric determination of zinc in biological fluids. Clin. Chem. **14,** 6 – 11 (1968).

MALMFORS, T.: Studies on adrenergic nerves. Acta physiol. scand. **64,** Suppl. 248, 1 – 93 (1965).

MARTIN, H., ROKA, L.: Zur Frage des Heparin-Gehaltes der Blutmastzellen des Menschen. Acta haemat. (Basel) **10,** 26 – 31 (1953).

MARTIN, S. P., MCKINNEY, G. R., GREEN, R.: The metabolism of human polymorphonuclear leukocytes. Ann. N. Y. Acad. Sci. **59,** 996 – 1002 (1955).

MATHEWS, A. A.: A contribution to the chemistry of cytological staining. Amer. J. Physiol. **1,** 445 (1898).

MCMANUS, J. F. A.: Histological demonstration of mucin after periodic acid. Nature (Lond.) **158,** 202 (1946).

MCMANUS, J. F. A.: Some comparative aspects of histochemistry. Bull. int. Ass. med. Mus. **28,** 73 – 79 (1949).

MELI, P., DAVIES, L.: 1953. Cited in: J. H. MORRISON and S. KRONHEIM: The cytochemical demonstration of succinic dehydrogenase in mouse leukocytes. J. Histochem. Cytochem. **10,** 402 – 411 (1962).

MERKER, H.: Grundlagen zur klinisch-morphologischen Blutdiagnostik mit Hydrolasen. In: Zyto- und Histochemie in der Haematologie. Ed. H. MERKER. 9. Freiburger Symposion. Berlin-Göttingen-Heidelberg: Springer 1963.

MERKER, H.: Fermentreaktionen an Blutzellen und ihre Bedeutung in der Haematologie. In: Beiträge zur Inneren Medizin. Ed. W. KEIDERLING. Stuttgart: Schattauer 1964.

MERKER, H.: In: Handbuch der inneren Medizin. Vol. II/1 Berlin-Heidelberg-New York: Springer 1968.

MICHAELIS, L.: The nature of the interaction of nucleic acids and nuclei with basic dyestuffs. Cold Spring Harbor Symp. Quart. Rev. Biol. **12,** 131 – 142 (1947).

MICHELS, N. A.: The mast cells, In: Handbook of Hematology, Vol. I. H. DOWNEY (ed). New York: Hoeber Inc. 1938.

MOLONEY, W. C., MCPHERSON, K., FLIEGELMAN, L.: Esterase-activity in leukocytes demonstrated by the use of naphthol AS-D chloroacetate substrate. J. Histochem. Cytochem. **8,** 200 – 207 (1960).

MOMMSEN, H.: Über die elektrostatische Ladung von Zellen des menschlichen Blutes, ein Beitrag zur Frage der Azido- und der Basophilie. Folia haemat. (Lpz.) **34**, 50 – 64 (1927).

MORRISON, J. H., KRONHEIM, S.: The cytochemical demonstration of succinic dehydrogenase in mouse leukocytes. J. Histochem. Cytochem. **10**, 402 – 411 (1962).

MOWRY, R. W.: Alcian blue technics for the histochemical study of acidic carbohydrates. J. Histochem. Cytochem. **4**, 407 (1956 a).

MOWRY, R. W.: Alcian blue and alcian-blue-periodic acid Schiff stains for carbohydrates, p. 3. Dept. of Path., Univ. of Alabama, Med. Center. Birmingham (Alabama): Mimeo 1956 b.

MOWRY, R. W.: Histochemistry of carbohydrates. In: The Carbohydrates, pp. 624 – 640. W. Pigman, (ed.). New York: Academic Press 1957.

NACHLAS, M. M., TSOU, K. C., DE SOUZA, E., CHENG, C. S., SELIGMAN, A. M.: Cytochemical demonstration of succinic dehydrogenase by the use of a new p-nitrophenyl substituted ditetrazole. J. Cytochem. Histochem. **5**, 420 – 436 (1957).

NACHLAS, M. M., WALKER, D. G., SELIGMAN, A. M.: A histochemical method for the demonstration of diphosphopyridine nucleotide diaphorase. J. biophys. biochem. Cytol. **4**, 29 – 38 (1958 a).

NACHLAS, M. M., WALKER, D. G., SELIGMAN, A. M.: The histochemical localization of triphosphorpyridine nucleotide diaphorase. J. biophys. biochem. Cytol. **4**, 467 – 482 (1958 b).

NAEGELI, O.: Die Mastzellen des Blutes. In: Blutkrankheiten und Blutdiagnostik, pp. 200 – 205. Berlin und Leipzig: Springer 1919.

NAGAYO, M.: Studien über die Gewebsmastzellen. Zbl. allg. Path. path. Anat. **43**, 289 – 293 (1928).

NARTSISSOV, R. P.: Dihydroorotic acid dehydrogenase activity in blood cells of children. Lab. Delo **6**, 336 – 338 (1965).

NORBERG, K.-A.: Drug-induced changes in catecholamine levels in the sympathetic adrenergic cell bodies and terminals. Acta physiol. scand. **65**, 221 – 234 (1965).

NOVIKOFF, A. B., MASEK, R.: 1953. Cited in: Novikoff, A. B.: Effects of ribonuclease on ribonucleic acid and enzyme activities of microsomes isolated from rat liver homogenates. J. Histochem. Cytochem. **2**, 401 – 406 (1954).

NOVIKOFF, A. B., SHIN, W. Y., DRUCKER, J.: Cold acetone fixation for enzyme localization in frozen sections. J. Histochem. Cytochem. **8**, 37 – 40 (1960).

OKAMOTO, K.: Biologische Untersuchungen der Metalle. Trans. Soc. path. jap. **32**, 99 (1942).

ORTMAN, R., FORBES, W. F., BALASUBRAMANIAN, A.: Concerning the staining properties of aldehyde basic fuchsin. J. Histochem. Cytochem. **14**, 104 – 111 (1966).

PAPPENHEIM, A.: Allgemeine Leukozytologie der Entzündung. Folia haemat. (Lpz.), **3**, 564 – 569 und **9**, 642 – 643 (1906 – 1910).

PAPPENHEIM, A., NAKANO, J.: Beiträge über Beziehungen zwischen Vitalfärbung, Supravitalfärbung und Oxydasereaktion. Folia haemat. (Lpz.) **14**, 260 – 294 (1912).

PATON, W. D. M.: Histamine by compounds of simple chemical structure. Pharmacol. Rev. **9**, 269 – 328 (1957).

PARWARESCH, M. R., LENNERT, K.: Zur Differenzierung der Blutbasophilen und Gewebsmastzellen nach dem Reifegrad ihrer Granula. Eine Modifikation der Toluidinblau-pH-Reihe. Histochemie **19**, 262 – 271 (1969).

PARWARESCH, M. R., DANNENBERG, K., LEDER, L.-D.: Der Nachweis von Naphthol-AS-D-Chloracetat-Esterase in normalen basophilen Granulopoiesezellen. Klin. Wschr. **48**, 1008 – 1009 (1970).

PARWARESCH, M. R., LEDER, L.-D., DANNENBERG, K. E. G.: On the origin of human basophilic granulocytes. Acta haemat. (Basel) **45,** 273 – 279 (1971).

PEARSE, A. G. E.: Intracellular localization of dehydrogenase system using monotetrazolium salt and metal chelation of their formazan. J. Histochem. Cytochem. **5,** 515 – 527 (1957).

PEARSE, A. G. E.: Histochemistry, Theoretical and Applied, 2nd ed., pp. 124, 179, 255 – 261, 271 – 273, 286, 609 – 627. Boston: Little Brown & Co. 1960.

PEARSE, A. G. E., ALMEIDA, D. F.: Extension of the limits of cellular pathology: The role of enzyme histochemistry. J. clin. Path. **11,** 520 – 534 (1958).

PEARSE, A. G. E., SCARPELLI, D. G., HESS, R.: A cytochemical study of the dehydrogenases of mitochondria and mitochondrial particulates by a monotetrazolium-cobalt chelation method. J. biopoys. biochem. Cytol. **7,** 243 – 249 (1960).

PEARSE, A. G. E., HESS, R.: Substantivity and other factors responsible for formazan patterns in dehydrogenase histochemistry. Experientia (Basel) **17,** 136 – 141 (1961).

PEARSE, L., CASEY, A. E.: Studies in blood cytology of rabbit; blood counts in normal rabbits. J. exp. Med. **51,** 83 – 97 (1930 a).

PEARSE, L., CASEY, A. E.: Studies in blood cytology of rabbit; consecutive neutrophile, basophile and eosinophile observations on groups of normal rabbits. J. exp. Med. **52,** 145 – 166 (1930 b).

PIETTE, M., PIETTE, C.: Cytologie-coloration métachromatique et coloration „acide périodique réactif de schiff", appliquées aux granulocytes basophilés du sang humain normal. C. R. Acad. Sci. (Paris) **242,** 2775 – 2777 (1956).

PIOCH, W.: Über die Darstellung saurer Mucopolysaccharide mit dem Kupferphthalocyaminfarbstoff Astrablau. Virchows Arch. **330,** 337 – 346 (1957).

PISCHINGER, A.: Die Lage des isoelektrischen Punktes histologischer Elemente als Ursache ihrer verschiedenen Färbbarkeit. Z. Zellforsch. **3,** 169 – 197 (1926).

PISCHINGER, A.: Über die isoelektrischen Punkte der Muskelbestandteile. Pflügers Arch. Physiol. **217,** 205 – 209 (1927).

QUAGLINO, D., HAYHOE, F. G.: Acetone fixation for the cytochemical demonstration of dehydrogenases in blood and bone marrow cells. Nature (Lond.) **187,** 85 (1960).

QUAGLINO, D., HAYHOE, F. G., FLEMANS, R. J.: Cytochemical observations on the effect of phytohemagglutinin in short-term tissue cultures. Nature (Lond.) **196,** 338 – 340 (1962).

QUINTARELLI, G., SCOTT, J. E., DELLOVO, M. C.: The chemical and histochemical properties of Alcian blue. II. Dye binding of tissue polyanions. Histochemie **4,** 86 – 98 (1964 a).

QUINTARELLI, G., SCOTT, J. E., DELLOVO, M. C.: The chemical and histochemical properties of Alcian blue. III. Chemical blocking and unblocking. Histochemie **4,** 99 – 112 (1964 b).

QUINTARELLI, G., DELLOVO, M. C.: The chemical and histochemical properties of Alcian blue. IV. Further studies on the methods for the identification of acid glycosaminoglycans. Histochemie **5,** 196 – 209 (1965).

RABENOVITCH, M., MOTA, I., YONEDA, S.: Note on the histochemical localization of glycogen and pentose polynucleotides in the visual cells of the chick (*Gallus gallus*). Experientia (Basel) **10,** 187 – 188 (1954).

RASCOVIC, D., GEREBTZOFF, M. A.: Cytochemical localization of zinc in blood and bone marrow cells. Acta histochem. (Jena) **3,** 165 – 175 (1963).

REVEL, J. P.: Electron microscopy of glycogen. J. Histochem. Cytochem. **12,** 104 – 114 (1964).

RHEINGOLD, J. J., WISLOCKI, G. B.: Histochemical methods applied to hematology. Blood **3,** 641 – 655 (1948 a).
RHEINGOLD, J. J., WISLOCKI, G. B.: Histochemical methods applied to hematology. Bull. New Engl. med. Cent. **10,** 133 – 137 (1948 b).
RILEY, J. F.: The relationship of the tissue mast cells to the blood vessels in the rat. J. Path. Bact. **65,** 461 – 469 (1953).
RILEY, J. F.: The Mast Cells. Edinburgh and London: E. S. Livingstone Ltd. 1959.
RILEY, J. F., WEST, G. B.: Histamine in tissue mast cells. J. Physiol. (Lond.) **117,** 72 (1952).
RILEY, J. F., WEST, G. B.: Mast cells and histamine in normal and pathological tissues. J. Physiol. (Lond.) **19,** 44 (1953 a).
RILEY, J. F., WEST, G. B.: The presence of histamine in tissue mast cells. J. Physiol. (Lond.) **120,** 528 – 537 (1953 b).
RILEY, J. F., WEST, G. B.: Tissue mast cells. Studies with a histamine liberator of low toxicity (compund 48/80). J. Path. Bact. **69,** 269 – 282 (1955 a).
RILEY, J. F., WEST, G. B.: Histamine liberation in the rat and mouse. Arch. int. Pharmacodyn. **102,** 304 – 313 (1955 b).
RITZÉN, M.: Quantitative fluorescence microspectrophotometry of 5-hydroxytryptamine formaldehyde products in models and in mast cells. Exp. Cell. Res. **45,** 178 – 194 (1967).
RITZÉN, M., HAMMARSTRÖM, L., ULLBERG, S.: Autoradiographic distribution of 5-hydroxytryptamine and 5-hydroxytryptophan in the mouse. Biochem. Pharmacol. **14,** 313 – 321 (1965).
RUTENBURG, A. M., COHEN, R. B., SELIGMAN, A. M.: Histochemical demonstration of arylsulfatase. Science **116,** 539 – 543 (1952).
SALVI, F.: Comportamento delle mastzellen e delle sostanze cromotrope diffuse nell apparato genitale feminile. Minerva ginec. **4,** 634 – 646 (1952).
SAMPSON, D., ARCHER, G. T.: see page 26.
SCARPELLI, G. D., PEARSE, A. G. E.: Physical and chemical protection of cell constituents and the precise localization of enzymes. J. Histochem. Cytochem. **6,** 369 – 376 (1958).
SCHAEFER, H. E., FISCHER, R.: Der Peroxydasenachweis an Ausstrichpräparaten sowie an Gewebsschnitten nach Entkalkung und Paraffineinbettung. Klin. Wschr. **46,** 1228 – 1230 (1968).
SCHAEFER, H. E., HÜBNER, G., FISCHER, R.: Vergleichende morphologische und cytochemische Untersuchungen an den Blutbasophilen der Nager. Haemat. Bluttransfus. **8,** 256 – 259 (1969).
SCHAEFER, H. E., KÄUFER, C., FISCHER, R.: Vergleichende fermentcytochemische Untersuchungen an Blut- und Knochenmarkszellen bei Laboratoriumstieren. Virchows Arch. Abt. B **4,** 310 – 334 (1970).
SCHAUER, A., WERLE, E.: Zur histochemischen Darstellung des Histamins der Mastzellen. Z. ges. exp. Med. **131,** 100 – 104 (1959).
SCHAYER, R. W.: Relationship of stress-induced histidine decarboxylase to circulatory homeostasis and shock. Science **131,** 226 – 227 (1960).
SCHAYER, R. W.: Histidine decarboxylase in mast cells. Ann. N. Y. Acad. Sci. **103,** 164 – 178 (1963).
SCHÖNBERG, W. D.: Über die Bildung und Rückbildung des subepithelial abgelagerten Amyloids der menschlichen Bläschendrüsen. Frankfurt. Z. Path. **59,** 477 – 494 (1948).
SCHUBERT, J. F. C., KATZENMEYER, F.: Der zytochemische Nachweis der Leucinaminopeptidase in menschlichen Blut- und Knochenmarksausstrichen. In: Zyto-

und Histochemie in der Haematologie. 9. Freiburger Symposion. Ed.: H. MERKER. Berlin-Göttingen-Heidelberg: Springer 1963.
SCHUBERT, J. F. C., MARTIN, H.: Beobachtungen an sieben Kranken mit „Blutmastzell-Leukämie". Klin. Wschr. **46,** 929 – 936 (1968 a).
SCHUBERT, J. F. C., MARTIN, H.: Beobachtungen bei Blutmastzellenleukämien. Blut **18,** 35 – 39 (1968 b).
SCHUBERT, M., LEVINE, A.: A qualitative theory of metachromasia in solution. J. Amer. chem. Soc. **77,** 4197 – 4201 (1955).
SCHUBERT, M., HAMERMAN, D.: Metachromasia; chemical theory and histochemical use. J. Histochem. Cytochem. **4,** 159 – 189 (1956).
SCHÜMMELFELDER, N., STOCK, K. F.: Die Bestimmung des Umladebereiches (isoelektrischer Punkt) von Gewebselementen mit dem Fluorochrom Acridinorange. Z. Zellforsch. **44,** 327 – 338 (1956).
SCHULTZE, W. H.: Zur Differentialdiagnose der Leukämien. Münch. med. Wschr. **56,** 167 – 169 (1909).
SCHWARZ-KARSTEN, H.: Über Blutfärbung mit gepufferten Farblösungen. Dtsch. med. Wschr. **53,** 1820 – 1821 (1927).
SCOTT, H. R., CLAYTON, B. P.: A comparison of the staining affinities of aldehyde-fuchsin and the Schiff reagent. J. Histochem. Cytochem. **1,** 336 – 352 (1953).
SCOTT, J. E., QUINTARELLI, G., DELLOVO, M. C.: The chemical and histochemical properties of Alcian blue. I. The mechanism of Alcian blue staining. Histochemie **4,** 73 – 85 (1964).
SCOTT, J. E., DORLING, J.: Differential staining of acid glycosaminoglycans (mucopolysaccharides) by Alcian blue in salt solutions. Histochemie **5,** 221 – 233 (1965).
SELYE, H.: see page 26.
SHEEHAN, H. L.: The staining of leucocyte granules by Sudan black B. J. Path. Bact. **49,** 580 – 581 (1939).
SHELLEY, W. B., JUHLIN, L.: Histamine chromatography and electrophoresis: the o-phthalaldehyde fluorogram. J. Chromat. **22,** 130 – 138 (1966).
SHELLEY, W. B., ÖHMAN, S., PARNES, H. M.: Mast cell stain for histamine in freeze-dried embedded tissue. J. Histochem. Cytochem. **16,** 433 – 439 (1968).
SHIBATA, A., *et al:* see page 26.
SHORE, P. A., BURKHALTER, A., COHN, V. H.: A method for the fluorometric assay of histamine in tissues. J. Pharmacol. exp. Ther. **127,** 182 – 186 (1959).
SINGER, M.: The staining of basophilic components. J. Histochem. Cytochem. **2,** 322 – 331 (1954).
SMITH, C.: Glycogen in basophilic leucocytes in human blood smears. Proc. Soc. exp. Biol. (N. Y.) **72,** 209 – 210 (1949).
SMITH, G. L., JENKINS, R. A., GOUGH, F.: A fluorescent method for the detection and localization of zinc in human granulocytes. J. Histochem. Cytochem. **17,** 749 – 750 (1969).
SMITH, L. H., BAKER, F. A.: Pyrimidine metabolism in man. I. The biosynthesis of orotic acid. J. clin. Invest. **38,** 1044 – 1052 (1959).
SPATZ, M.: Bismarck brown as a selective stain for mast cells. Techn. Bull. Reg. med. Technol. **30,** 141 – 143 (1960).
SPICER, S. S.: A correlative study of the histochemical properties of rodent acid mucopolysaccharides. J. Histochem. Cytochem. **8,** 18 – 36 (1960).
SPICER, S. S., MEYER, D. B.: Histochemical differentiation of acid mucopolysaccharides by means of combined aldehyde fuchsin-alcian blue staining. Amer. J. clin. Path. **33,** 453 – 460 (1960).

Spicer, S. S., Leppi, T. J., Stoward, P. J.: Suggestions for a histochemical terminology of carbohydrate-rich tissue components. J. Histochem. Cytochem. **13,** 599 – 603 (1965).

Staemmler, M.: Untersuchungen über Vorkommen und Bedeutung der histiogenen Mastzellen im menschlichen Körper unter normalen und pathologischen Veränderungen. Frankfurt. Z. Path. **25,** 391 – 435 (1921).

Steedman, H. F.: Alcian blue 8 GS: a new stain for mucin. Quart. J. micr. Sci. **91,** 477 – 479 (1950).

Storti, E., Perugini, S.: Criteri citochimici applicati alla diagnostica delle leucosi acute. Minerva pediat. **2,** 272 – 276 (1949).

Storti, E., Perugini, S.: Ricerche istochimiche sui lipidi delle cellule del sangue e degli organi emopoietici dell uomo normale. Studia Ghisleriana. Studi med. Biol. **1,** 313 – 337 (3. Serie) (1951 a).

Storti, E., Perugini, S.: Cytochemical researches on the lipids of the hematic cells with particular attention to those of acute leukosis. Acta haemat. (Basel) **5,** 321 – 333 (1951 b).

Sylvén, B.: Metachromatic dye-substrate interactions. Quart. J. micr. Sci. **95,** 327 – 358 (1954).

Szirmai, J. A., Balazs, E. A.: Metachromasia and the quantitative determination of dye binding. Acta histochem. (Jena) **1,** 56 – 79 (1958).

Szmigielski, St., Litwin, J.: The histochemical study of zinc content in granulocytes in normal adults in hematologic disorders. Blood **25,** 56 – 62 (1965).

Takamatsu, H.: 1938 Cited in: Takamatsu 1939. Histologische und biochemische Studien über die Phosphatase. I. Histochemische Untersuchungsmethodik der Phosphatase und deren Verteilung in verschiedenen Organen und Geweben. Trans. Soc. path. jap. **29,** 492 – 498 (1939).

Takamatsu, H.: Histologische und biochemische Studien über die Phosphatase. I. Histochemische Untersuchungsmethodik der Phosphatase und deren Verteilung in verschiedenen Organen und Geweben. Trans. Soc. Path. jap. **29,** 492 – 498 (1939).

Tokué, K.: The oxidase and peroxidase reaction in different leucocytes of the blood. Tohoku J. exp. Med. **12,** 445 – 459 (1929 a).

Tokué, K.: see page 27.

Undritz, E.: In: K. Lennert und H. Lindner. Colloquium: Cytochemie der Mastzellen. Proc. 8th Congr. Europ. Soc. Haemat., pp. 40 – 94 Wien 1961.

Valentine, W. N., Lawrence, J. S., Pearse, M. L., Beck, W. S.: Relationship of basophil to blood histamine in man. Blood **10,** 154 – 159 (1955).

Vialli, M.: Osservazioni sull'uso dell'Alcian blue 8 GS nello studio dei mucopolisaccharidi. Boll. Soc. ital. Biol. sper. **27,** 597 – 599 (1951).

Vickerstaff, T.: Physical Chemistry. Springfield: Ch. C. Thomas 1954.

Walker, D. G., Seligman, A. M.: Formalin fixation in the cytochemical demonstration of succinic dehydrogenase of mitochondria. J. biophys. biochem. Cytol. **9,** 415 – 427 (1961).

Watanabe, I., Donahue, S., Hoggatt, N.: Method for electron microscopic studies of circulating human leukocytes and observations on their fine structure. J. Ultrastruct. Res. **20,** 366 – 382 (1967).

Weissmann, N., Carnes, W. H., Rubin, P. S., Fisher, J.: Metachromasia of toluidine-blue induced by nucleic acids. J. Amer. chem. Soc. **74,** 1423 – 1426 (1952).

Weitzel, G.: Chemie und Physiologie biogener Zink-Verbindungen. Angew. Chem. **68,** 566 – 573 (1956).

WEITZEL, G., FRETZDORFF, A. M.: Zink in den Augen von Säugetieren. Z. physiol. Chem. **292,** 221 – 231 (1953).
WEITZEL, G., FRETZDORFF, A. M.: Zink-Imidazol-Verbindungen. Z. physiol. Chem. **305,** 1 – 20 (1956).
WERMEL, E., SASSUCHIN, D.: Untersuchungen über die Kernsubstanzen und die Methoden ihrer Darstellung. II. Über die Natur des Volutins und der Mastzellen-Granula. Z. Zellforsch. **6,** 424 – 439 (1927).
WILLANDER, O.: 1937. Cited in: Complete blood analysis of heparinized blood. Acta med. scand. **94,** 258 – 266 (1938).
WILTSHAW, E., MOLONEY, W. C.: Histochemical and biochemical studies on leukocytes: alkaline phosphatase activity. Blood **10,** 1120 – 1131 (1955).
WISLOCKI, G. B., DEMPSEY, E. W.: Observations on the chemical cytology of normal blood and hemopoietic tissues. Anat. Rec. **96,** 249 – 279 (1946).
WISLOCKI, G. B., BUNTING, H., DEMPSEY, E. W.: Metachromasia in mammalian tissues and its relationship to mucopolysaccharides. Amer. J. Anat. **81,** 1 – 37 (1947).
WISLOCKI, G. B., RHEINGOLD, J. J., DEMPSEY, E. W.: The occurrence of the periodic acid-Schiff reaction in various normal cells of blood and connective tissue. Blood **4,** 562 – 568 (1949).
WOLMAN, M.: A histochemical method for the differential staining of acid tissue components (particularly ground substance polysaccharides). Bull. Res. Coun. Israel E, 27 – 31 (1956).
WOLSTENHOME, G. E. W., O'CONNOR, C. M.: Histamine. Boston: Little Brown & Co. 1956.
ZUCKER-FRANKLIN, D.: Electron microscopic studies of human granulocytes: structural variations related to function. Seminars Hemat. **5,** 109 – 133 (1968).
ZURWEHME, H., MITZKAT, J., ODRIOZOLA, J. POLIWODA, H.: Histochemie von Enzymen des energieliefernden Stoffwechsels in den Zellen der Granulopoiese. Klin. Wschr. **48,** 828 – 829 (1970).

VI. Comparative Studies on the Morphology of Blood Basophils

This chapter of mast cell and basophil research has long been the subject of extensive work (MICHELS, 1938; UNDRITZ and STEINEMANN, 1963). Phylogenetically these cells display special features. On the one hand, there appears to be a reciprocal quantitative relationship between the two types of basophilic granulated cells, yet on the other hand, it is extremely difficult to distinguish between them in many animal species. In the higher vertebrates, especially in mammals, the number of blood basophils is minimal. In the higher apes the count remains below 1% of total leukocytes. According to PONDER *et al.* (1929), higher counts – up to 20% – can be detected only among chimpanzees. Ruminants have counts of up to 3% of total leukocytes. KNOLL (1930) reported in camelids values up to 9.3%. Further investigations of basophil counts have been made in pigs (KNOLL, 1932 a, b), dogs (JOLLY, 1900; MAXIMOW, 1910; 1913), and llamas (PONDER *et al.,* 1929). Among the ruminants, the highest values were displayed by the llamas with

37%. Although dogs and cats possess numerous tissue mast cells, their basophil counts are low.

Lower vertebrates, such as birds, reptiles and fish, have also been investigated, especially by the earlier authors. For chickens, BURNETT (1908), SCHMEISSER (1916), and FORKNER (1929) gave values between 1 and 3.6%. Other birds were found to have counts up to 23%. For frogs, the values reported vary between 5 and 23%, with the majority of authors quoting around 20% (FREIDSOHN, 1910; MICHELS, 1923; KLIENEBERGER and CARL, 1927). Reptiles, for example snakes, display a relatively high number of basophil granulocytes (GRÜNBERG, 1901; MICHELS, 1922; 1923). Fish are reported to have very few or no blood basophils (ROMIEU, 1924; LÖWENTHAL, 1927; 1930; MICHELS, 1938).

Rodents, such as mice, rats, guinea pigs and rabbits, are of special significance in this connection, as they are the most popular experimental animals. Whether rats and mice have any blood basophils at all has been repeatedly debated (DUNN, 1963). Earlier works often reported the presence of basophils in the blood of these animals (JOLLY, 1900; WEIDENREICH, 1908; MAXIMOW, 1910; 1913). SCHERMER (1958) reported the occurrence of basophil granulated cells in limited numbers in rat and mouse blood. Recent results by SCHÄFER *et al.* (1969) have to a great extent supported these findings. We have also found in the blood of rats and mice cells which reveal a faint toluidine-blue metachromasia. In contrast, one can see in these animals numerous extremely large tissue mast cells, which are distributed throughout the whole body with special prevalence in mesenterium, subcutis and tongue. These cells desquamate at the slightest irritation and can thus be isolated in large numbers. They are for this reason very suitable for cytomorphological and cytophysiological investigations.

Blood basophils in guinea pigs make up approximately 3% of total leukocytes; their granules are, in contrast to those of almost all other laboratory animals, water-insoluble and hence easy to handle and suitable for both electron-microscopic and immunologic studies (WINQVIST, 1963; SPICER *et al.*, 1968).

The basophil granulocytes of rabbits are in many ways similar to those of man; they possess extremely water-soluble granules and there seems to be good functional conformity between the two types of blood basophils. In addition, rabbit basophils display a relatively constant quantitative behavior with minor fluctuations. KLIENEBERGER and CARL (1927) reported values up to 5%, PEARSE and CASEY (1930 a, b) 9.9%, SCARBOROUGH (1930) up to 12% BUSHNELL and BANGS (1930) 3.58%, CHENG (1930) up to 8.1%, and BESSMANS and LAMBIN (1931) 11.06%. According to MICHELS (1938), rabbits possess only a very few tissue mast cells and the blood basophil count ranges from 4 to 12%.

The best investigations of blood basophils in invertebrates based upon modern hematological concepts have been carried out by UNDRITZ (1946), STEINEMANN-HUSSEIN (1962) and UNDRITZ and STEINEMANN (1963). They differentiated basophils with water-soluble granules from those with water-insoluble granules in *Ascidia mentula, Ciona intestinalis* and *Phallusia mam-*

millata. The cells with soluble metachromatic grains were referred to as basophil granulocytes.

Numerous investigations have also been carried out on *Ascidia chordata* (review by KNOLL, 1893; JORDAN, 1938; MICHELS, 1938; STEINEMANN-HUSSEIN, 1962). BÉTANCÈS (1921) was able to verify the appearance of blood basophils in *Astacus (deuterostomia).* Basophil granulated cells have also been observed in insects. *Carausius morosus, Truxalia nasuta,* and various cicades such as *Mantis religiosa, Philium sprurium* and *Cyphocrania gigas* have further been mentioned in this connection. In the orthoptera, blood basophils account for up to 13% of the leukocytes. KELLY *et al.* (1961) examined 29 leguanes from the group *Phyrnosoma cornutum* and were able to identify 8% of the leukocytes as being basophil granulocytes.

As early as 1938 MICHELS pointed out that a reciprocal relationship exists between the number of basophils and the number of tissue mast cells, and numerous more recent phyologenetic investigations have confirmed this assertion (BOSEILA, 1959; SELYE, 1965). Fish are often offered as an example of this, as they have either a very small basophil count (LÖWENTHAL, 1930) or none at all (DRZEWINA, 1905; PAPPENHEIM, 1909; WEIDENREICH, 1911; WERZBERG, 1911; MICHELS, 1923; JORDAN and SPEIDEL, 1924; ROMIEU, 1924; BOLTON, 1933). DRZEWINA (1905) maintained that she did not observe one single blood basophil during investigations on 69 different species of fish and WERZBERG (1911) obtained similar results. Conversely, fish possess many tissue mast cells (MICHELS, 1923; ROMIEU, 1924; LÖWENTHAL, 1930). As a rule, mammals also have very few blood basophils and a high tissue mast cell count. In rats and mice, the ratio favors tissue mast cells to the extreme. Rabbits, many birds, and lizards have a high blood basophil count (5 – 40%) and possess a very limited number of tissue mast cells. Guinea pigs, cats, and high vertebrates have a preponderance of tissue mast cells. Although a large number of animals cannot be fitted into this scheme, the rule appears to apply to most species.

While the blood basophil count displays large fluctuations along the phylogenetic line, cell size also differs greatly from one species to another. Most animals have blood basophils averaging between 10 and 15 µm in size, but in *Chrysemys picta,* and *Cryptobranchus alleghaniensis* huge forms up to 100 µm have been reported (MICHELS, 1938). The size and shape of the granules also varies from species to species. In guinea pigs, the granules are water-insoluble and of uniform size and are distributed throughout the cytoplasm. Rats and mice have tiny, inconspicuous, strongly water-soluble granules in their basophil equivalents. The blood basophils of pigs, camels, and horses possess especially large and striking granules.

Comparative cytochemical investigations on blood basophils (Table 9) have been carried out by a few authors (ACKERMAN, 1963; SHUBICH, 1966; WETZEL *et al.,* 1967; FISCHER and SCHÄFER, 1968; SCHÄFER *et al.,* 1969; SCHÄFER *et al.,* 1970).

According to ACKERMAN (1963), blood basophils from guinea pig, rabbit, and man have largely similar behavior: they display no activity to alkaline phosphatase, naphthol AS-D chloroacetate esterase, amino peptidase or per-

Table 9. Cytochemical behavior of normal blood basophils in different species

Reactions	Man	Rabbit	Guinea Pig	Cat
Alkaline phosphatase	–	–	–	–
Acid phosphatase	+ + +	+ +	+ +	
LEDER's esterase	–	–	+ + + +	+ +
Nonspecific esterases	+	+	+	+
Peroxidase	– / +	– / +	–	–

oxidase. SCHÄFER *et al.* (1970) reported that blood basophils in rats were not indentifiable with the alkaline phosphatase reaction. In the mouse these cells reacted negatively with the same enzyme. Basophil granulocytes from guinea pigs, rabbits, and cats also showed no enzyme activity. A negative peroxidase reaction was observed in the blood basophils of rats, guinea pigs, and cats. Blood basophils from rats yielded a weak positive reaction to naphthol AS-D chloroacetate esterase. Like ACKERMAN (1963), SCHÄFER *et al.* also could not detect any naphthol AS-D chloroacetate esterase activity in blood basophils from rabbits (Fig. 16) although basophils from guinea pigs gave a strongly positive reaction. The latter finding is contrary to ACKERMAN's. In our experiments, too, guinea-pig blood basophils were strongly positive to naphthol AS-D chloroacetate esterase (Fig. 17).

Blood basophils from cats and murides contain chloroacetate esterase in their granules as well. The intensity of this enzyme is obviously stronger in blood basophils than in neutrophil granulocytes in the following species: *Trionomous delarolus, Mieretus clelhrionomys gloerolus, Microtus alvaris, Microtus agrestis, Arvicola terrestris,* and the mediterranean murides: *Acomys minus, Acomys tracheranus demitiatus,* also in the F_1 hybrids of both *acomys* species. Only in *acomys artel* and its hybrids did the peroxidase reaction turn out positive. Blood basophils in many types of murides can be distinguished from the peroxidase-positive neutrophils and eosinophils simply on the basis of the missing peroxidase activity. Alkaline phosphatase can be detected in the blood basophils of all murides whose neutrophils display a positive reaction (FISCHER and SCHÄFER, 1968; SCHÄFER *et al.*, 1969).

In a thorough investigation of alkaline phosphatase in the leukocytes of various species, JAIN (1968) considered blood basophils only in rabbits; he also found a negative reaction. WETZEL *et al.* (1967) reported similar results. According to these authors, blood basophils from rabbits possess neither alkaline nor acid phosphatase. SPICER *et al.* (1968) studied the phosphatase content of blood basophils electron microscopically. They established that a limited activity of acid phosphatase can occasionally be observed in the dilated vesicles of the Golgi apparatus. In respect to alkaline phosphatase, however, only negative results were obtained.

The chemical make-up of basophil granules has often been studied in rabbits (HORN and SPICER, 1964; WETZEL *et al.*, 1967; BAINTON *et al.*, 1968 a,

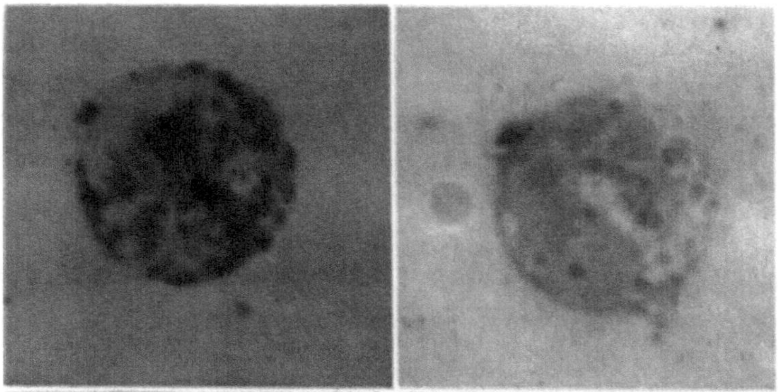

Fig. 16

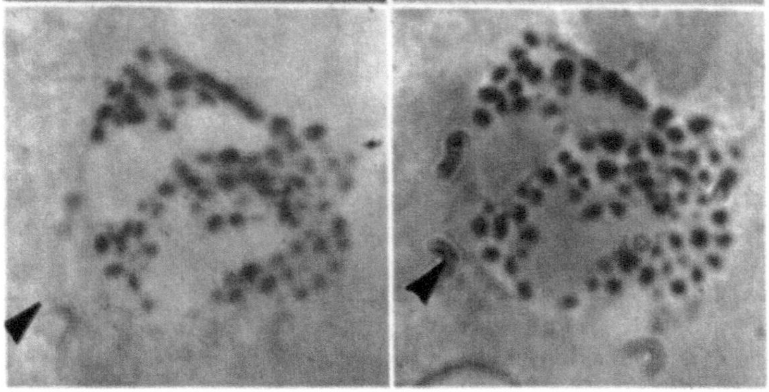

Fig. 17

Fig. 16. Rabbit basophil stained with toluidine blue (left) and subsequently subjected to the naphthol AS-D chloroacetate esterase reaction (right). ×2,000

Fig. 17. Guinea pig basophil stained with toluidine blue (left) and subsequently subjected to the naphthol AS-D chloroacetate esterase reaction (right). ×2,000

b). Basophil granules contain abundant sulfated glycosaminoglycans and incorporate considerable amounts of radiosulfate. The presence of heparin in the basophils of rodents, and especially of rabbits, has been verified by numerous workers (Laves and Thoma, 1950; Jorpes *et al.*, 1953; Horn and Spicer, 1964; Bainton and Farquhar, 1966.)

Most of the authors who have studied the granulogenesis of blood basophils agree with the view that basophil granules are derived from precursors in the Golgi field. However, other modes of development of basophil granules have not been completely excluded.

References

Ackermann, G. A.: see page 55.

Bainton, D. F., Farquhar, M. G.: Origin of granules in polymorphonuclear leukocytes. Two types derived from opposite faces of the Golgi complex in developing granulocytes. J. Cell. Biol. **28,** 277 – 301 (1966).

Bainton, D. F., Farquhar, M. G.: Differences in enzyme content of azurophil and specific granules of polymorphonuclear leukocytes. I. Histochemical staining of bone marrow smears. J. Cell. Biol. **39,** 286 – 298 (1968 a).

BAINTON, D. F., FARQUHAR, M. G.: Differences in enzyme content of azurophil and specific granules of polymorphonuclear leukocytes. II. Cytochemistry and electron microscopy of bone marrow cells. J. Cell Biol. **39**, 299 – 317 (1968 b).

BESSEMANS, A., LAMBIN, P.: Les modifications de la formule leucocytaire du lapin au cours de son infection par Tréponéma pallidum ou Tréponéma euniculi. Rev. belge Sci. méd. **3**, 717 – 729 (1931).

BETANCES, L.-M.: Les cellules du sang de *l'Astacus fluviatilis*. Arch. Anat. micr. (Paris) **18**, 1 – 45 (1921).

BOLTON, L.: Basophilic (mast) cells in alimentary canal of salmonoid fishes. J. Morph. **54**, 549 – 582 (1933).

BOSEILA, A. W. A.: The basophil leucocyte and its relationship to the tissue mast cells. Copenhagen: Munksgaard 1959.

BURNETT, S.: The Clinical Pathology of the Blood of Domesticated Animals. Ithaca: Taylor and Carpenter 1908.

BUSHNELL, L., BANGS, E.: A study of the variations in number of blood cells of normal rabbits. J. infect. Dis. **39**, 291 – 301 (1930).

CHENG, S.: Leukocyte counts in rabbit. Amer. J. Hyg. **11**, 449 – 533 (1930).

DRZEWINA, A.: Contribution à l'étude du tissu lymphoïde des Ichthyopsidés. Arch. d. zool. expér. et gén. **3**, 145 – 151 (1905).

DUNN, T. B.: Round table discussion. In: Mast cells and basophils. Ed. J. Padawer. Ann. N. Y. Acad. Sci. **103**, 441 – 492 (1963).

FISCHER, R., SCHAEFER, H. E.: Artspezifische Unterschiede der alkalischen Phosphatase in den Blutzellen verschiedener Muridenarten. 13. Tag. Dtsch. Ges. Haematologie. Ulm 1968.

FORKNER, C.: see page 23.

FREIDSOHN, A.: Zur Morphologie des Amphibienblutes. Zugleich ein Beitrag zu der Lehre von der Differenzierung der Lymphocyten. Arch. mikr. Anat. **75**, 435 – 472 (1910).

GRÜNBERG, C.: Beiträge zur vergleichenden Morphologie der Leukozyten. Virchows Arch. **163**, 303 – 342 (1901).

HORN, R. G., SPICER, S. S.: Sulfated mucopolysaccharide and basic protein in certain granules of rabbit leucocytes. Lab. Invest. **13**, 1 – 15 (1964).

JAIN, N. C.: Alkaline phosphatase activity in leukocytes of some animal species. Acta haemat. (Basel) **39**, 51 – 59 (1968).

JOLLY, J.: Clasmatocytes et mastzellen. C. R. Soc. Biol. (Paris) **52**, 609 – 611 (1900).

JORDAN, H. E., Comparative hematology. In: H. Downey: Handbook of Hematology, Vol. 2. New York: HOEBER Inc. 1938.

JORDAN, H. E., SPEIDEL, S.: Studies on lymphocytes. III. Granulopoiesis in the salamander, with special reference to the monophyletic theory of blood cell origin. Amer. J. Anat. **33**, 485 – 505 (1924).

JORPES, E., ODEBLAD, F., BOSTRÖM, H.: An autoradiographic study on the uptake of S35-labelled sodium sulphate in the mast cells. Acta haemat. (Basel) **9**, 273 – 276 (1953).

KELLY, J. W., BOSEILA, A. W. A., KAVAZOS, L. F., FEAGANS, W. M.: Hematology of the horned lizard, especially blood basophils and tissue mast cells. Acta haemat. (Basel), **26**, 378 – 384 (1961).

KLIENEBERGER, C., CARL, W.: Die Blutmorphologie der Laboratoriumstiere. Leipzig: Barth 1927.

KNOLL, W.: Das Blutbild der Cameliden. Folia haemat. (Lpz.) **42**, 350 – 358 (1930).

KNOLL, W.: Das morphologische Blutbild der Säugetiere. I. Allgemeine und spezielle Morphologie der kernhaltigen Blutzellen der Säugetiere. Z. mikr. anat. Forsch. **30,** 116 – 150 (1932 a).

KNOLL, W.: Untersuchungen über die Morphologie des Säugetierblutes. Folia haemat. (Lpz.) **47,** 201 – 219 (1932 b).

LAVES, W., THOMA, K.: see page 61.

LOEWENTHAL, N.: Du taux relatif des globules blancs éosinophiles et basophiles dans le sang. Rev. méd. Suisse rom. **47,** 457 – 464 (1927).

LOEWENTHAL, N.: Nouvelles observations sur les globules blancs du sang chez les animaux vértebrés. Arch. anat. histol. embryol. **11,** 245 – 332 (1930).

MAXIMOW, A.: Untersuchungen über Blut und Bindegewebe. III. Die embryonale Histogenese des Knochenmarkes der Säugetiere. Arch. mikr. Anat. **76,** 1 – 107 (1910).

MAXIMOW, A.: Untersuchungen über Blut und Bindegewebe. VI. Blutmastzellen. Arch. mikr. Anat. **83,** 247 – 289 (1913).

MICHELS, N. A.: Genèse hétéroplastique et homoplastique des labrocytes (Mastzellen) chez le vertébrés inférieurs. C. R. Soc. Biol. (Paris) **87,** 111 (1922).

MICHELS, M.: The mast cell in the lower vertebrates. Cellule **33,** 339 – 462 (1923).

MICHELS, N. A.: The mast cell. In: Handbook of Hematology. Ed. H. Downey, Sect. IV, **2,** 231 – 372. New York: Paul B. Hoeber Inc. 1938. Repr. in Ann. N. Y. Acad. Sci. **103,** 275 – 354 (1963).

PAPPENHEIM, A.: Einige interessante Tatsachen und theoretische Ergebnisse der vergleichenden Leukocytenmorphologie. Folia haemat. (Lpz.) **8,** 504 – 563 (1909).

PEARSE, L., CASEY, A. E.: see page 65.

PEARSE, L., CASEY, A. E.: see page 65.

PONDER, E., JEAGER, J., CHARIPPER, H.: Studies in comparative haematology, I – III. Quart. J. exp. Physiol. **19,** 115 – 272 (1929).

ROMIEU, M.: Contribution à l'étude des mastocytes des poissons osseux. C. R. Soc. Biol. (Paris) **91,** 655 – 657 (1924).

SCARBOROUGH, R.: Blood picture of normal laboratory animals. Yale J. Biol. Med. **3,** 63 – 80 (1930).

SCHAEFER, H. E., HÜBNER, G., FISCHER, R.: see page 66.

SCHAEFER, H. E., KÄUFER, C., FISCHER, R.: see page 66.

SCHERMER, S.: Die Blutmorphologie der Laboratoriumstiere. Leipzig: J. A. Barth 1958.

SCHMEISSER, H. C.: Leukemia of the fowl: spontaneous and experimental. Johns Hopk. Hosp. Rep. **17,** 551 – 586 (1916).

SELYE, H.: see page 26.

SHUBICH, M. G.: A cytochemical study of leukocyte alkaline phosphatase activity in experimental animals. Tsitologiya **8,** 420 – 421 (1966).

SPICER, S. S., HORN, R. G., WETZEL, B. K.: see page 27.

STEINEMANN-HUSSEIN, A.: Morphologie des Evertebratenblutes. Inaugural-Diss. Zürich 1962.

UNDRITZ, E.: see page 68.

UNDRITZ, E., STEINEMANN, A.: Die Blutkörperchen der Ascidien. Schweiz. med. Wschr. **41,** 1477 – 1482 (1963).

WEIDENREICH, F.: Zur Kenntnis der Zellen mit basophilen Granulationen in Blut- und Bindegewebe. Folia haemat. (Lpz.) **5,** 135 – 155 (1908).

WEIDENREICH, F.: Leukocyten und verwandte Zellformen. Wiesbaden: Bergmann 1911.

WERZBERG, A.: Studien zur vergleichenden Haemozytologie einiger poikilothermer Vertebraten. Folia haemat. (Lpz.) **11**, 17 – 193 (1911).
WETZEL, B. K., SPICER, S. S., HORN, R. G.: Fine structural localization of acid and alkaline phosphatases in cells of rabbit blood and bone marrow. J. Histochem. Cytochem. **15**, 311 – 334 (1967).
WETZEL, B. K., HORN, R. G., SPICER, S. S.: see page 28.
WINQVIST, G.: see page 28.

B. The Origin of Blood Basophils

I. Literature Review

From the turn of the century two great hematological schools have dominated the literature concerning genesis and origin of blood basophils. On the one side are EHRLICH, NAEGELI, SCHRIDDE, ZIEGLER, TÜRK, and SABIN and on the other PAPPENHEIM, WEIDENREICH, and GRAWITZ. Repetitions, uncritical acceptance of hypotheses, and confusions in terminology all combine to impede an exact analysis of their work today. As there are already several works that aim to cover the history of this part of hematology (MICHELS, 1938; SABIN, 1940; SELYE, 1965), we limit ourselves in the following pages to works that have been of decisive importance for an understanding of the cytogenesis of blood basophils.

Blood basophils were recognized and distinguished from other leukocytes and particularly from tissue mast cells, by EHRLICH (1879; 1880). EHRLICH (1898) believed these cells to be an independent type of granulocytes and, like neutrophils and eosinophils, of myeloid origin. PAPPENHEIM (1900) and WEIDENREICH (1900) opposed this view and there followed a long argument about the origin of blood basophils. PAPPENHEIM (1901; 1904; 1905; 1914; 1920) alternately viewed blood basophils as being either immature eosinophils or degenerated "mucoid" lymphoid cells (most lymphocytes, pseudolymphocytes). His thesis was based on the assumption that basophils would not occur in bone marrow; they were vacuolated, difficult to stain and small in number. His view was supported by his students PRÖSCHER (1909), BENACCHIO (1911), KARDOS (1911), and SZECSI (1912) and further by BLUMENTHAL (1905), WEIDENREICH (1908 a, b), GRAWITZ (1911), GRAHAM (1920), and POPPER (1922), who could find no peroxidase activity in these cells. JORDAN and FILLIPIN (1913), JORDAN (1919; 1926), and JORDAN and SPEIDEL (1923; 1924; 1929) as well as TOKUE (1929) went on propagating the degeneration theory of PAPPENHEIM. The degeneration theory was firmly refuted by EHRLICH (1879; 1891; 1898) and further opposed by HIRSCHFELD (1898), JOLLY (1900), TÜRK (1900; 1904; 1905; 1912), LEVADITI (1902), MICHAELIS (1902), BRUCKNER (1904), DUCATI and CAVALIERI (1905), MAXIMOW (1905; 1906; 1907; 1910; 1913), HELLY (1906), and NAEGELI (1909; 1919; 1931). It eventually became established that blood basophils originate from bone marrow, where their generative line and mitotic forms regularly occur. They represent a special form of granulocytes and as such are involved in myeloproliferative diseases.

II. Detection of Blood Basophils and Their Precursors in Normal Human Bone Marrow

The usual panchromic staining techniques (MAY-GRÜNWALD-GIEMSA; WRIGHT, KARDOSCH) are sufficient for recognizing mature basophils and some of their immature forms. The demonstration of their early precursors, however, is not always possible with these methods. Hence, most of the so-called myelographs do not mention basophil precursor cells.

Table 10. Distribution of different maturation stages of the basophilic cell line in normal bone marrow expressed as a percentage of total nucleated cells

Author	Pro-myelo-cyte	Myelo-cyte	Meta-myelo-cyte	Band-form	Segmented
ARINKIN (1929)	–	–	–	–	0.1 – 0.7
ESCUDERO and VARELA (1932)	–	0.2	–	–	–
HOLMES and BROWN (1933)	–	–	–	–	0.3
NORDENSON (1935)	–	0.0 – 0.5	–	–	0.0 – 0.75
SEGERDAHL (1935)	–	–	–	–	0.14
YOUNG and OSGOOD (1935)	–	–	–	0.0 – 0.6	0.0 – 0.2
PICENA (1937)	–	0.1	–	–	0.2
KLIMA (1938)	–	–	–	–	–
WEIL and PERLES (1938)	–	–	–	–	–
REVOL (1938)	–	–	–	–	–
HENNING and KEILHACK (1939)	–	0.1	0.1	0.1	–
FIESCHI (1940)	–	0.1	–	–	–
KIENLE (1943)	–	–	–	–	–

Data available on this special question are rare and incomplete. The basophil cell line has been reported to account for 0.03% (MURAKAMI *et al.*, 1969) or 0.05 to 0.1% (OPITZ and WEICKER, 1954; ROHR, 1960) of all bone marrow cells. The ratio of basophils to marrow leukocytes has been said to average 0.3 ± 0.03% (JUHLIN, 1963) or 1.0% (MCDONALD *et al.*, 1966). It has proved even more difficult to assess early basophil precursors in bone marrow specimens, since no reliable histochemical method is yet available. Other criteria used for estimating the maturity of individual myeloid cells, like the extent of nuclear segmentation, do not apply to the basophil line. The

Table 11. Reported incidence of different maturation stages of the basophilic cell line as a percentage of the total of non-erythropoietic cells in human bone marrow

Author	Pro-myelocyte	Myelocyte	Meta-myelocyte	Bandform	Segmented
TEMPKA and BRAUN (1932)	–	0.0 – 0.3	0.0 – 0.1	0.0 – 0.16	0.2 – 0.3
MARKOFF (1936)	–	0.05	0.05	–	0.5
SCHNETZ and GREIF (1938)	–	0.1 – 0.2	0.01 – 0.0	–	0.15 – 0.2
DE WEERDT (1939)	–	0.8	–	0.2	–
HEILMEYER (1955)	–	–	–	–	1.0
ROHR (1960)	–	–	–	–	0.0 – 1.0
PARWARESCH and NOTTBOHM (1975)	0.09	0.1	0.04	0.06	0.11

usual panchromic techniques do not allow a clear differentiation between azurophil granules and early basophil granules. Further difficulties arise from the extreme rarity and water-solubility of the specific basophil granules. The few data given in the literature on the number of basophil precursors are reviewed in Tables 10 and 11.

We believe that the myelogenic origin of blood basophils is well supported by much indirect evidence; nevertheless, there are still differing views on the origin of basophils (SCHLEICHER, 1968). It is true that no final and complete description of the ascendance of blood basophils from their precursors has yet been achieved. With few exceptions (UNDRITZ, 1952), the general consensus is that blood basophils originate from promyelo cytes (TÜRK, 1904; NAEGELI, 1909; 1919; DOWNEY, 1914; 1915; RINGOEN, 1923; etc.). These claims rest on observations with the panchromatic stain by means of which transitional stages between the azurophil granulated promyelocyte and the specific granulated myelocytes have been described. The cells are said to contain both promyelocytic azure granules and metachromatic basophil granules alongside one another. Such statements ignore the fact that, while the panchromatic staining procedure is excellent for portraying the azure granules in promyelocytes, it is not suitable for distinguishing the water-soluble immature metachromatic basophil granules. Special fixation methods are required to preserve the morphological integrity of the early immature basophil granules (PARWARESCH and LENNERT, 1967). Furthermore, with the panchromatic techniques promyelocyte granules take on a reddish violet color, which is very similar to that of the basophil granules. It seems impossible, therefore, to make a reliable distinction in individual cases between the two types of granules in one and the same cell. In our experience the few metachromatic granules present in the early immature basophils cannot be adequately identified with the usual panchromatic staining.

We describe below some attempts to achieve a reliable assessment of the basophil population of normal human bone marrow in order to establish a cytological sequence for the maturation process of the basophil cell line, as has already been done for the neutrophil and eosinophil granulocytes. It would also be valuable to determine whether it is possible to make an exact distinction between basophil promyelocytes, myelocytes, metamyelocytes, bandforms, and polymorphonuclear forms, as in the neutrophil cell line. Furthermore, blood basophils should be precisely identified by a reliable method in order to ascertain the actual population in bone marrow and the quantitative composition of their precursors.

A selective demonstration of the basophil precursors present in bone marrow is easily accomplished with the use of such widely applied basic dyes as toluidine blue or other stains that have an affinity for basophils, such as aldehyde fuchsin. However, it is still not possible to determine the precise degree of cell maturity on the basis of purely morphological criteria. Along with the typical cytomorphology, the myeloid system is distinguished by its highly specific reactivity to LEDER's esterase and myeloperoxidase, two enzymes that occur specifically in the myelogenous cells.

The demonstration of myeloperoxidase in basophils has proved very problematical, due to the lability of the peroxidase and solubility of basophil granules. As a result, either the enzyme activity is abolished by the fixative, or the inadequately prepared granules dissolve in the course of the enzyme-cytochemical reaction. The susceptibility of the myeloperoxidase reaction to artifacts led us to study the enzyme naphthol AS-D chloroacetate esterase in the basophil cell line. It was shown that this enzyme is regularly present in basophil precursors (PARWARESCH *et al.*, 1970; 1971). Here, too, difficulties arose in identifying blood basophils by their metachromatic properties and then testing for their enzyme content. Numerous useful fixatives caused inactivation of the otherwise very stable and widely heat-resistant enzyme. Special fixing solutions had therefore to be developed to overcome these problems. It was ascertained in preliminary investigations that a dilute solution of N-cetylpyridinium chloride produced no obvious decrease in the intensity of the naphthol AS-D chloroacetate esterase activity as measured in 100 promyelocytes and 100 polymorphonuclear neutrophils before and after a 30 min treatment with the fixing solution.

Once the presence of naphthol AS-D chloroacetate esterase in the basophil cell line was established, it became possible to find the characteristic enzyme activity at various stages of maturity.

1. Qualitative Findings

a) Application of Basic Dyes

The metachromatic structures of the blood basophils were successfully stained with a 0.1% aqueous solution of toluidine blue at various pH levels. A pH of 4.2 was found to be optimal during preliminary testing for the demonstration of a wide spectrum of cells in the basophil cell line. Although almost all blood basophils in the peripheral blood can be visualized within the range pH 2.8 to 3.4, the best value for human bone marrow lies in the less acidic region of pH 4.2. The cytochemical basis of this shift in the toluidine blue pH series has been extensively described in Section A. V. 3. The basophil population in bone marrow consists predominantly of immature cells with immature metachromatic granules which preferentially stain in the higher pH region. (CASTIGLIONI, 1947; PEARSE, 1949; SALVI, 1952; ASTALDI *et al.*, 1954; SCHUBERT, 1955; LENNERT and SCHUBERT, 1959; LENNERT and BACH, 1961; LENNERT and LINDNER, 1962; PARWARESCH and LENNERT, 1969). At pH 4.2, toluidine blue selectively stains the metachromatic substances in both mature and immature basophils.

Mature basophil granules show a strong, light pink metachromasia. The granules are rounded and well defined. The irregularly segmented nuclei are stained a faint blue. The intergranular cytoplasm usually remains colorless (Fig. 18).

The immature basophils display an irregular arrangement of the metachromatic substances. The extent of the metachromasia increases with increasing maturity. The granules are seldom optically dense and well-defined from their surroundings. In more mature precursor stages, the classic, age-dependent nuclear form, analogous to the neutrophils, is only occasionally observed. Less mature precursor stages, on the other hand, regularly show a rounded or lightly oval, relatively large, faint bluish nucleus. The intergranular cytoplasm is not seen to contain any vacuoles in either the mature or immature precursor stages. Mitoses of basophil precursors occur only in the promyelocytic and myelocytic stages. Mitotic forms are easily discernable with this technique.

The criteria for distinguishing between mature and immature basophils are subjective in many ways. For example, the theory advanced in so many hematological reports, that the size of the cells is an important feature, has frequently turned out to be of little help. It is well known that large, immature precursor cells can divide into two daughter cells of the same age. These then display the morphological characteristics of the parent cells, but are markedly smaller. Since the morphology of the blood cells does not change significantly shortly before or shortly after mitosis, the evidence of size does not always closely correspond to the degree of maturity. Furthermore, there are other factors that influence cell size in smear preparations, for example, thickness of the smear, cell content, and plasma impurities. Neither does the form of the nucleus, as just mentioned, impart any reliable information. The segmentation tendency of basophils is much more limited than that of neutrophils. Segmented nuclei are often twisted, so that they can appear as compact, rounded, oval, or bandformed.

In conclusion, it has been established that fixing with N-cetylpyridinium chloride effects optimum stabilization of the water-soluble structures present in basophils and their precursors. Staining with aqueous toluidine blue solution at pH 4.2 gives a selective demonstration of all of the basophil granulopoietic cells which, because of their metachromatic properties, stand out markedly from the other cellular constituents. A rough differentiation between mature and immature cells is possible in many cases, although it is

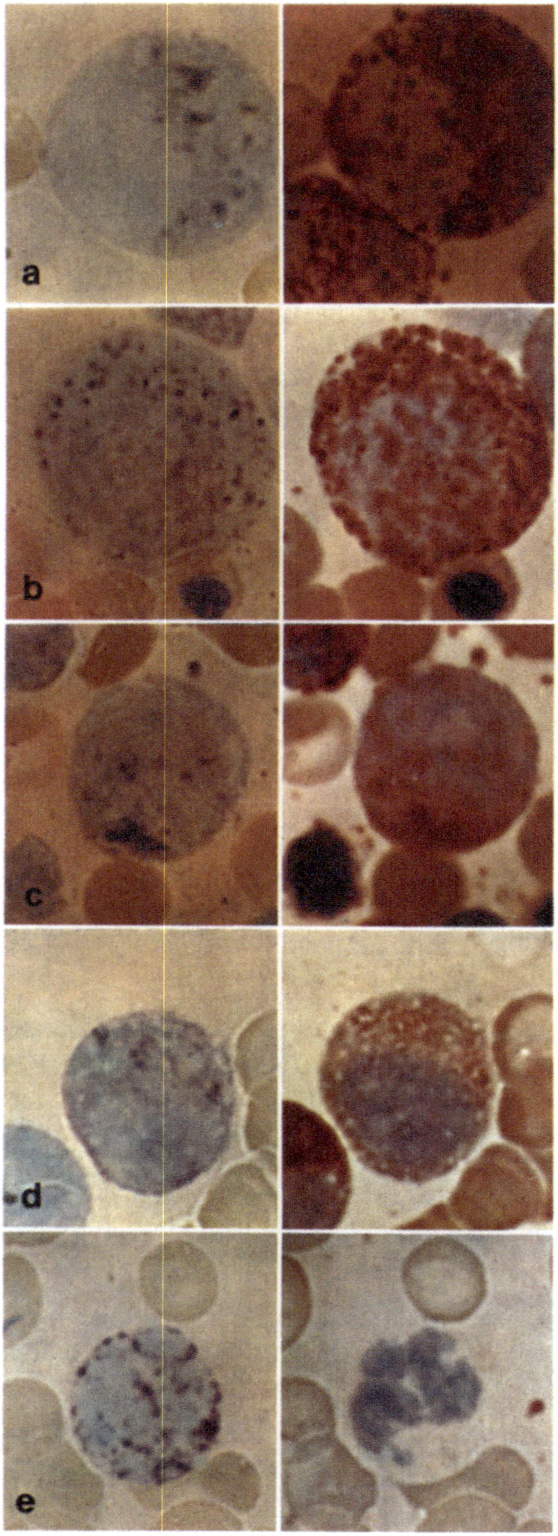

Fig. 18. Demonstration of normal basophilic granulopoietic cells. Left: Toluidine blue, pH 4.2. Right: The same cells subjected to the naphthol AS-D chloroacetate esterase reaction. Note the considerable decrease in the enzyme activity from the promyelocyte to the polymorphonuclear stage of basophil. Normal marrow smear. (a) basophilic promyelocyte, (b) basophilic myelocyte, (c) basophilic metamyelocyte, (d) rod-nuclear basophil, (e) polymorphonuclear basophil, ×1,500

not possible with this technique to arrive at definite conclusions as to the individual degree of maturity. Mitoses in basophil precursors are observed in every smear, and are by no means a rarity. The typical mitotic phases can be well defined. Metachromasia is usually not influenced by mitotic activity.

b) Detection with the Naphthol AS-D Chloroacetate Esterase Reaction

In agreement with LAMBERS and BAUER-SIC (1963), ACKERMAN (1963), LEDER (1967), and LANGNER and STEIGLEDER (1966), we, too, could detect no activity to LEDER's esterase in mature blood basophils. We were unable to detect in 5000 blood basophils taken from 50 healthy individuals a single positive reaction in mature basophils. This finding justifies the statement that blood basophils, taken under normal or non-leukemic conditions and examined by the usual methods, never demonstrate a naphthol AS-D chloroacetate hydrolyzing enzyme. This conclusion can be broadened to the effect that all blood basophils that yield a negative enzyme reaction must be regarded under physiological conditions as mature, polymorphonuclear basophil granulocytes. Although mature blood basophils display no enzyme activity, PARWARESCH *et al.* (1970) reported on the occurrence of typical activity of this enzyme at the different maturity stages of the basophil precursors.

Since the first description of this chloroacyl-splitting enzyme by GOMORI (1953), many investigations have been conducted concerning this enzyme reaction. The intensity and the pattern of the enzyme reactivity in different cells of the peripheral blood and bone marrow have been dealt with by a number of authors (MOLONEY *et al.,* 1960; BAGUENA-CANDELA and FORTEZA-BOVER, 1961; LÖFFLER, 1961 a; 1962; SCHÜMMELFEDER, 1961; SCHWEINITZ and BRAUNS, 1961; LAMBERS and BAUER-SIC, 1963; LEDER and NICOLAS 1963; MERKER, 1963; WULFF, 1963; FISCHER *et al.,* 1964; LEDER, 1967 and 1970; PARWARESCH *et al.,* 1970; 1971).

In order to clarify the results obtained with this technique, we must go more closely into the behavior of this enzyme. The reaction was carried out according to a method given by LEDER (1964). Cells reacting positively take up a luminous red colour in a predominantly fine, granulated form. The intensity of the activity is always constant within a given cell type under normal conditions. No exceptions to this rule were found, either in the literature or in our own investigations. No activity was ever detected in erythropoietic cells, which were readily differentiated by means of their stained nuclei. This cell line, which regularly displays a distinct alpha-naphthyl acetate esterase activity and a more limited naphthol AS-D acetate esterase activity, showed after complete inactivation of these enzymes through preceding fixation a negative naphthol AS-D chloroacetate esterase reaction. Lymphocytes and plasma cells, which occasionally display a weak nonspecific esterase activity, never show a positive naphthol AS-D chloroacetate esterase reaction. Megakaryoblasts, megakaryocytes, and thrombocytes, which also demonstrate a strong nonspecific esterase activity, never in our experiments showed naphthol AS-D chloroacetate esterase activity. The reticulum cells, which display the strongest alpha-naphthyl acetate esterase activity (LÖFFLER, 1961 b), always gave a negative enzyme reaction. The same proved to be true for the vascular endothelium. In contrast, tissue

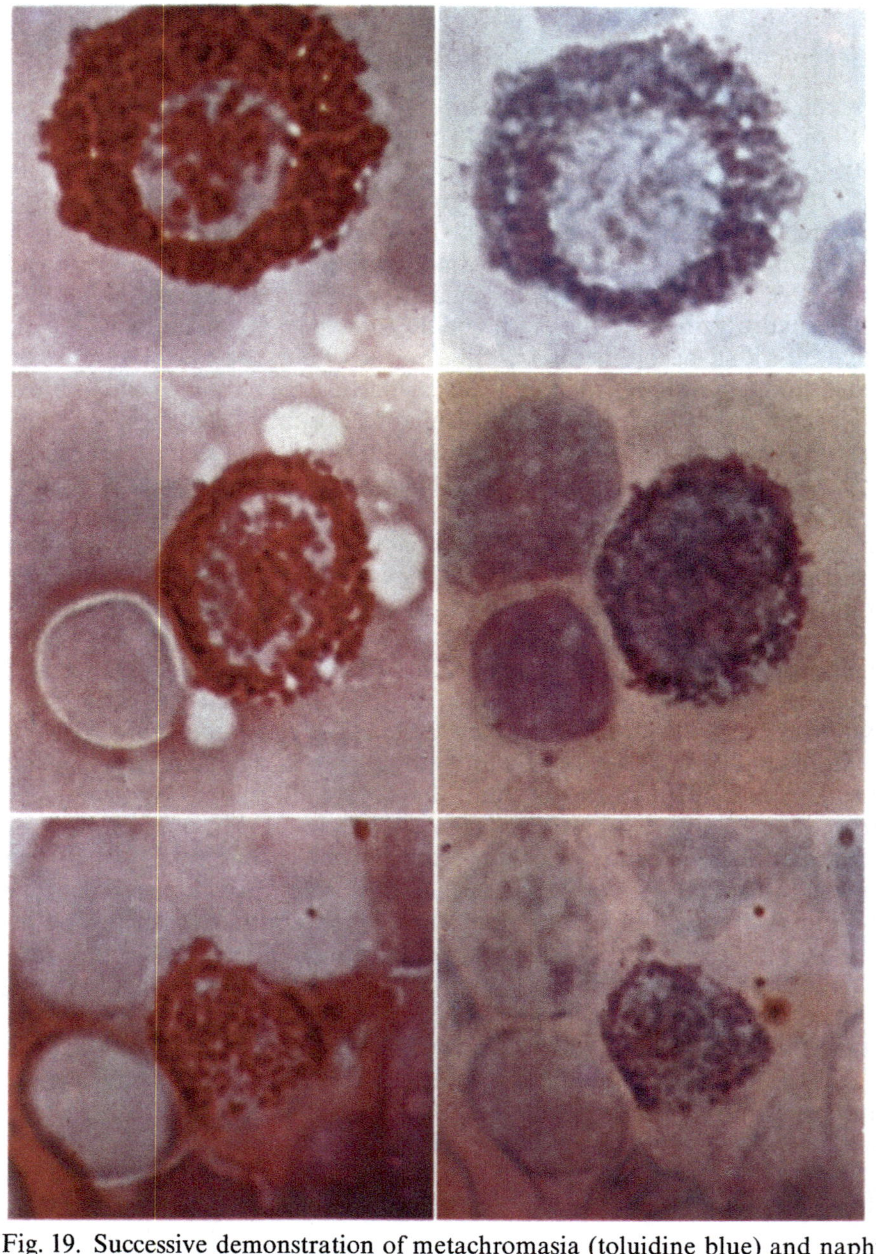

Fig. 19. Successive demonstration of metachromasia (toluidine blue) and naphthol AS-D chloroacetate esterase reaction at various maturity stages of human tissue mast cells in bone marrow smears. ×1,800

mast cells display a strong activity to naphthol AS-D chloroacetate esterase (Fig. 19).

The behavior of the naphthol AS-D chloracetate esterase reaction in the granulopoietic cells is of special interest. A characteristic intensity is observed not only in mature granulocytes. Their precursor stages also regularly display typical activities which can be used to indicate the degree of cell maturity, as can be demonstrated by direct measurements.

In the following section we discuss the behavior of LEDER's esterase and its qualitative characteristics in the various granulopoietic cells. We distinguish the following five morphologically distinct stages of maturity of the granulopoietic cells: promyelocytes, myelocytes, metamyelocytes, bandforms and polymorphonuclear granulocytes (HEILMEYER, 1951; ROHR, 1960; ACKERMAN, 1964; BEGEMANN, 1969).

Promyelocytes are large cells with rounded or oval nuclei containing a relatively compact chromatin structure. Nucleoli can only occasionally be clearly recognized. The cytoplasm shows moderate basophilia. The younger cells possess exclusively the typical azurophil granules which are distributed evenly throughout the entire cytoplasm. With appropriate methods, secondary granules can be recognized in the more mature promyelocytes.

Myelocytes, which we, contrary to some authors, do not further subdivide, are usually somewhat smaller than promyelocytes and have a light, eccentric nucleus. The nucleus is round-to-oval or kidney-shaped, with a compact chromatin structure. Nucleoli can often be detected. Cytoplasm basophilia is less than in the promyelocytes. A limited number of secondary granules is easily recognized. Promyelocytes and myelocytes are the predecessor cells of the granulocyte series and possess the ability to divide. Their mitotic forms are often observed in bone marrow specimens. Panchromatic stains, however, do not successfully distinguish them.

Metamyelocytes are the same size as myelocytes. The shrinking of the indented nucleus in neutrophil granulocytes is the manifestation of a strong tendency to segmentation. The chromatin displays a coarsely layered, optically dense structure. A characteristic feature of granulopoiesis is its segmentation tendency, which is more or less pronounced in all its cytogenetic derivatives. The band-nuclear granulocytes display a marked narrowing of their nuclei with a beginning segmentation (ROHR, 1960) but without any shrinkage of the intersegmental bonds. Their differentiation from metamyelocytes is often difficult, due to the smooth transitional state which exists between the two forms. Differentiating between the polymorphonuclear granulocytes proceeds without difficulty. Polymorphonuclear neutrophils generally display 3 to 4 segments, and eosinophils often possess a 2-segmented nucleus. Exceptions, however, are not rare. Determining the number of segments in mature blood basophils is often difficult, due to the twisted and coiled form of its nucleus and the variable sizes of the segments. The above morphological criteria are based, to a large extent, upon panoptic staining.

Neutrophil granulopoietic cells give a positive naphthol AS-D chloroacetate esterase reaction. Promyelocytes regularly show the strongest activity, with a markedly granular reaction product. Myelocytes display a more limited enzyme activity with a similar granular pattern. The intensity diminishes with the maturation of the neutrophil line. Metamyelocytes and band forms react more weakly. The reaction product is coarsely granular, luminous red, and sharply defined. The intensity of the polymorphonuclear neutrophils is much more limited than that of their predecessor cells. Under

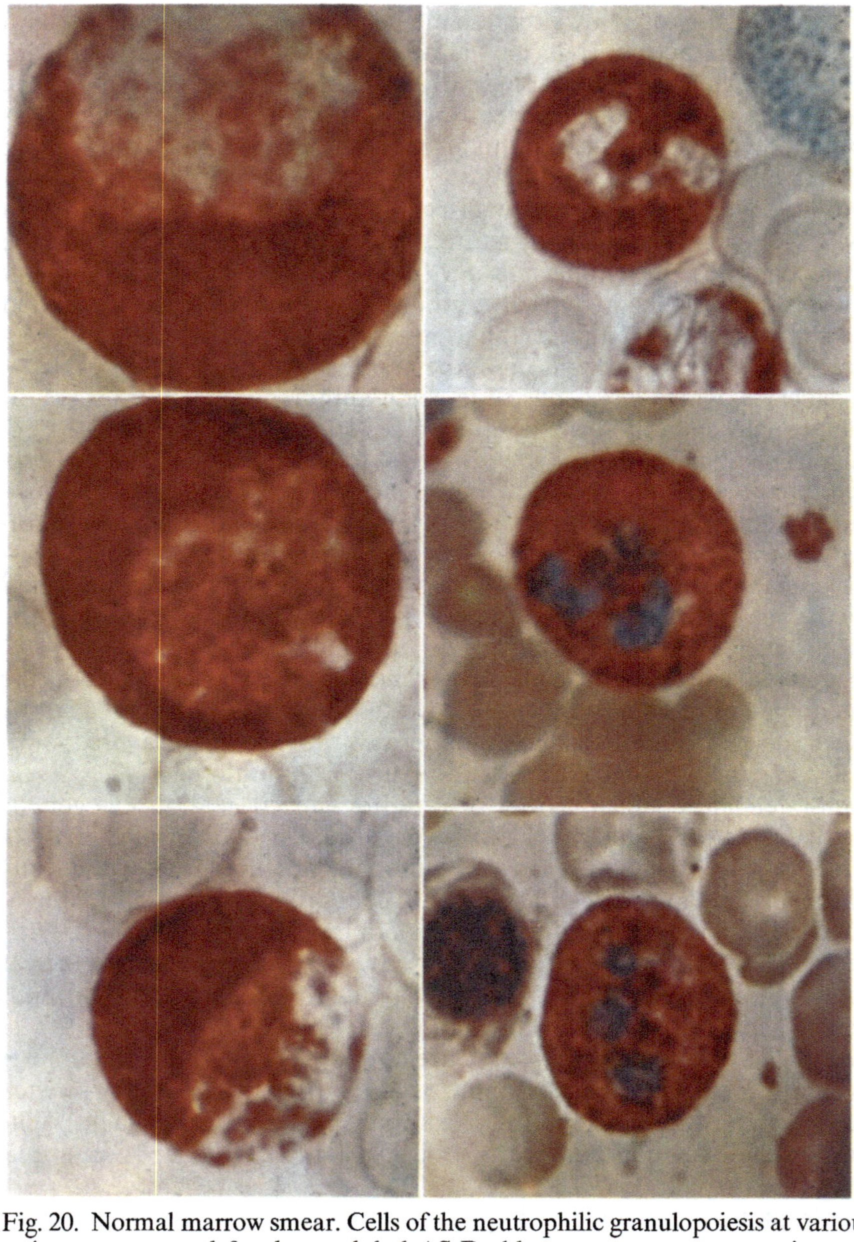

Fig. 20. Normal marrow smear. Cells of the neutrophilic granulopoiesis at various maturity stages treated for the naphthol AS-D chloroacetate esterase reaction. ×2,000

physiological conditions, we never observed enzyme-negative polymorphonuclear neutrophils, either in the peripheral blood or in the bone marrow (Fig. 20).

LEDER (1970) and LEDER and PAPE (1970 a, b) have recently investigated the behavior of the eosinophil cell line to the naphthol AS-D chloroacetate esterase. Eosinophils have been found to give a negative reaction in the polymorphonuclear, band-nuclear, metamyelocytic, myelocytic, and to a great extent even in the promyelocytic maturation stages. Using the p-dimethylaminobenzaldehyde nitrite reaction (ADAMS, 1957), which gives selective staining of the eosinophil granules at all stages, combined with the naphthol AS-D chloroacetate reaction, these authors could find promyelocytes with just detectable eosinophil granules and with a clear activity to the esterase reaction (Fig. 21). The enzyme activity subsided with increasing eosinophil granulation or with increasing maturation of the bone marrow eosinophils. It should be noted in this connection that the activity of this enzyme reaction in the various myeloid cells and their developing stages is valid only under physiological conditions. In myeloproliferative diseases exceptions, in the form of an enzyme persistence or enzyme defect have repeatedly been reported (LEDER, 1970).

On the basis of common morphological criteria and the typical reactivity to the peroxidase, alpha-naphthyl acetate, naphthol AS-D chloroacetate, and naphthol AS acetate esterase reactions, one can, according to LEDER (1967) distinguish a cell type that falls between myelocytes and mature monocytes and displays the criteria typical of a transitional cell called large monocyte or promonocyte. As the promonocyte develops from the promyelocyte and matures into the blood monocyte, it sustains heavy losses of naphthol AS-D chloroacetate esterase activity in the same way as the other granulocytes. Mature monocytes do occasionally display enzyme activity with slight granular reaction product, but the reaction of monocytes to naphthol AS-D chloroacetate esterase may increase considerably under certain prerequisites and topical tissue conditions, as can also its ability to divide (THIEDE *et al.*, 1970; PARWARESCH *et al.*, 1971).

In order to study the naphthol AS-D chloroacetate esterase activity in blood basophils and their precursors, bone marrow smears from healthy individuals were fixed in a methanol-formol mixture containing N-cetylpyridinium chloride and stained in an aqueous toluidine-blue solution at ph 4.2. Cells with typical metachromasia were photographed and marked without reference to their morphological particulars. After a short destaining at pH 4.8, the smears were subjected to the naphthol AS-D chloroacetate esterase reaction. The marked cells were again searched out and tested for enzyme activity. The same cells were photographed twice, once following toluidine-blue staining, and once after the enzyme reaction.

Mature basophil granulocytes with strong, well-defined, optically impervious metachromatic granules were always found to be enzyme-negative with the applied technique. Rod-nuclear stage of basophils, which display metachromasia, demonstrate a very weak enzyme activity. The metamyelocytes displayed a clearly positive, granular enzyme pattern. The me-

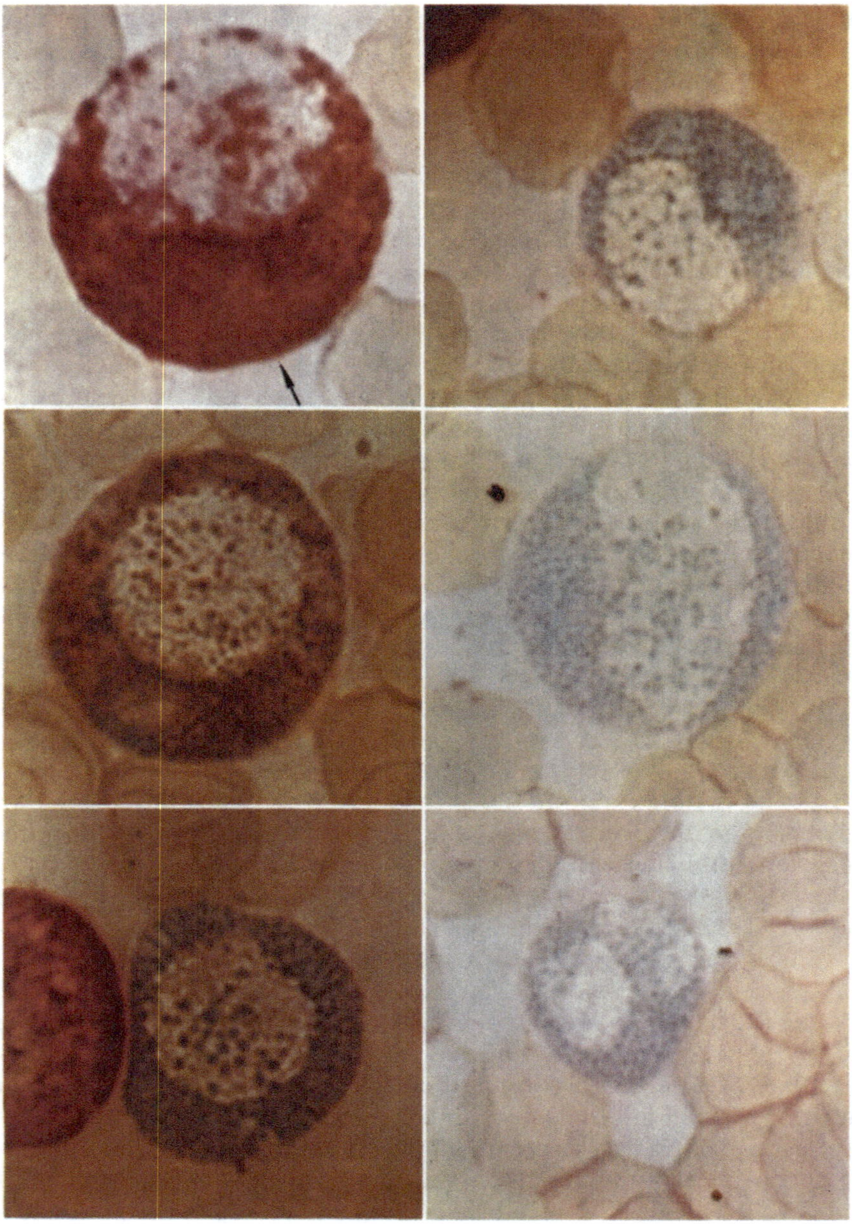

Fig. 21. Normal marrow smear. Cells of the eosinophilic granulopoiesis at various maturity stages with combined ADAMS stain (grey-green) and naphthol AS-D chloroacetate esterase (red). Note the positivity of both reactions in the promyelocyte with its already distinctly visible specific granules (*arrow*). ×2,000

tachromatic granulation here was, however, definitely weaker than that of the rod-nuclear and polymorphonuclear basophils. The basophil myelocytes were metachromatically granulated to varying intensities – less so, on the average, than the more mature forms. The esterase reaction was strongly positive and corresponded with the reaction intensity in the neutrophil myelocytes. The youngest predecessor cells of the basophil series exhibited only a slight degree of metachromasia. Their enzyme content was high and corresponded to that of the nonspecific promyelocytes.

Within the basophil maturation line, the activity to the naphthol AS-D chloroacetate esterase reaction decreases in a gradual, smooth manner. Metachromasia develops quickly and more erratically, so that on the basis of the extent of metachromasia alone no reliable determination of the degree of cell maturity can be made. We had the impression that each stage of maturity of the basophil granulopoiesis reveals a characteristic intensity of the enzyme reaction (Fig. 18). Therefore we conducted a quantitative, cytophotometric investigation, which is described in the following section.

2. Quantitative Findings

a) Cytophotometric Determination of the Naphthol AS-D Chloroacetate Esterase Activity in Basophil Granulopoietic Cells

To provide quantitative support for our impression, we conducted a second experiment in which we measured the esterase activity cytophotometrically (Parwaresch and Sadighi, 1971). The first step was identification of the basophil cell line with specific basic dyes (toluidine blue). The same cells were then restained with the enzyme reaction, the intensity of which was measured with the filter-graduated integrating microdensitometer (type DN 2, Bahr and Strout Ltd), at a wavelength of 4800 Å. The extinction values were recorded relatively and expressed in terms of working units (WU). As a control, a cell-free region of the slide in the immediate vicinity of the cells was measured. The random test samples fell into 5 separate groups. Each item represents an average value of 3 measurements. In order to compare the different groups with one another, a variance analysis was performed and the H-test applied as an overall test of the medians of the independent random samples. The WHITE test for independent random samples was used to verify the data specifically (Lienert, 1962). Basophil granulopoietic cells demonstrate varying enzyme intensities according to their degree of maturity. This difference could be statistically ascertained. The calculated median values never overlapped (Fig. 22). The basophil promyelocytes regularly displayed the highest values, ranging from 64 to 75 WU. Most promyelocytes indicated an enzyme activity between 65 and 72 WU, with a median between 70 and 71.

The enzyme content of basophil myelocytes lay very near to that of promyelocytes, but without ever quite reaching it. Their median values lay between 54 and 65 WU, i.e. considerably lower than the promyelocyte values. The minimum values of the metamyelocytes lay very near to the maximum values of the rod-nuclear stage of basophils but the median values were well separated from each other.

The polymorphonuclear basophils were always enzyme-negative, nevertheless displaying an absorption of 5 to 17 WU. A control test on 100 nucleated enzyme-negative bone marrow cells revealed a similar but somewhat wider distribution of 4 to 21 WU. Thus, the mature blood basophils, as expected, display an absorption which is located within the borderline value for control cells. The median value lay between 9 and 11 WU. The variance analysis revealed a marked heterogeneity, and a comparison of the median values yielded significant ($p < 0.01$) differences between all groups. The WHITE test for independent control samples revealed a value for critical $z = 2.58$, with a margin of error for all $p < 0.01$. The results of the cytochemical investigations were confirmed by those of the cytophotometric studies. As in cytological findings, promyelocytes produced the highest values and 85% of them displayed an enzyme activity between 67 and 71 WU. Myelocytes yielded a statistically significant difference of a somewhat more limited enzyme content, 79% of them giving values between 53 and 57 WU. Similarly, metamyelocytes and rod-nuclear basophils had a far lower enzyme content. The median values of their curves lay 6 WU from each other, although the extreme values overlapped.

In agreement with the control values, the mature blood basophils were always enzyme-negative. The absorption recorded fell without exception within the extreme values for the absorption of nonreactive cells.

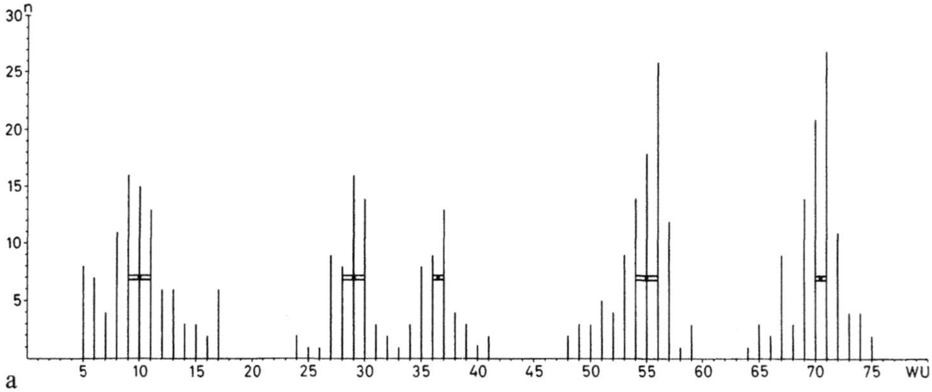

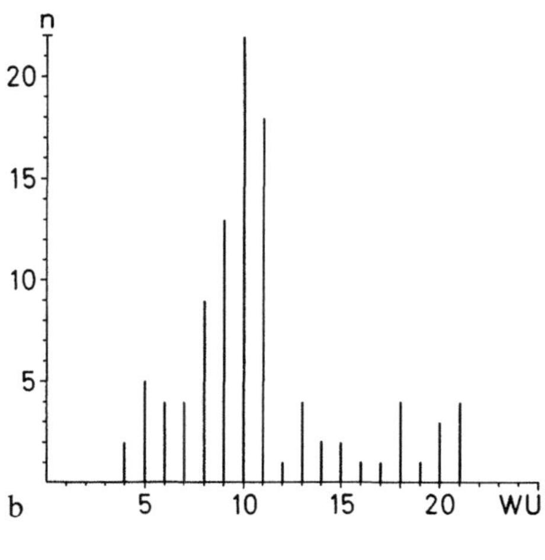

Fig. 22 a and b. (a) Cytophotometric measurement of the naphthol AS-D chloroacetate esterase activity in cells of the basophilic granulopoiesis at various maturity stages. Ordinate: Number of cells counted. Abscissa: Absorption spectra of the cells of a definite maturity stage in terms of arbitrarily chosen working units (*WU*); left to right: polymorphonuclear basophils, rod-nuclear basophils, metamyelocytes, myelocytes, promyelocytes. Medians are depicted as horizontal parallel lines. (b) Basic extinction curve of 100 nucleated bone marrow cells with a negative naphthol AS-D chloroacetate esterase reaction

b) The Quantitative Composition of Basophil Granulopoietic Cells in Human Bone Marrow

Once the selective demonstration of basophil granulopoietic cells had been achieved and their degree of maturity more exactly defined, we attempted (PARWARESCH and NOTTBOHM, 1975) to determine the number of cells at each of the various stages of maturity within the basophil population. We used for this investigation fresh normal sternal smears showing an even cell distribution. In order to limit the large possibility of error inherent in the panchromatic stain techniques, we used specific cytochemical methods for the reliable identification of the different marrow cells.

The monocytes and their precursors were recognized by a combined application of LEDER's esterase and the naphthol AS-D acetate esterase reactions. The eosinophil cell line was demonstrated with the ADAMS or light green stain. The neutrophil series were identified by their high activity to the naphthol AS-D chloroacetate esterase reaction. The cells of the basophil granulopoiesis were demonstrated by the successive application of toluidine blue and the naphthol AS-D chloroacetate esterase reaction. Lymphocytes, capillary endothelium, plasma cells, and reticulum cells were easily recognized by their typical morphology.

Table 12. Distribution of different maturation stages of basophils in the bone marrow of 10 healthy subjects expressed as a percentage of total basophils

N	Segmented	Bandform	Meta-myelocyte	Myelocyte	Pro-myelocyte	Mitoses
1	43.50	7.14	8.44	24.02	16.88	5.84
2	14.00	10.00	18.00	33.00	25.00	4.00
3	23.37	7.79	15.58	27.27	25.97	0.00
4	11.65	21.35	12.62	31.06	23.30	1.94
5	18.64	13.07	14.61	27.67	26.15	5.83
6	31.40	12.39	12.39	20.66	23.14	3.30
7	30.68	28.40	3.40	10.22	27.27	2.27
8	32.18	18.39	6.89	24.13	18.39	3.44
9	43.03	15.18	8.86	20.25	12.65	3.79
10	18.03	21.31	11.47	24.59	24.59	4.91
$\bar{X}$	27.30%	14.70%	11.30%	24.50%	22.20%	3.70%
±S	11.35%	6.87%	4.39%	6.41%	4.77%	1.76%
RANGE	11.65 to 43.50	7.14 to 28.40	3.40 to 15.58	10.22 to 33.00	12.65 to 27.27	0.00 to 5.84

In the 10 normal subjects examined, blood basophils and their precursors made up an average of 0.39 ± 0.15 (0.14 to 0.61) % of the bone-marrow leukocytes. The frequency distributions of the various maturity stages within the total basophil population is shown in Table 12. There is a high percentage of basophil precursors capable of mitosis (promyelocytes and myelocytes). Together, they make up about 50% of the total basophil population of bone marrow. This finding is further supported by the high incidence of mitotic forms. About 4% of all bone marrow basophils were found to be in mitosis. Metamyelocytes and rod-nuclear basophils make up about one fourth of the bone marrow basophils, and polymorphonuclear basophils represent an equal amount.

III. Evidence of Basophil Descent from Promyelocytes

Despite a few opinions to the contrary (SCHLEICHER, 1968), most authors agree upon the myelogenic origin of blood basophils, which is supported by a good body of findings:

Cells of the basophil granulopoiesis and their mitotic forms can always be detected in normal bone marrow (JOLLY, 1900; MAXIMOW, 1913). EHRLICH (1898) established that they increase in almost all cases of myeloproliferative diseases. The basophil cell line exhibits the specific properties of granulocytes; they contain the cytogenetic information for producing peroxidase and naphthol AS-D chloroacetate esterase. They have a segmented nucleus and, like other polymorphonuclear leukocytes, represent a final developmental stage incapable of further division.

We accept these results as providing sufficient evidence of the myelogenic origin of blood basophils. A complete portrayal of the cytogenetic ascendence of blood basophils has, however, not yet been achieved.

A surveying of the literature reveals that the sequence of development described for the basophil granulocytes has been founded more upon inferences drawn by analogy with the developmental process of neutrophils than upon methodologically sound, well-founded results (DANTCHEV, 1952).

The uncertainty associated with a pure, cytologically corroborated deduction concerning basophils emerges clearly from the views of such an experienced cytologist as UNDRITZ (1952), who maintained that the basophil series was autonomous and completely independent of the other granulocyte series in the sense of a strict polyphyletism. He believed that the basophil series begins with its own basophil blasts and did not consider as proven the existence of hybrid forms, i.e. 'transitional forms' between unspecific promyelocytes and basophil myelocytes. Judged in light of the panoptic stains, these observations are correct; the WRIGHT or PAPPENHEIM staining techniques as used in routine diagnostics are, however, not suited for the separation of metachromatic granules from azure granules.

Our search for criteria to allow reliable identification of both promyelocyte granules and metachromatic granules showed the successive application of toluidine blue and the naphthol AS-D chloroacetate esterase reaction to one and the same cell to be satisfactory. It enabled us to demonstrate all stages of development of cells occurring between the toluidine blue-negative, strongly esterase-positive 'unspecific promyelocytes' and the toluidine blue-positive, completely esterase-negative, mature basophil granulocytes. The results of this experiment provide further evidence of the broad, manifold cytogenetic potency of the promyelocyte. Even though this cell displays morphologically well-developed characteristics as a differentiated cell, it nevertheless develops into four different cells forms. This clearly shows that the level of differentiation achieved tells us very little about the level of determination or about the 'still-possible', potency in the future. To view the strongly naphtol AS-D chloroacetate esterase-positive promyelocytes as being mature (SCHMALZL, 1968) thus seems unwarranted. There is, moreover, no basis for disputing in principle (LÖFFLER, 1969) the ability of the promyelocytes to differentiate in various directions.

In general, it is maintained (DANTCHEV, 1952) that the number of azure granules diminishes as unspecific promyelocytes turn into specific ones, or into specific myelocytes. They finally disappear completely, whereas the specific granules continually increase. However, according to our findings, such a mode of granule development cannot be accepted as correct. A precise comparison of micrographs of the same cell with both reactions applied revealed cytotopographic agreement between the metachromatic material and the positive chloroacetate esterase reaction. This comparison demonstrated that the specific granules do not merely arise separately from or in the vincinity of azure granules; instead, they seem to develop directly out of them. Wether all or only some of the azure granules transform into metachromatic granules remains obscure. It must be borne in mind that form promyelocyte to mature basophil granulocyte, many mitoses occur. It is thus possible that the compact azure granulation of the original promyelocytes becomes distributed among a large number of daughter cells. Furthermore, it appears possible that the azure granule count decreases due to fusion, since the secondary granules (SPICER and MEYER, 1960) have sizes of the order of 0.2 μm, thus far exceeding the size of the azure granules. Naphthol AS-D chloroacetate esterase-positive granules occur up to the rod-nuclear state in the basophil cell line. This finding shows that the promyelocytic (azurophil) or 'primary' granules are contained in relatively mature precursors of blood basophils, a conclusion that is further supported by ultrastructural findings.

This theory of the development of basophil granules from azure granules has a good parallel in the development of eosinophil granules. As the eosinophil maturation progresses the pure naphthol AS-D chloroacetate esterase-positive azure granules in eosinophilic promyelocytes yield in ever-stronger amounts a positive para-dimethylaminobenzaldehyde nitrite reaction, which is specific for eosinophil granules (LEDER *et al.*, 1970; LEDER and PAPE, 1970). Cells containing azure granules positive to the naphthol AS-D chloroacetate esterase reaction were never found clearly separated from dimethyl aminobenzaldehyde nitrite-positive eosinophil granules in the same cell. Eosinophil granules thus also seem to arise out of azure granules.

Similar findings have been achieved with the electron microscope in connection with the development of neutrophil granulocytes. Intermediate or transitional forms between azure granules and neutrophil granules at various stages of maturity have been found (BESSIS and THIERY, 1961). We cannot, therefore, on the basis of our findings and the results obtained on eosinophils and neutrophils, support the view that basophil granules develop as secondary granules alongside azure granules. We believe that basophil granules arise from azure granules, parallel with the specific granules of these two cell types.

Our findings further support the view that cell size is not a reliable criterion for determining degree of maturity. Since mitosis lasts about 30 to 60 min, giving rise to two daughter cells which are only 30 to 60 min behind the precursor cell with respect to maturity, the daughter cells are markedly smaller than the mother cell. Thus we may expect to find in bone marrow smears cells that present large variations in size but are similar in all other respects (BOLL, 1966; LEDER, 1967). Taken as a whole, our findings support NAEGELI's theory of dualism. We must reject polyphyletic theory in the sense of UNDRITZ (1952), in which eosinophil, basophil, neutrophil, and monocytic cell series are derived completely distinctly from one another.

It is also more logical to reconcile the variety of hemopathologic findings with the assumption that the various types of granulocytes and monocytes develop out of one cell, an unspecific promyelocyte. A large increase in basophil granulocytes is found in most cases of the myeloid leukemias, where usually neutrophils predominate. The same is true of a similar increase in eosinophils or monocytes in the chronic myeloid leukemias. If we assume a common origin for the affected cells, such findings are obvious and simple to explain, whereas on the basis of a polyphyletic origin, such phenomena would be hard to understand. For instance, it has frequently been suggested that in myeloproliferative diseases there is a reactive increase in eosinophils, basophils, or monocytes. In the same way, labels such as 'the coreaction of the one or the other cell line' are offered. If one accepts that all the above-mentioned cell types have a common parent cell, such hypotheses become superfluous. In Chapter D we present evidence that the so-called coreacting cells are simply neoplastic proliferating cells derived from a common progenitor cell, which has been affected by the leukogenic agent (DAMESHEK and GUNZ, 1964; PARWARESCH *et al.*, 1970)

To summarize: the combination of two methods used by us has proved advantageous for the study of the origin of the blood basophils. Toluidine blue at pH 4.2 stains metachromatic granules that permit assessment of the entire basophil population of the bone marrow. The naphthol AS-D chloroacetate esterase reaction, on the other hand, demonstrates the azure granules of the promyelocytes. Metachromatic precursors of the basophil granulocytes display various degrees of naphthol AS-D chloroacetate esterase activity, the intensity of which is subject to regular variations according to the actual degree of maturity. All transitional forms between the nonmetachromatic, strongly naphthol AS-D chloroacetate esterase-positive 'unspecific' myelocytes, and the strongly metachromatic but completely esterase-negative mature basophils are detectable. The findings justify the conclusion that basophil granulocytes, like monocytes, neutrophils, and eosinophils, are derived from a common promyelocyte. This means that in the typical morphology, and especially in the highly characteristic granules, a certain differentiation of promyelocytes is expressed, which does not, however, preclude further differentiation steps. Our findings support the dualistic view of the genesis of white blood cells, the concept of which is portrayed in Fig. 23.

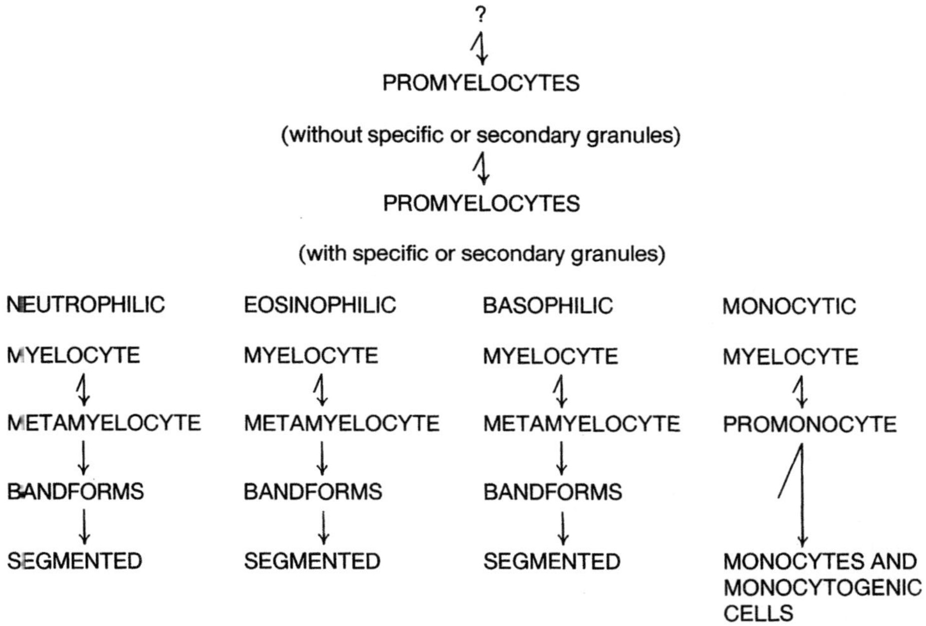

Fig. 23. Derivation of myelogenous cells from a "common" promyelocyte with azurophilic granules only

References

Ackerman, G. A.: see page 55.

Ackerman, G. A.: see page 55. Ed. H. R. Bierman.

Adams, C. W. M.: A p-dimethylaminobenzaldehyde-nitrite method for the histochemical demonstration of tryptophane and related compounds. J. clin. Path. **10,** 56 – 62 (1957).

Astaldi, G., Rondanelli, E. G., Bernadelli, E.: see page 56.

Baguena-Candela, R., Forteza-Bover, G.: Incidence of leukemia in the Spanish Levant during the years 1959 – 1960. Med. esp. **45,** 455 – 459 (1961).

Begemann, H.: Klinische Haematologie. Stuttgart: Georg Thieme Verlag 1969.

Benacchio, G. B.: Gibt es bei Meerschweinchen und Kaninchen Mastmyelocyten und stammen die basophil gekörnten Blutmastzellen aus dem Knochenmark? Folia haemat. (Lpz.) **2,** 253 – 270 (1911).

BESSIS, M., THIÉRY, J.-P.: Electron microscopy of human white blood cells and their stem cells. Int. Rev. Cytol. **12**, 199 – 241 (1961).
BESSIS, M., THIÉRY, J.-P.: Study by electronic microscope on human leukemia. I. Granulocytic leukemia. Nouv. Rev. franç. Hémat. **1**, 703 – 728 (1961).
BLUMENTHAL, R.: La filiation des globules blancs et la valeur biologique de leurs granulations chez l'homme. Ann. Soc. roy. Sci. méd. nat. Brux. **14**, 85 – 97 (1905).
BOLL, I.: Granulocytopoese unter physiologischen und pathologischen Bedingungen. In: Experimentelle Medizin. Pathologie und Klinik, Bd. 17. Berlin-Heidelberg-New York: Springer 1966.
BRUCKNER, I.: Beiträge zum Studium der EHRLICHschen Zellen (Mastzellen) im menschlichen Blute. In: Riv. de chir. (1904). Abstr. in: Folia haemat. (Lpz.) **1**, 404 – 405 (1904).
CASTIGLIONI, G. G.: Osservazioni sulla cromotropia delle mastzellen. Proposta di un metodo di colorazione. Ann. Biol. norm. pat. **1**, 71 – 76 (1947).
DAMESHEK, W. F., GUNZ, F.: Leukaemia. London: Grune and Stratton 1964.
DANTCHEV, D.: Particularités morphologiques dans la formation des granulocytes éosinophiles et basophiles. Sang **23**, 439 – 445 (1952).
DOWNEY, H.: Heteroplastic development of eosinophil leucocytes and haematogenous mast cells in bone marrow of guinea-pig. Anat. Rec. **8**, 135 – 137 (1914).
EHRLICH, P.: see page 23.
EHRLICH, P.: Methodologische Beiträge zur Physiologie und Pathologie der verschiedenen Formen der Leukocyten. Z. klin. Med. **1**, 553 – 560 (1880).
EHRLICH, P.: Färbeanalytische Untersuchungen zur Histologie und Klinik des Blutes. Berlin: Hirschwald 1891.
EHRLICH, P.: Diskussionsbemerkungen zum Vortrage Engels. Dtsch. med. Wschr. **37**, 274 (1898).
FISCHER, R., LORBACHER, F., KÄUFER, C.: Untersuchungen zur enzymhistochemischen Differenzierung von leukaemischen Erkrankungen am Schnittpräparat. Virchows Arch. path. Anat. **337**, 525 – 534 (1964).
GOMORI, G.: see page 59.
GRAHAM, G.: see page 59.
GRAWITZ, E.: Klinische Pathologie des Blutes, 4. Aufl. Leipzig: Thieme 1911.
HEILMEYER, L., BEGEMANN, H.: Handbuch der inneren Medizin, Bd. II: Blut und Blutkrankheiten. Berlin-Göttingen-Heidelberg: Springer 1951.
HELLY, K.: see page 24.
HIRSCHFELD, H.: Zur Kenntnis der Histogenese der granulierten Knochenmarkszellen. Virchows Arch. **153**, 335 – 347 (1898).
JOLLY, J.: see page 74.
JOLLY, J.: Sur les Plasmazellen du grand epipoloom. C. R. Soc. Biol. (Paris) **52**, 1104 – 1105 (1900 b).
JORDAN, H. E.: The histology of the blood and the red bone marrow of the leopard frog *Rana pipieus.* Amer. J. Anat. **25**, 437 – 480 (1919).
JORDAN, H. E.: On the nature of the basophilic granulocytes of the blood and tissues. Anat. Rec. **33**, 89 – 106 (1926).
JORDAN, H. E., FILLIPIN, J. C.: Haematopoiesis in Chelonia. Folia haemat. (Lpz.) **15**, 1 – 24 (1913).
JORDAN, H. E., SPEIDEL, C. C.: Studies on lymphocytes. I. Effect of splenectomy, experimental hemorrhage and a hemolytic toxin in the frog. Amer. J. Anat. **32**, 155 – 167 (1923).
JORDAN, H. E., SPEIDEL, C. C.: see page 74.

JORDAN, H. E., SPEIDEL, C. C.: Blood-cell formation in the horned toad, *Phrynosoma solare.* Amer. J. Anat. **43,** 77 – 102 (1929).

JUHLIN, L.: Basophil leucocyte differential in blood and bone marrow. Acta haemat. (Basel) **29,** 89 – 95 (1963).

KARDOS, E.: Über die Entstehung der Blutmastzellen aus dem Knochenmark. Folia haemat. (Lpz.) **2,** 271 – 372 (1911).

LAMBERS, K., BAUER-SIC, P.: Hydrolytische Enzyme in der klinischen Diagnostik. In: Zyto- und Histochemie der Hämatologie. 9. Freiburger Symposion. Ed. H. MERKER. Berlin-Göttingen-Heidelberg: Springer 1963.

LANGNER, R., STEIGLEDER, G. K.: see page 61.

LEDER, L.-D.: see page 62.

LEDER, L.-D.: Der Blutmonocyt. Berlin-Heidelberg-New York: Springer 1967.

LEDER, L.-D.: Diagnostic experiences with the naphthol AS-D chloroacetate esterase. Blut **21,** 1 – 8 (1970).

LEDER, L.-D., NICOLAS, R.: see page 62.

LEDER, L.-D., PAPE, B.: Der Nachweis von Naphthol-AS-D-Chloracetat-Esterase in normalen eosinophilen Vorstufen. Klin. Wschr. **48,** 885 – 887 (1970 a).

LEDER, L.-D., PAPE, B.: Der Nachweis von Übergangsformen zwischen Promyelocyten und eosinophilen Myelocyten. Klin. Wschr. **48,** 1009 –1010 (1970 b).

LEDER, L.-D., STUTTE, H. J., PAPE, B.: Zur selektiven Darstellung von eosinophilen Granulocyten und ihren Vorstufen in Ausstrichen und Schnitten. Klin. Wschr. **48,** 191 (1970).

LENNERT, K., BACH, G.: see page 62.

LENNERT, K., LINDNER, J.: Cytochemistry of mast cells. Proc. 8th Congr. europ. Soc. Haemat. Vienna 1961, Bd. III (1962).

LENNERT, K., SCHUBERT, J. F. C.: see page 62.

LEVADITI, C.: Contributions à l'étude des mastzellen et de la mastzellen-leucocytose. Thèse pour le doctorat en médecine. Faculté de Médecine de Paris. Paris: C. Naud (Ed.) **1,** 78 (1902).

LIENERT, G. A.: Verteilungsfreie Methoden in der Biostatistik. Meisenheim am Glan: A. Hain 1962.

LÖFFLER, H.: Cytochemischer Nachweis von unspezifischer Esterase in Ausstrichen. Beiträge zur Technik und Ergebnisse im Blutausstrich des Menschen. Klin. Wschr. **39,** 1220 – 1227 (1961 a).

LÖFFLER, H.: Untersuchungen über die Aktivität der alkalischen Phosphatase und der unspezifischen Esterase in den Retikulumzellen des Knochenmarks. Ein Vergleich zwischen Knochenmark und Lymphknoten. Folia haemat. (Frankfurt) **6,** 1 – 3 (1961 b).

LÖFFLER, H.: see page 63.

LÖFFLER, H.: Cytochemische Klassifizierung der akuten Leukosen und malignen Lymphome. Int. Arbeitstagung über Chemo- und Immunotherapie der Leukosen und malignen Lymphome. Wien 1969.

MAXIMOW, A.: Beiträge zur Histologie der eitrigen Entzündung. Beitr. path. Anat. **38,** 301 – 353 (1905).

MAXIMOW, A.: Über die Zellformen des lockeren Bindegewebes. Arch. mikr. Anat. **67,** 680 – 757 (1906).

MAXIMOW, A.: Experimentelle Untersuchungen zur postfoetalen Histogenese des myeloiden Gewebes Beitr. path. Anat. **41,** 122 – 166 (1907).

MAXIMOW, A.: see page 75.

MAXIMOW, A.: see page 75.

McDonald, J. R., Cruickshank, C. N., Dodds, E.: Cited by J. R. Cooper and C. N. Cruickshank: Improved methods for direct counting of basophil leukocytes. 1966. J. clin. Path. **19,** 402 (1966).

Merker, H.: see page 63.

Michaelis, L.: see page 25.

Michels, N. A.: see page 63.

Moloney, W. C., McPherson, K., Fliegelman, L.: see page 63.

Murakami, I., Ogawa, M., Amo, H., Ota, K.: H^3-thymidine autoradiograph. III. Eosinophils and basophils. Acta haemat. jap. **32,** 384 – 390 (1969).

Naegeli, O.: Die weißen Blutkörperchen. In: Nothnagel: Spezielle Pathologie und Therapie. Wien-Leipzig: A. Hoelder 1909.

Naegeli, O.: Die Mastzellen des Blutes. In: Blutkrankheiten und Blutdiagnostik. S. 200 – 205. Berlin und Leipzig: Springer 1919.

Naegeli, O.: Blutkrankheiten und Blutdiagnostik. Lehrbuch der morphologischen Haematologie. Berlin: Springer 1931 (re-published).

Opitz, A., Weicker, A.: In: Brock, J. (Ed.). Biologische Daten für den Kinderarzt. 2. edn., Vol. 1. Berlin: Springer 1954.

Pappenheim, A.: Von den gegenseitigen Beziehungen der farblosen Blutzellen zueinander. I. und II. Teil, Bd. 159 (1900).

Pappenheim, A.: Wie verhalten sich die Unna'schen Plasmazellen zu Lymphocyten? Virchows Arch. **166,** 424 – 484 (1901).

Pappenheim, A.: Zusatz zu der Mitteilung von Pröscher über experimentelle Leukocytosen. Fol. haemat. (Berlin) **1,** 686 – 688 (1904).

Pappenheim, A.: Erwiderung auf die „kritischen Bemerkungen“ von Türk in Nr. 4 der Folia haematologica. Folia haemat. (Berlin) **2,** 671 – 676 (1905).

Pappenheim, A.: Die Zellen der leukaemischen Myelose. Jena: Fischer 1914.

Pappenheim, A.: Haematologische Bestimmungstafeln. Leipzig: Hirschfeldt (Klinkhardt posthumes) 1920.

Parwaresch, M. R., Leder, L.-D., Dannenberg, K. E. G.: see page 65.

Parwaresch, M. R., Lennert, K.: see page 25.

Parwaresch, M. R., Lennert, K.: see page 64.

Parwaresch, M. R., Sadighi, R.: Cytophotometrische Messung der Aktivität von Naphthol-AS-D-Chloracetat-Esterase in den normalen menschlichen basophilen Granulopoiesezellen. Virchows Arch. Abt. B. Zellpath. **6,** 88 – 96 (1970).

Parwaresch, M. R., Nottbohm, F.: Quantitative Verteilung von Zellen basophiler Granulopoiese in Sternalpunktaten blutgesunder Menschen. Klin. Wschr.: **53,** 661 – 667 (1975).

Pearse, A. G. E.: The nature of Russell bodies and Kurloff bodies. Observations on the cytochemistry of plasma cells and reticulum cells. J. clin. Path. **2,** 81 – 90 (1949).

Popper, M.: Contribution à l'étude des ferments oxydants dans les leucocytes. C. R. Sod. Biol. (Paris) **87,** 41 (1922).

Pröscher, F.: Über experimentelle basophile Leukocytose beim Kaninchen. Folia haemat. (Berlin) **7,** 107 – 115 (1909).

Ringoen, A.: see page 26.

Rohr, K.: Das menschliche Knochenmark. Stuttgart: Georg Thieme 1960.

Sabine, J. C.: The history of the classification of human blood corpuscles. II. The two great schools of hematology: the primitive stem cell and its interpretation. Bull. Hist. Med. I, **8,** 696 – 720 (1940), II, **8,** 785 – 805 (1940).

Salvi, F.: see page 66.

SCHLEICHER, E. M.: Reticulohistiocytic origin of the blood basophil in human marrow. Acta haemat. (Basel) **40,** 162 – 165 (1968).
SCHMALZL, F., BRAUNSTEINER, H.: Cytochemische Darstellung von Esteraseaktivitäten in Blut- und Knochenmarkszellen. Klin. Wschr. **46,** 642 – 650 (1968).
SCHUBERT, J. F. C.: Differenzierungsmethode metachromatischer Zellen nach ihrem Säuregrad. Experientia (Basel) **12,** 346 – 347 (1955).
SCHÜMMELFEDER, N.: Probleme der Fermentcytochemie. Folia haemat. (Frankfurt) **6,** 117 – 144 (1961).
SCHWEINITZ, H. A., BRAUNS, M. T.: Cytochemische Untersuchungen über den Bestand hydrolysierender Fermente in menschlichen Knochenmarkszellen. Proc. 8th Congr. Europ. Soc. Haemat., Part I/44, Vienna 1961.
SELYE, H.: see page 26.
SPICER, S. S., MEYER, D. B.: see page 67.
SZÉCSI, St.: Experimentelle Studien über Serosa-Exsudatzellen. Folia haemat. (Berlin) **13,** 1 – 23 (1912).
THIEDE, A., SONNTAG, A.-G., LEDER, L.-D., MÜLLER-HERMELINK, H. K., MÜLLER-RUCHHOLTZ, W.: Lymphknotenveränderungen nach lokaler Injektion heterologer Antithymocyten- und Antimakrophagenseren. Verh. dtsch. Ges. Path. **54,** 218 – 221 (1970).
TOKUÉ, K.: see page 27.
TÜRK, W.: Vorlesungen über klinische Haematologie. Pt. I, Wien (1904), Braunmüller.
UNDRITZ, E.: Atlas of Haematology, p. 49. Basel: Sandoz 1952.
WEIDENREICH, F.: Über Bau und Verhornung der menschlichen Oberhaut. Arch. mikr. Anat. **56,** (1900).
WEIDENREICH, F.: Beiträge zur Kenntnis der granulierten Leukocyten. V. Fortsetzung der Studien über das Blut und die blutbildenden und -zerstörenden Organe. Arch. mikr. Anat. **72,** 209 (1908 a).
WEIDENREICH, F.: see page 75.
WULFF, H. R.: Histochemical studies of leukocytes from an inflammatory exsudate. Acta haemat. (Basel) **30,** 159 – 167 (1963).

C. Biochemistry and Function of Blood Basophils

I. Heparin in Blood Basophils

1. Evidence of Heparin in Basophil Granules

Two methodological procedures in particular have been used for the identification of substances occurring in basophil granules. By far the largest group of workers used cytochemical methods (EHRLICH, 1879; PAPPENHEIM, 1906; HERWERDEN, 1919; STAEMMLER, 1921; MAXIMOW, 1927; NAGAYO, 1928; WERMEL and SASSUCHIN, 1928; WISLOCKI and DEMPSEY, 1946; ASTALDI *et al.*, 1953; SCHUBERT, 1955; 1958; LENNERT and SCHUBERT, 1959; 1960; LENNERT and PARWARESCH, 1968). Only a limited number of authors have applied direct analytical methods for the identification of the substances occurring in blood basophils.

The numerous cytochemical works on the metachromatic granules of the tissue mast cells and blood basophils have revealed the acid glycosaminoglycan nature of these structures. Further papers supplied evidence that substances in these granules are more or less identical with the anticoagulant substance described by MCLEAN (1916) and HOWELL and HOLT (1918) as heparin (JORPES *et al.*, 1937; JORPES *et al.*, 1948; JORPES and GARDELL, 1948; BEHRENS and TAUBERT, 1952; JORPES *et al.*, 1953; ASBOEHANSEN, 1953; MARTIN and ROKA, 1953; AMANN and MARTIN, 1961). Evidence of the high degree of sulfation of these substances in blood basophils was put forward by THOMA and WIERCINSKI (1950). These authors were able to induce blood and bone marrow basophilia in guinea pigs by repeated intraperitoneal application of bovine serum. Extract obtained from basophil suspensions resembled heparin in its ability to inhibit blood coagulation. Prothrombin time was further found to be prolonged with increasing basophil count. With a basophil count of 0 to 5 cells per view field, the prothrombin time was 14 to 23 sec; with a cell count of 6 to 12 cells per field, this time was extended to 24 to 28 sec.

As early as 1948, LAVES thought it probable that some highly esterified polysaccharidic acids of the type of mucoitin sulphuric acid were present in basophil granules. ROKA and MARTIN (1950) succeeded in obtaining from the osmotically cytolyzed leukocytes a lyophylizate that induced a marked prolongation of the recalcification and prothrombin time of normal plasma. They also found that this substance either occurs in very limited quantities or is completely absent in immature cases of myeloid leukemias. In contrast, the leukocytes in cases of well-differentiated myeloid leukemia have a higher content of the substance. Similar extracts from erythrocytes and lymphocytes did not show this property.

In 1952 BEHRENS and TAUBERT reported a new method of separating basophils from other leukocytes. This made blood basophils accessible to direct biochemical analysis for the first time. They tested the effect of extracts from basophil concentrates on blood coagulation. The extraction was processed in a 0.5% sodium bicarbonate solution in a boiling water bath to inactivate the heat-sensitive substances with thrombokinase-like activities. Heparin is not significantly influenced by temperatures of this level. The addition of 50 μl of the extract prolonged coagulation time from 4 to 26 min. A simultaneously conducted control test of a similarly obtained extract of neutrophil, erythrocyte and lymphocyte concentrates proved ineffective.

The results hitherto available provide a rough physicochemical and biological characterization of the anticoagulant: a heat-stable, polysulfuric acid ester, reacting metachromatically to toluidine blue and having an effect similar to antithrombin. The coagulation-inhibiting factor from basophil extracts could be hydrolyzed with hyaluronidase from *Clostridium Welchii*. These characteristics are to a very large extent in accord with those of heparin, as obtained by analytical methods (ROKA and MARTIN, 1950; LAVES and THOMA, 1950). The view that heparin occurred in basophil granules was by no means universally accepted (KOLLERS, 1947; HEILMEYER, 1951). Definite evidence of its occurence was presented by MARTIN and ROKA (1953) in a case of basophil leukemia. Acetone-dried leukocyte fractions suspended in plasma yielded the same anticoagulatory activity as heparin. This factor proved to be heat- and acid-resistant. It lost its antithrombin and antithrombokinase effect upon neutralization with clupein methyl ester chlorohydrate. The presence of heparin sulfate in human blood basophils has since been repeatedly demonstrated by other workers using mainly cytochemical methods (NINNI and BELLONI, 1953). ASTALDI *et al.* (1953), using similar cytochemical methods, maintained that the mucopolysaccharides of leukemic basophil granules are hyaluronic acid and not heparin.

The question of the heparin content of blood basophils was taken up again in 1961 by AMANN and MARTIN. Using the technique of WESTPHAL *et al.* (1952), they transferred the acidic mucopolysaccharide fraction of an extract of lyophylized leukocyte concentrates into the aqueous phase of an aqueous phenol mixture. After several days of dialysis and vaporizing, the sample was concentrated, lyophylized again, and subjected to 14 days of trypsin digestion. The extract obtained was then tested for its anticoagulatory effect. The recalcification time and the thrombin clotting time were found to be much prolonged.However, the thromboplastin time remained almost unchanged. The anticoagulation factor proved to be heat-stable and could be inhibited with protamine sulfate. Chromatographic analyses in a mixture of N-butanol, N-propanol, glacial acetic acid, and water (15 : 25 : 2 : 58) for 18 h established that the basophil extracts were identical with heparin (AMANN, 1957). In view of these considerations, toluidine blue or a 0.2% methylene green and 0.1% azocarmine B in 6% acetic acid in methanol, as given by GIBLAN and BAROLLIER (1956), were applied for the visualization of the migrating acid glycosaminoglycan fractions. It has been shown that blood basophils are very like tissue mast cells with respect to their histamine and heparin content (JORPES *et al.,* 1937; SCHÜRER, 1946; JÜRGENS and STUDER, 1948; JULÉN *et al.,* 1950; ZOLLINGER 1950). Although there is little doubt about the heparin content of basophil granules, the possibility that glycosaminoglycans other than heparin may also occur in these granules has not been completely eliminated.

Even heparin itself cannot be regarded as an homogeneous compound. Differences in molecular weight, in degree of polymerization, and in sulfate content may give rise to chromatographic and electrophoretic heterogeneity. Differences in its anticoagulatory and lipolytic properties have also repeatedly been reported.

2. Biochemical-Functional Significance of Heparin

Heparin represents a sulfated glycosaminoglycan (acid mucopolysaccharide) from an equimolar amount of glucosamine (2-amino-2-desoxy-D-glucose) and glucuronic acid (BRIMACOMBE and WEBBER, 1964). An alpha-1,4-glycosidic bond exists between the glucosamine and the glucuronic acid. WALTON *et al.* (1966) believe heparin to have a nonbranching 1,4-glycosidic chain. The C-6 hydroxy group of glucosamine and C-2 of glucuronic acid are esterified with sulfo groups. However, sulfate groups can also be bonded with other C atoms. The hexosamine groups can appear in either a sulfated or acetylated form (JAQUES *et al.,* 1968; CIFONELLI, 1968). Similarly, different degrees of sulfation per unit of disaccharide are found according to the technique used and the tissue at hand (WALTON, 1955; CIFONELLI and DORFMAN, 1962; LINKER and HOVINGH, 1965; WALTON *et al.,* 1966; KORN, 1967; YOSHIZAWA, 1969; MEYER, 1969; MUIR, 1969).

The molecular weight of heparin and consequently the chain length also appear to vary with the number of sulfate groups present. The molecular weight is reported to range between 10,000 and 20,000. A direct, physical determination is somewhat difficult due to its strongly polyanionic character. Results vary according to the ionic strength of the samples used. By the light dispersion method in a 0.05 to 1.0 M sodium chloride solution, BARLOW *et al.* (1961) obtained values around 16,000. With the sedimentation-diffusion method (1 M NaCl) deviations of $\pm 15\%$ from the light dispersion method were found (JENSEN *et al.,* 1948; PATAT and ELIAS, 1959; LAURENT, 1961). According to BRASWELL (1963) values obtained with the sedimentation method are 30% lower than the actual values. For commercial heparin, he reported values ranging from 20,000 to 28,000. No definite agreement has been obtained concerning number of recurring monomer units. According to WALTON (1955), the heparin chain is composed of about 52 monomer units.

The number of sulfate groups is of decisive importance for some of the biological effects of heparin. In earlier investigations, 2.5 to 3 sulfate groups per disaccharide unit were found. Later investigations showed that the number of sulphate groups was not constant. Generally, averages of 5.2, 5.5, and 6.5 sulfate groups per tetrasaccharide unit were calculated (JORPES, 1935; JAQUES *et al.*, 1942; WOLFROM *et al.*, 1943; JORPES and GARDELL, 1948; DURNAT *et al.*, 1962; WOLFROM *et al.*, 1962; 1963; 1964).

The localization of individual sulfate groups is a special problem in the chemistry of heparin. With periodate oxidation and partial desulfation, certain clues were found that suggested that the free hydroxyl groups of C 6 of glucosamine and C 2 of glucuronic acid are esterified with sulfo groups. The discrepancy between the various heparin preparations is said to be mainly due to the different degree of sulfation of glucuronic acid at C 2 and of hexosamine at C 3. The amino groups can also appear as sulfate or acetylate. It is not clear whether these divergent findings are due to a genuine structural difference or to artefacts resulting from the analysis. In any case, under the conditions of acid hydrolysis the N-sulfate bonds are very labile (WALTON, *et al.*, 1966).

Heparin, with the properties listed, is a most unusual biologic compound and the strongest acid that occurs in the animal organism. In blood, heparin appears only in basophil granulocytes and by means of cytochemical methods is detected in the specific granules of basophils. The question as to how the strongly water-soluble heparin is bound to the granules has long remained unanswered because of due to the difficulties of handling blood basophils. Ultrastructurally, basophil granules behave like those of tissue mast cells, so that in studies of these relationships tissue mast cell granules were preferred as experimental models. Numerous findings have shown that the molecular linkage of acid glycosaminoglycans onto the cell structures proceeds through a similar, if not identical peptide chain. This is certainly true for chondroitin-4-sulfate, chondroitin-6-sulfate, keratan sulfate, and heparin. The amino acid serine occupies a key position, as was first recognized by MUIR (1958) and later confirmed by numerous other workers, in the attachment of glycosaminoglycans to the subcellular structures. SNELLMAN *et al.* (1951) used differential centrifugation to test the subcellular heparin fraction for protein content. They were able to isolate a rapidly moving, strongly water-soluble, floating fraction, which displayed a high antithrombin activity with some lipoprotein properties. Further investigations showed that the main constituent of this fraction is a polypeptide with a lipid portion. The lipid component is made up of lecithin, cholesterol, and neutral fats, apparently lacking a constant composition. The amount of lecithin in the fat fraction varied between 11 and 55%, with cholesterol contributing about 8%. The neutral fats averaged 37% of the total fat fraction. The protein component, to which the intragranular acid glycosaminoglycans appear to be attached, was identified as an oligopeptide with six amino acids (SNELLMAN *et al.*, 1951). In the electrophoretically obtained polypeptide fraction, cysteine, threonine, tyrosine, glycine, and leucine could be detected by chromatography. In addition, tryptophane was also found, the ratio of tyrosine to tryptophane being 5.5 : 1. Arginine was occasionally found in similarly obtained fractions. Later investigations supported these findings to varying extents (JACOBS and MUIR, 1963; BRIMACOMBE and WEBBER, 1964; MUIR, 1964; ASHWELL, 1964; FILTON JACKSON *et al.*, 1965; GOTTSCHALK,

1965; NEUFELD and GINSBURG, 1965; QUINTARELLI and SCOTT, 1966; SCHILLER, 1966; LINDAHL, 1969).

Large amounts of serine were found to be present in heparin preparations treated with papain. In gel filtrates serine comprised up to 20% of the total amino acid contents, thereby making up the largest portion. After graduated proteolysis with pronase, leucine amino peptidase, and carboxy peptidase, serine was the only identifiable amino acid left. Serine accounted for over 96% of the total amino acids (MUIR, 1958) in an isolated fraction obtained through high voltage electrophoresis. Studies on chondroitin-4-sulfate (RODÉN and ARMAND, 1966; RODÉN and SMITH, 1966; KLEINE and HILZ, 1968; KLEINE *et al.,* 1968) led to the assumption of a galactose-xylose-serine bonding between heparin and the structure proteins. By the method of enzymatic detection of xylose with D-xylose-isomerase and of galactose with D-galactose dehydrogenase obtained from *pseudomonas saccharophila* (DONDOROFF, 1962; SLEIN, 1962), followed by paper chromatographic analysis of heparin hydrolysates (several hours in 1 M HCl), LINDAHL and RODÉN (1965) found up to 86 μM of galactose per gram of heparin (corresponding to 5.3 M/100 M glucosamine). In all investigations, the amount of galactose found was equivalent to, or exceeded the amount of serine present. In the different heparin samples examined, 1 mole of serine was found for every 26, 31, or 53 monomer units, respectively. The serine content was approximately 1 mole per mole of heparin. The compound xylosylserine was also clearly detected in the corresponding hydrolysates by LINDBERG and SILVANDER (1965).

TOMINAGA *et al.* (1965) isolated from normal urine xylosylserine, which represents the end-product of acid glycosaminoglycan catabolism. Serine-xylose and galactose could also be detected chromatographically. The different values obtained for galactose and serine can to some extent be attributed to methodological difficulties. The fact that compounds such as xylosyl-serine and galactosyl-xylosyl-serine could be detected separately, and that at the same time free oxidizable groups were detected, was the reason for assuming a glycosidic linkage. The sequence was given as Glc US-Gal-Gal-Xyl-Ser (GREGORY *et al.,* 1964; LINDAHL *et al.,* 1965). This compound displayed a cationic migration in a pyridine acetic acid buffer solution at pH 2, but not at pH 6. For this reason the conclusion was drawn that the amino groups and the carboxyl groups of serine are free, and that hydroxyl group bonding takes place. This finding agrees well with those of ANDERSON *et al.* (1965), who found that in the alkali degradation of acid glycosaminoglycan-peptide chains, only the serine hydroxyl group participates in the xylosyl-serine bonding. The hydrolytic splitting of galactose, which takes place in a biphase process, so indicating the presence of two galactose molecules, provides further confirmation of the mentioned concept of the molecular arrangement of polysaccharide-protein samples. RODÉN and ARMAND (1966) provided reliable evidence of the participation of glucuronosyl-D-galactose. They were able to isolate from chondroitin-4-sulfate extract, after 4 h of hydrochloric acid hydrolysis, adsorption of the remaining cations to Dowex 50, and final fractionation by gel filtration over Sephadex G-25, highly purified glucuronosyl-galactose. Chemically pure glucuronosyl-D-galactose samples were used as a control.

On the basis of the results achieved by LINDAHL and RODÉN (1965), LINDAHL (1966 a, b, c) and HORWITZ and DORFMAN (1968) the following molecular arrangement for heparin is widely accepted:

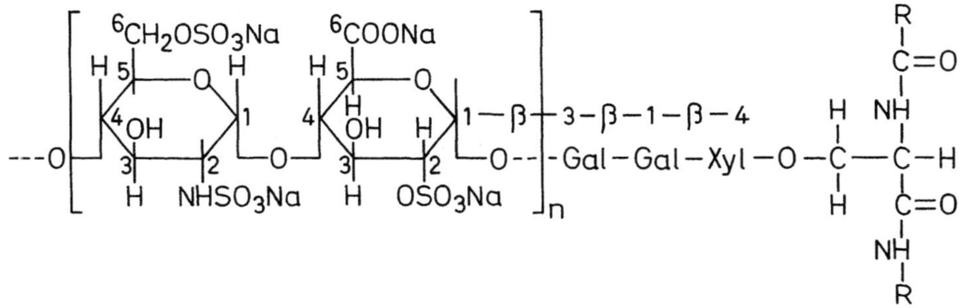

Similar groups have also been established for the other glycosaminoglycans (LINDAHL and RODÉN, 1965; FRANSSON 1967, 1968 a, b; FRANSSON and RODÉN, 1967).

Although the chemical composition of the bonding between heparin and the structure proteins like Gal-Gal-Xyl-Ser is now widely accepted (HELTING, 1971), there is still no unambiguous concept of the nature of the serine-bound peptide chain. The original findings of SNELLMAN *et al.* (1951) had to be modified on the basis of later results concerning the amino acid sequence of the connecting peptide fragment. SNELLMAN *et al.* (1951) believed there to be covalent bonding between glycosaminoglycans and certain peptide chains. SERAFINI-FRACASSINI *et al.* (1967; 1968) claimed that the protein component of heparin accounted for 13.21% and that of chondroitin-4-sulfate for 14.2% of the total dry weight. The authors were able to detect 22 different amino acids in the protein component.

Electron-optically, periodic structures about 30 Å in diameter were observed in the granules of tissue mast cells and blood basophils. These granules also contain areas of varying optical density. SERAFINI-FRACASSINI *et al.* (1969) attempted to compare the electron-optical findings on tissue mast cell granules with those on isolated heparin-protein preparations. In both experimental models, they found well-ordered fibrils 1200 Å in length with 20 to 25 coarse-grained areas 30 Å in diameter. These findings were in agreement with the model proposed by MATHEWS and LOZAITYTE (1958) of a central protein axis with lateral deposits of acid glycosaminogylcan chains, in so far that the observed rhythm was due to the absence of bismuth deposits. In this technique the heparin molecules appear somewhat larger than the corresponding chondroitin-4-sulfate chains. These authors think this can be explained by the fact that the high degree of sulfation of heparin causes a stronger accumulation of bismuth. Corresponding heparin-protein models in solution yield a somewhat larger particle diameter of

34.5 Å (STIVALA *et al.*, 1968). The lower values obtained with the electron microscope are thought to be caused by shrinkage due to dehydration.

The results of biochemical investigations on the molecular configuration of acid glycosaminoglycans in metachromatic granules are in broad agreement with the electron-microscopic findings. There is also close agreement between the light-microscopic cytochemical findings and the results of direct analysis. However, most of these investigations have been carried out on either tissue mast cell granules or model substrates. While it is probable that the structural arrangement of these substances in basophil granules presents a similar, if not identical, pattern at molecular level, we are not entitled to assume that the analogy is complete. Our conception of the substructural organization of the intragranular acid glycosaminoglycans in blood basophils is founded upon indirect evidence. Blood basophil and tissue mast cell granules are electron-microscopically similar. This similarity can be traced almost up to the molecular level of the resolution. We know that the tissue mast cells contain the same glycosaminoglycan-protein groups as other tissues. This finding has been verified by electron microscope studies, chemical analyses, and combined procedures. However, no direct chemical analyses of blood basophil granules have yet been carried out.

a) Biological Properties of Heparin and its Structure-Action Relationships

The best-known biological property of heparin is its anticoagulant activity. Heparin also exerts a clearing effect upon the 'exogenous lipoproteins' in serum and is said to possess a limited cytostatic or antimitotic effect. Being a strong polyanion, heparin has a marked affinity for basic organic substances such as proteins and biogenic amines. The strongly acid character of heparin appears to be responsible for the majority of its biological properties.

The anticoagulant effect of heparin can be completely inhibited by the addition of an organic base, such as protamine. Organic bases like albumin, protamine, lysozyme, and other basic proteins yield both *in vivo* and *in vitro* mostly insoluble salt complexes with heparin. In blood, heparin is transported as a protein complex also with a salt-type bonding. The polyanionic nature of heparin determines the substructural bonding and stabilization of histamine in mast cell and basophil granules (AMANN and WERLE, 1956; WERLE and AMANN, 1956; HAGEN, 1961; KOBAYASHI, 1962). We will discuss in more detail the significance of heparin for the local concentration of amines in metachromatic granules.

We do not yet have a clear idea about the structure-action relationships of heparin relative to its numerous biological properties. The degree of sulfation and the shape of the macromolecule, as well as the chain length are believed to be important. WOLFROM *et al.* (1953) maintained that the degree of sulfation of heparin has no bearing upon its anticoagulant activity. Acid glycosaminoglycans with a larger number of sulfate groups than normal heparin prove to be less effective than heparin. The chemical addition of sulfate groups to a highly active sodium heparinate up to an end sulphur content of 14.4% produced a 50% decrease in anticoagulant activity. This would seem to indicate that the anticoagulant activity of heparin is not substantially dependent upon the number of ester sulfate groups (WOLFROM and McNEELY, 1945). On the other hand, there is a direct relationship between the number of sulfate groups and the lipolytic activity of heparin, and various differently sulfated dextran samples display increasing lipolytic activity, depending upon the number of their sulfate groups (ROBINSON *et al.*, 1959).

The anticoagulant effect of heparin may be at least partially related to the N-sulfate groups. For example, chistosan sulfate, with its N-sulfate groups, displays a marked anticoagulant activity, whereas modified chistosan sulfate, which possesses only N-sulfate groups, exerts no anticoagulant effect. Acid hydrolysis of the amino groups of heparin leads to a loss of anticoagulant effect. After 48 h of acid hydrolysis of a 2% barium-heparin solution in 11% acetic acid at 68±2° C, WOLFROM and McNEELY (1945) found an almost complete loss of anti-coagulant properties. This loss was observed in the heparin samples after the hydrolysis of half of the amino groups. Although these results are not in any way generally recognized, the anticoagulant property of heparin is at least to some extent related to the presence of N-sulfate groups. However, there appears to exist a critical optimum for the number of sulfate groups. Any large deviations from this number induce a considerable decrease in anticoagulant activity. According to the investigations of LAURENT (1961), the biological properties of heparin are influenced by its chain length and therefore also by its molecular weight. PATAT and ELIAS (1959) reported an increase in activity with a lengthening of the chain. In later studies, BARLOW *et al.* (1961) were not able to find such a connection between molecular weight and the anticoagulant activity of heparin.

By appropriate manipulations of the heparin molecule, it is possible to produce compounds in which only one of the properties of heparin is markedly present. NOMINE *et al.* (1961) and FOSTER *et al.* (1961; 1963) were able, through methanolysis and acid hydrolysis, to arrest the antilipemic activity of heparin. Similar effects have also been achieved by gamma-irradiation of heparin (ADAMS *et al.*, 1961; FOSTER *et al.*, 1961; 1963). Some heparin compounds, such as derivatives of N-(3,5-dinitro-benzoyl) and N-(3,5-dimethylbenzoyl), possess, along with a full-blown antilipemic property only a very weak anticoagulant effect. Heparin preparations which possess 30% succinyl-substituted N-sulfate groups also show normal lipolytic activity but only a minimal anticoagulant effect (BROWN *et al.*, 1962). FOSTER *et al.* (1963) were successful in producing selective inhibition of the anticoagulant properties of heparin through periodate oxidation. Alkali hydrolysis and subsequent oxidation by hydrogen peroxide also lead to inhibition of the anticoagulant effect. Since most of these treatments are accompanied by an alteration of the heparin molecule, numerous authors have expressed the opinion that it is the macromolecular structure of heparin that is responsible for its anticoagulant effect. There are some findings suggesting that the heparin chain is helical. This hypothesis is supported by the fact that the alpha-D-(1,4) configuration, in contrast to the beta-glycosidic linkages, is helical. A certain stabilization may be achieved through intramolecular $NH\text{-}SO_2\text{-}O$ bonds. Such an explanation would also fit in well with the observation that the anticoagulant activity dependens upon a critical number of N-sulfate groups.

b) Anticoagulant Activity of Heparin

The anticoagulant property of heparin was reported in the earliest works on this substance (McLean, 1916), yet the mechanism and the actual sites of reaction are still not fully understood. Some antithrombin activity has been detected, but it only reaches its full capabilities in association with a coinhibitor protein. The compound thus formed by heparin and thrombin has a much more limited ability to stimulate coagulation than pure thrombin preparations (Marquard and Walzman, 1959). Jaques and Beel (1959) believe the importance of the activity of heparin lies in its ability to suppress thromboplastin. These authors were able to eliminate the anticoagulant activity of heparin by adding thromboplastin. Similar notions concerning the mode of action of heparin have been held by Biggs *et al.* (1953) and Douglas (1956). Further evidence that the anticoagulant activity of heparin is at least partially due to thromboplastin suppression was obtained from *in-vitro* experiments by Douglas (1956). He ascertained that the normal consumption of coagulation factors V and VIII halts upon the addition of heparin. According to the results of O'Brien (1960) heparin should also bind with the Christmas factor (factor IX), neutralizing it to ineffectiveness. Biggs and MacFarlane (1962), however, were not able to support these findings. The question of the sites of heparin action in the coagulation system appears to be very complex. However, it seems to be unanimously accepted that heparin participates in the prothombin-thrombin system and in the production of the prothrombin transformation factor ('thrombokinase').

A closer examination of the relationship between heparin and blood coagulation does not fall within the scope of this monograph. We have presented these data on the anticoagulant action of heparin only for the purpose of demonstrating the nature of its principal mode of action and in order to compare this with other effects of heparin, for example, that of serum lipolysis. Numerous findings show that both the anticoagulant activity of heparin and its lipolytic action can be attributed to its high affinity for basic proteins.

c) Blood Basophils and Heparin-Induced Serum Lipolysis

The investigations of Hahn (1943) and Korn (1958) have shown that the initial step of lipid assimilation is triggered by heparin. Evidence of the presence of heparin in tissue mast cells (Jorpes, 1946) and in blood basophils (Laves and Thoma, 1950; Behrens and Taubert, 1952; Martin and Roka, 1953) raised the question of the part these cells play in intravascular fat processing.

In this section, we discuss first the significance of endogenous heparin in serum lipolysis, then the role of basophil granulocytes in the lipolytic serum system.

Under normal conditions of nutrition 1 to 2 g of fat per kg of body weight is taken in daily in the form of triglycerides (FREDRICKSON *et al.,* 1958; 1967); after intestinal emulsification and partial hydrolysis, these fats are taken up by the intestinal mucosal epithelium as follows: 50% as free fatty acids and glycerol, 40% as monoglycerides, and 10% as di- and triglycerides. These last are probably taken up through a pinocytotic activity of the intestinal mucosal epithelium. The resorbed fat is stabilized for transport in an aqueous (plasma) medium through a process of re-esterification and the attachment of certain polypeptides (apoproteins) to the large lipid aggregates (FREDRICKSON *et al.,* 1967). The fats pass into the lymphatic vessels as so-called 'exogenous particles' or chylomicrons (GAGE and FISH, 1924), reaching the blood via the thoracic duct. If the triglyceride concentration exceeds 20 meq per liter of serum (590 mg/100 ml), the opalescence and light-dispersal properties of the chylomicrons induce a milky cloudiness in the plasma (ALBRINK *et al.,* 1955; KRAUP, 1963). Most of the triglycerides are transported in the chylomicrons and very-low-density lipoprotein (VLDL).

Under physiological conditions, postprandial hyperlipidemia normalizes within about 5 h. HAHN (1943) showed that an intravenous heparin injection will clear alimentary hyperlipemia within a few minutes. Numerous other authors supported his findings with investigations on humans and animals (GOFMAN *et al.,* 1954; SPITZER *et al.,* 1956; NAVEL, 1957). The fact that heparin *in vitro* develops no clearing properties, together with the finding that, in contrast, plasma from an animal treated with heparin can cause rapid clearing of a turbid hyperlipemic serum sample *in vitro* (ANDERSON *et al.,* 1950) shows that the clearing effect of heparin must be associated with some other lipolytic factors. Later investigations showed that exogenous heparin activates a further clearing system, leading to hydrolysis of the chylomicron triglycerides (BROWN *et al.,* 1953; KORN and QUIGLEY, 1955; 1957) and rapid clearing of the lipemic serum accompanied by a rise in glycerol and unesterified fatty acids (ROBINSON and FRENCH, 1957).

The lypolytic activity of serum after an injection of heparin was attributed to an enzyme system, called by KORN and QUIGLEY (1955; 1957) the post-heparin clearing factor, or lipoprotein lipase. The ester bondings of the triglyceride present in VLDL and chylomicrons appear to be the specific substrate of lipoprotein lipase. Ester-cholesterol is not affected. Lipoprotein lipase has not yet been isolated. It is probable that the heparin-induced (post-heparin) lipolytic activity of serum is triggered by several synergetic enzymes (GRETEN *et al.,* 1968). Lipoprotein lipase is heat-labile and migrates electrophoretically with alpha-globulin. In the fractionation after KOHN, the activity is bound with fractions III/1-3. The highest lipolytic activity is determined at 37° C with pH of 7.2 to 7.6, although KRAUP (1963) determined this optimum to be at 40° C with pH between 8.5 and 9.0.

The relationship between heparin and lipoprotein lipase is also not completely clear. There is some evidence that heparin constitutes the prosthetic group of the enzyme. Very small amounts of heparin lead to a clearing of hyperlipemic serum. As little as 0.1 μg heparin per ml plasma triggers serum lipolysis (ZÖLLNER, 1963). Within certain limits, the more heparin is present, the greater the lipolytic activity (ROBINSON and FRENCH, 1957). A fall in activity is caused by the inactivation of heparin in the liver (SPITZER and SPITZER, 1956). According to ZÖLLNER (1963), the breakdown or elimination rate of the clearing factor, expressed in terms of heparin concentration, is about 0.2 μg/ml/h. The activity of the clearing factor is inhibited by a surplus of heparin or by the addition of protamine. The origin of the clearing factor itself is not known. It is a complex system, which only attains full activity through the combined action of several separate factors (possibly several enzymes). It must be assumed that at least one component originates in the immediate vicinity of the blood vessels (capillary endothelium, fat cells). Two facts support this view: (a) exogenous heparin has no effect under *in vitro* conditions, and (b) the activity of the clearing factor rapidly appears *in vivo*.

The possibility that endogenous heparin plays a part in the lipolytic process has often been discussed, but it has not yet been unanimously accepted. The activity of lipoprotein lipase is weak and there are considerable technical difficulties in its assessment; moreover, the concentration of heparin in serum is extremely low. The known methods of measuring lipoprotein lipase activity are prone to considerable errors. If the optical density is taken as a criterion for serum lipolysis, there is every likelihood that minor lipolytic reactions, which are not necessarily accompanied by a marked clearing effect, will be overlooked (WILLS, 1965). Also, the large fluctations in the individual optical density of various sera present a parameter which is very difficult to standardize, and which can lead to large errors (SCHÖLL, 1963). The regular control of the level of glycerin in the incubation medium during the lipolysis is also subject to large errors. The increase in glycerin concentration, especially in the earlier phase of the lypolytic reaction, does not run parallel to serum lipolysis. In this technique, glycerin is determined as trivalent alcohol. The mono- or diester intermediate products of a partial hydrolysis of triglycerides cannot be determined in this way. Far better results are achieved by measuring the fatty acid level. In this way, the lipoprotein lipase activity is determined by assessing the increase in fatty acid concentration in the incubation medium. Titrimetric methods (DOLE, 1963; GORDON and CHERKES, 1956; GORDON, 1957; SHAFRIR, 1958; TROUT *et al.*, 1960, CORVILAIN *et al.* 1961; HARTMANN, 1963) or manometric methods (SAILER *et al.*, 1961; KRAUP, 1963; SAILER and SANDHOFER, 1963) are appropriate.

The determination of the heparin level in serum is no more reliable. ZÖLLNER (1963), using a relatively sensitive method, was not able to detect any endogenous heparin in plasma. Since, with this method, it is possible to determine heparin concentrations down to about 0.15 μg/ml, he held the significance of endogenous heparin for the physiological serum lipolysis to be very questionable. In view of the fact that an injection of as little as 0.1 μg/ml heparin leads to a detectable clearing, this objection can be rejected. In the meantime, it has become possible through isotope dilution experiments, to determine normal heparin concentrations down to 0.06 μg/ml.

Having reviewed the methodical difficulties, we will now discuss the findings which indicate the role of endogenous heparin in the clearing process. The rapid elimination of large chylomicrons (Sf> 400) and of pre-beta-lipoproteins (Sf 10 – 400 and d < 1.063) with a biological half-life of only a few minutes indicates the existence of an efficient, intravasal lipolytic system (LALLA and GOFMAN, 1954; NESTEL, 1964; FREDRICKSON *et al.,* 1967). Our present knowledge of the submicroscopic composition of the capillary walls hardly permits the concept of their massive permeation by large particles of the dimensions given for exogenous fatty aggregates, i.e. 0.1 to 3 μm (BENNET *et al.,* 1959). WASSERMANN (1963) attempted, during activated serum lipolysis, to study the permeation of chylomicrons electron-microscopically. He was able to demonstrate the chylomicrons adhering to the inner surface of the capillary endothelia, but he did not succeed in detecting them in the perivascular space. He concluded from this that the chylomicrons were not able to leave the intravasal space without some alteration in their structure. An exception to this appears to occur in the liver (FELTS, 1962). FAWCETT (1955) found in the sinusoidal endothelia pores up to 1 μm in diameter, which may be involved in the transmission of chylomicrons.

The problem was to demonstrate that physiological clearing is also initiated by a heparin-induced lipolysis. Conclusive evidence was presented by the works of ENGELBERG (1956), ROBINSON and FRENCH (1957), FREDRICKSON *et al.* (1958) and WILLS (1965), who were able to demonstrate that some clearing activity occurred, even without the addition of exogenous heparin. This finding has sometimes been put forward as evidence against the participation of endogenous heparin. The ability to extract lipoprotein lipase without the addition of heparin does not exclude the presence of a small amount of endogenous heparin that is still sufficient for lipolysis. As KORN (1958) demonstrated, the clearing factor activity can be suppressed immediately by bacterial heparinase. The fact that the protamine effect is similar to that of Tween 80 and Triton A 20 may also be viewed as further evidence of the participation of endogenous heparin. A significant delay in lipemic clearing can be achieved by intravenous injection of protamine (BROWN, 1952; SPITZER, 1953; BRAGDON and HEVEL, 1954), or Tween 80, Triton A 20, or other surfactants known to suppress lipolysis (KELLNER *et al.,* 1951). The reactions that result in postprandial lipolysis resemble those of heparin-activated lipolysis *in vitro.* The essential difference is simply that under *in-vivo* conditions heparin is continually being inactivated in the liver and must be replaced from appropriate sources. In addition, the rapid elimination of free fatty acids from the serum favors the reaction. Serum albumin plays an important role in this context.

HAVEL and GORDON (1960) found a significant fall in clearing factor activity in a group of patients with endogenous hypertriglyceridemia. FELTS (1962) determined a linear relationship between the activity of lipoprotein lipase and the amount of labeled triglycerides (palmitate-1-^{14}C) assimilated.

After an injection of doubly labeled lipoproteins (^{3}H-glycerin and ^{14}C-palmitate) with an initial ratio ^{14}C : ^{3}H of 1 : 1, the ratio was found to be 1 in the liver, 11 in the heart muscle, and 16 in the fat tissue (FELTS, 1962). These findings were substantially confirmed by other authors (BORGSTRÖM and JORDAN, 1959; HAVEL and GOLDFIEN, 1961). They provide reliable evidence that glycerol and free fatty acids separately pass through the capillary walls, at least in heart muscle and fat tissue. The passage of intact lipoprotein-triglycerides through the sinusoidal endothelia of the liver appears to be possible and may represent an exception due to the special anatomical structure of this organ (LAURELL, 1950; ROUILLER, 1956; HAMPTON, 1958; STEIN and SHAPIRO, 1960; HAVEL *et al.,* 1962).

The above-mentioned results, as well as numerous other investigations carried out with labeled lipids and chylomicrons, present evidence that the peripheral fatty tissue can directly assimilate the triglycerides of chylomicrons after previous hydrolytic splitting. The high speed of assimilation of the chylomicrons depends upon the activity of an efficient lipolytic system in which endogenous heparin plays an important role. Heparin increases the clearing factor activity. It is further involved in the liberation of lipoprotein lipase. It is also possible that the long-chained polyanion makes up a part of the lipolytic enzyme.

Heparin is present in both tissue mast cells and blood basophils. Therefore postprandial lipolysis must cause depletion of heparin in its physiologic reservoirs, the tissue mast cells and blood basophils. The tissue mast cells with 20 to 60 μg heparin per 10^6 cells are more practical for research purposes (BRAUNSTEINER and THUMB, 1963). Their count and granule content have been studied in humans relative to increasing age, degree of atherosclerosis, frequency of arterial thrombosis, and heart infarction. The tissue mast cell count was measured in the skin, heart muscle, and the various layers of the vascular wall. Similar studies were made on rats fed with cholesterol. After reviewing the contradictory results in the literature, we examined the tissue mast cell count in the myocardium, mesenterium, and lips of rats after a 13-week period of cholesterol feeding. The number of tissue mast cells was found to be depressed in most of the organs studied during chronic hyperlipidemia (PARWARESCH and PETERSEN, 1969). However, it is still not known how chronic hyperlipidemia influences the tissue mast cell count in different organs and to what extent. Furthermore, results obtained from rats cannot be applied without reservations to humans, as there are considerable differences between the two species in tissue mast cell count and fat metabolism. Tables 13 and 14 summarize the results that various authors have obtained from humans and rats. The results so far achieved show only that no definitive statement can be based upon these studies.

The results achieved by various authors working with blood basophils, have been largely in agreement. BRAUNSTEINER *et al.* (1965) detected an increase in the basophil count during hyperlipidemia. SHELLEY and JUHLIN (1961) described morphological changes in the blood basophil granule pattern after oral fat administration. These findings can be explained in the light of the heparin content of blood basophils and the findings of earlier

Table 13. Quantitative changes in human tissue mast cells (TMC) with respect to age and atherosclerosis

Author	TMC in cases of	tissues examined	change
Constantinides and Cairns (1954)	atherosclerosis	myocardium	decreased
	atherosclerosis	myocardium	decreased
Paterson and Mills (1958)	atherosclerosis + thrombosis, myocardial infarction	myocardium	decreased
Paterson and Mills (1958)	atherosclerosis without thrombosis or infarction	myocardium	none
Pomerance (1958)	atherosclerosis	coronaries adventitia	increased
Lempert *et al.* (1961)	atherosclerosis	myocardium	none
Fernex and Sternby (1964)	atherosclerosis	myocardium	decreased
Puchlev *et al.* (1966)	atherosclerosis	coronary and aortic intima	decreased
Puchlev *et al.* (1966)	atherosclerosis	coronary and aortic adventitia, aorta	increased
Hellström and Holmgren (1950)	old age	skin, myocardium	decreased
Cairns and Constantinides (1954)	old age	myocardium	decreased
Sundberg (1955)	old age	adventitia of large vessels, aortic	decreased
		adventitia	none
Pollak (1956)	old age	aortic intima	none
Pomerance (1958)	old age	adventitia of coronaries	none
Keller (1960)	old age	myocardium	decreased
Meyer (1961)	old age	coronaries	none

authors, who found that basophil leukocytosis accompanies metabolic disorders with secondary hyperlipidemia. Turin (1910) noted a marked increase in basophil count in cases of hypothyroidism with hyperlipidemia. His findings were later confirmed by numerous other authors (Inagaki, 1957; Braunsteiner *et al.*, 1959; Braunsteiner and Thumb, 1963; Grabener, 1967). Braunsteiner and Thumb (1958) detected basophil leukocytosis in diabetic hyperlipidemia as well. These findings gave rise to the hypothesis that there must be a connection between the serum triglyceride level and blood basophils. The results of Braunsteiner *et al.* (1965) indicating that the blood basophil count rises in postprandial hyperlipidemia were la-

Table 14. Quantitative changes in rat tissue mast cells (TMC) with respect to age and following dietary lipid administration

Author	TMC with respect to	Tissues Examined	Alterations
GRUNDBAUM *et al.* (1957)	dietary lipid and cholesterol administration	skin	none
FODOR *et al.* (1958, 1960)	dietary lipid and cholesterol administration	mesenterium	decreased
JENNINGS *et al.* (1960)	dietary lipid and cholesterol administration	mesenterium	none
WATSON (1961)	dietary lipid and cholesterol administration	myocardium	none
MARKEES and FERNEX (1963)	dietary lipid and cholesterol administration	mesenterium and myocardium	decreased
DOUGLAS *et al.* (1964)	dietary lipid and cholesterol administration	skin	decreased
PARWARESCH and PETERSEN (1969)	dietary lipid and cholesterol administration	skin and myocardium and mesenterium	decreased
BATES (1935)	increasing age	skin	decreased
WEBB (1936)	increasing age	skin	< 13th day increased > 13th day decreased
PADAWER and GORDON (1956)	increasing age	peritoneum	increased
CONSTANTINIDES and RUTHERDALE (1957)	increasing age	myocardium	decreased
KELLER (1960)	increasing age	skin	decreased
MARX *et al.* (1960)	increasing age	lung, kidney, thymus	increased

ter confirmed by KEHNSCHERPER and BLAU (1966) and LENNERT and PARWARESCH (1970).

The technical difficulties referred to in Section III make the reproduction of the results of SHELLEY and JUHLIN (1961) very problematical. More reliable, if more tedious, is the study of the shift in the basophil maxima reacting metachromatically on the toluidine-blue pH scale because of the emergence of basophils with a lower content of acidic glycosaminoglycans (LENNERT and SCHUBERT, 1960). PARWARESCH and LENNERT (1969), using this technique in a modified form gained some insight into the various functional and pathological changes that occur in blood basophils and tissue mast cells. The following experimental procedure was designed to detect cellular alterations in the blood basophils in the course of serum lipolysis.

Blood samples were taken from 10 young, helathy subjects of both sexes subsequent to a 12 h period of fasting. Hematologic controls and thorough lipid analyses were conducted to exclude abnormalities. Total lipid level was determined, without previous extraction, by means of the sulfo-phosphovanillin reaction according to ZÖLLNER and KIRSCH (1965). The same stock sera were subjected to discelectrophoresis in order to detect abnormalities in the lipoprotein pattern. Following an exhaustive extraction total lipids were measured as dry matter by the gravimetric technique of EGGE *et al.* (1970).

All determinations were repeated three times. Subjects who displayed abnormal lipid values were excluded. After the fasting values had been measured, each subject was given 2 g of butter per kg of body weight. In control experiments the same subjects were given, at different times, corresponding amounts of protein or carbohydrates. Since these substances do not induce changes in blood basophils (LENNERT and PARWARESCH, 1970), details will not be given. Nonalcoholic drinks were permitted during the course of the experiments. Blood was aspirated from the cubital vein at postprandial intervals of 1.5, 3, 4, 4.5, 5 and 5.5 h. In each case, 20 ml of venous blood was collected into a siliconized syringe. The syringe was then withdrawn while the needle was still in the cubital vein, and five blood smears were prepared. The blood samples were centrifuged (10 min at 200 g) and the serum was removed for lipid determination. The buffy coat was used for basophil-rich leukocyte concentrates for light-microscopic and electron-optical investigations (PARWARESCH, 1968). Blood smears from leukocyte concentrates were fixed (PARWARESCH and LENNERT, 1967) and stained in 0.1% aqueous toluidine blue solutions of increasing pH levels beginning with pH 2.8 (PARWARESCH and LENNERT, 1969). pH intervals of 0.2 were used throughout the staining procedure. In addition, the blood basophil count was determined directly according to COOPER and CRUICKSHANK (1966). The preparatory procedures used for the electron-optical investigations were those mentioned in Chapter A III. Assuming a normal distribution for the blood basophil counts and lipid values, the mean values were examined for significance by the t-test. To determine the staining maxima of the basophils on the toluidine-blue pH scale, the curve median ($\tilde{x}$) was calculated for each case, the average relationship and correlation with the corresponding regressions were calculated, and the respective correlation coefficients determined and tested for significance in their differences.

In one case, oral fat administration led after 3 h to a peak in the serum lipid curve; in 5 cases, the peak was reached 4 h postprandially, and in 6 cases after 4.5 h (Fig. 24). A comparison of postprandial with fasting values showed that the ascent of the lipids from the third postprandial hour on, became significant as compared to the initial values (tabular t-value of 2.821 at $p < 0.01$). The curve of basophil count showed an almost similar course (Fig. 24). The blood basophil count reached its maximum 4.5 h after fat intake, at which time it averaged 126.6 ± 31.46/μl. Here, too, the postprandial values were significantly higher than the initial values ($p < 0.01$).

The distance of each median determined for the toluidine-blue pH curves from the start line (pH 2.8) was employed as a quantitative measure for the shift to the right of the staining maxima of the basophils on the toluidine-blue pH scale (Fig. 24). The span *d* is limited by the position of pH 2.8

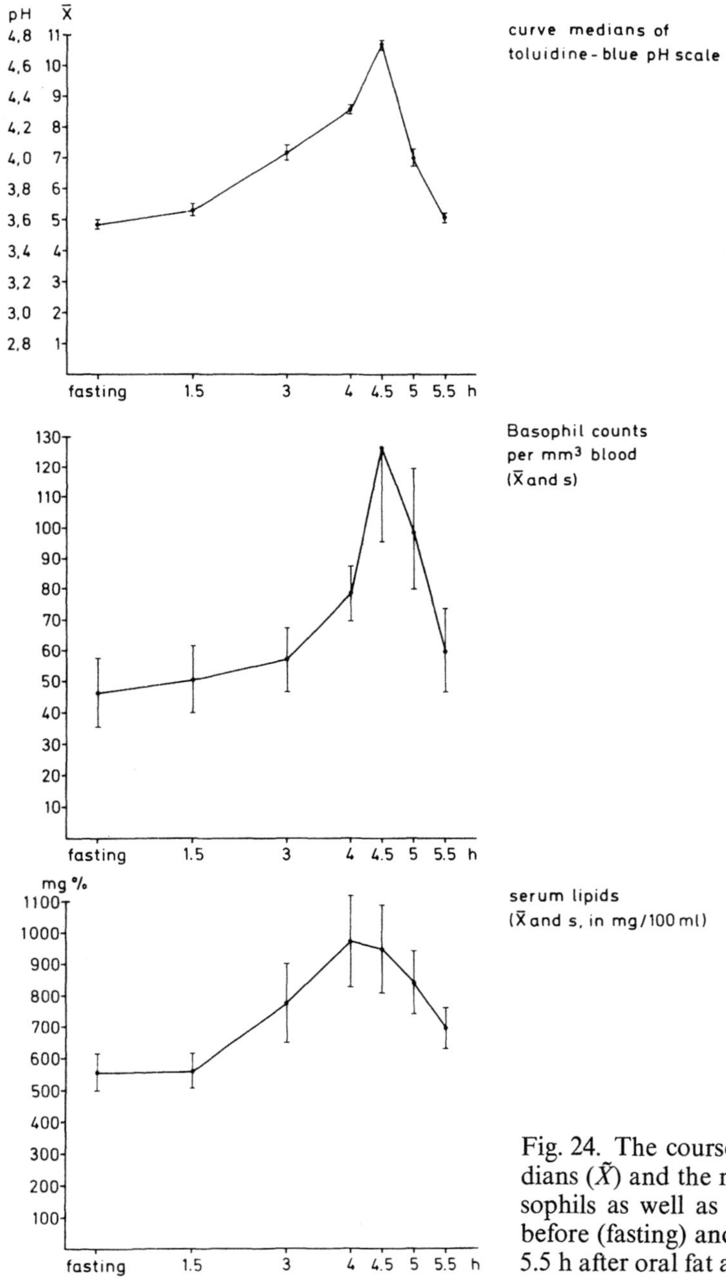

Fig. 24. The course of the curve medians ($\tilde{X}$) and the mean values of basophils as well as of the total lipids before (fasting) and 1.5, 3, 4.5, 5, and 5.5 h after oral fat administration

and the respective median value. Under identical experimental conditions, the values for *d* show a normal distribution. In our investigations, the values for *d* proved to be a reliable criterion, enabling us to draw conclusions concerning the histochemical properties of blood basophil granules. As compared to the initial values, the increase proved to be statistically highly significant (Fig. 24). We then attempted to express statistically the parallelity of the course of the increasing lipid values, the basophil count, and the extent of the shift of the staining maxima on the toluidine-blue pH scale expressed in terms of *d*-values. We therefore, compared the three parameters. After computing the regression grades and the correlation coefficients (r), we determined the extent of correlation between the sample values (Figs. 25 to 27).

There was a highly significant correlation between the values of the serum lipids and toluidine-blue pH median shifts (Fig. 25). A similar relationship was found between the lipid values and the basophil counts (Fig. 26). The significance boundary lay here, however, at $p < 0.05$. The correlation between the basophil curve and the toluidine-blue pH series curve (Fig. 27) was also highly significant. Fig. 28 illustrates schematically the correlative relationships between the parameters studied. Hyperlipidemia leads to an increase in basophil count, which is most probably the result of

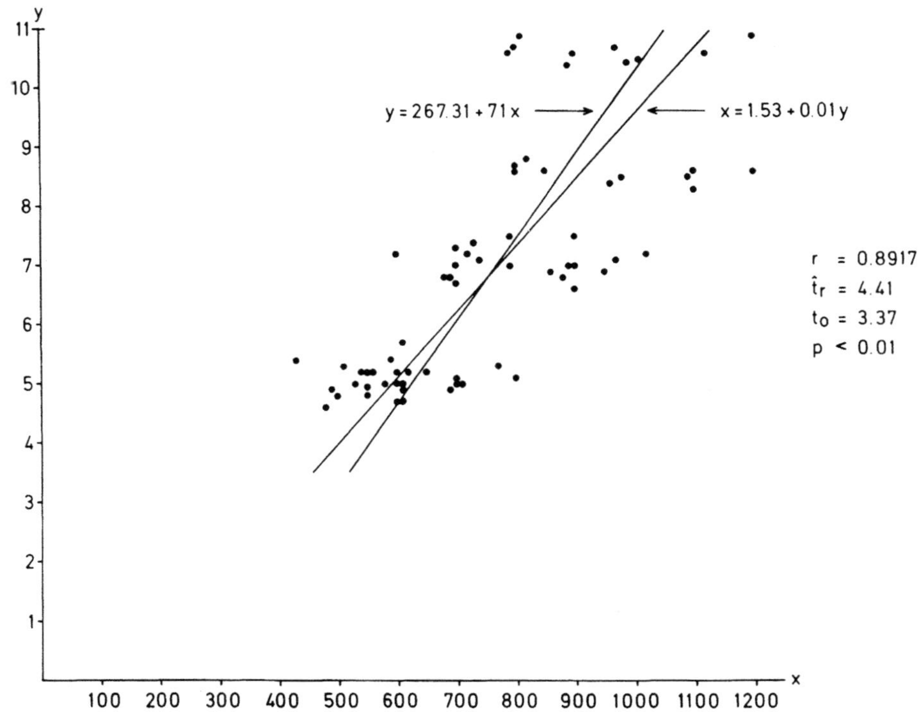

Fig. 25. Regression equation of the serum lipids (x axis) and the median values of the toluidine blue pH curves (y axis). Time-dependent course. *r*: estimated correlation coefficient, $\hat{t}$: tabular *t*-value, t_0: calculated *t*-value, *p*: probability

increased marrow output. The cells that are newly introduced into circulation display a different histochemical behavior on the toluidine-blue pH scale than the basophils in the pre-experimental state. Therefore, the toluidine-blue pH series represents an important criterion for determining the functional state of blood basophils. In a fasting condition, most basophils (70%) become stained at low pH levels. At these pH levels, the more strongly acidic glycosaminoglycans are preferentially metachromatically stained, since the acidity of the heparin chains changes according to the number of sulfo and carboxyl groups present (according to the degree of polymerization). Thus, granules stainable at low pH levels contain strongly polymerized and

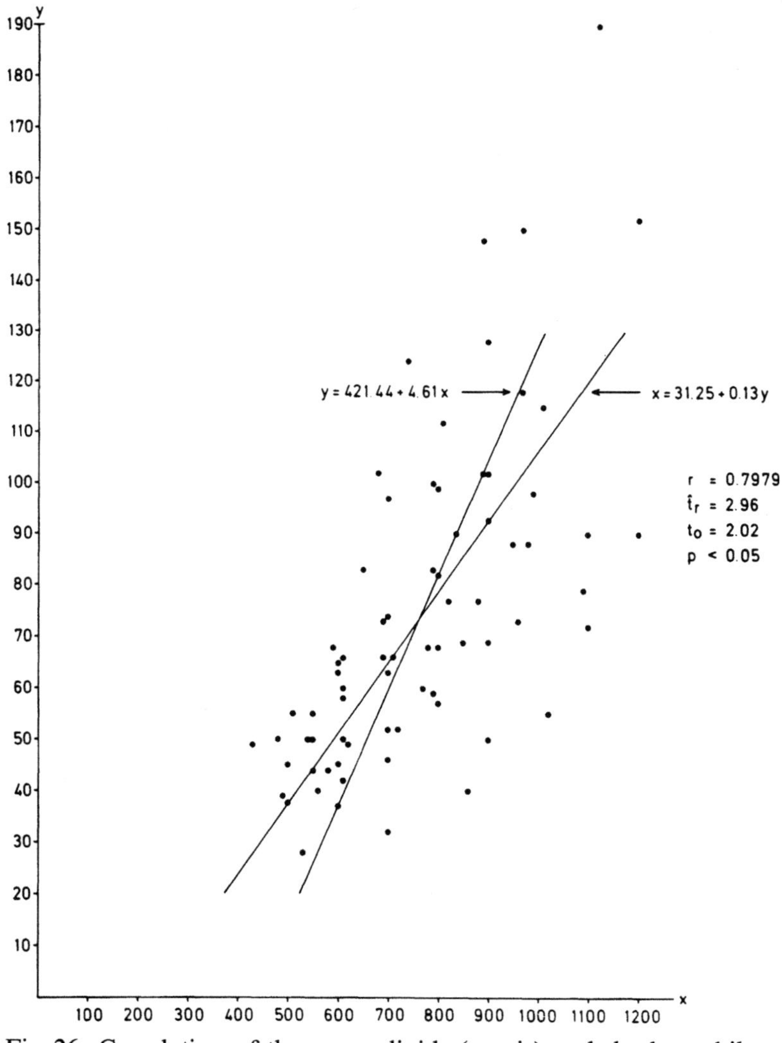

Fig. 26. Correlation of the serum lipids (x axis) and the basophil counts (y axis). Time-dependent course. *r*: estimated correlation coefficient, $\hat{t}$: tabular *t*-value, t_0: calculated *t*-value, *p*: probability

sulfated glycosaminoglycans and can be considered more mature. A shift of the curve maxima to higher pH levels would then correspond to a decrease in their acid content. This is typically observed in hyperlipidemia. After a maximum shift on the toluidine-blue pH scale 4.5 h after fat intake, a reverse tendency toward the more acidic pH region appears at a later time, and

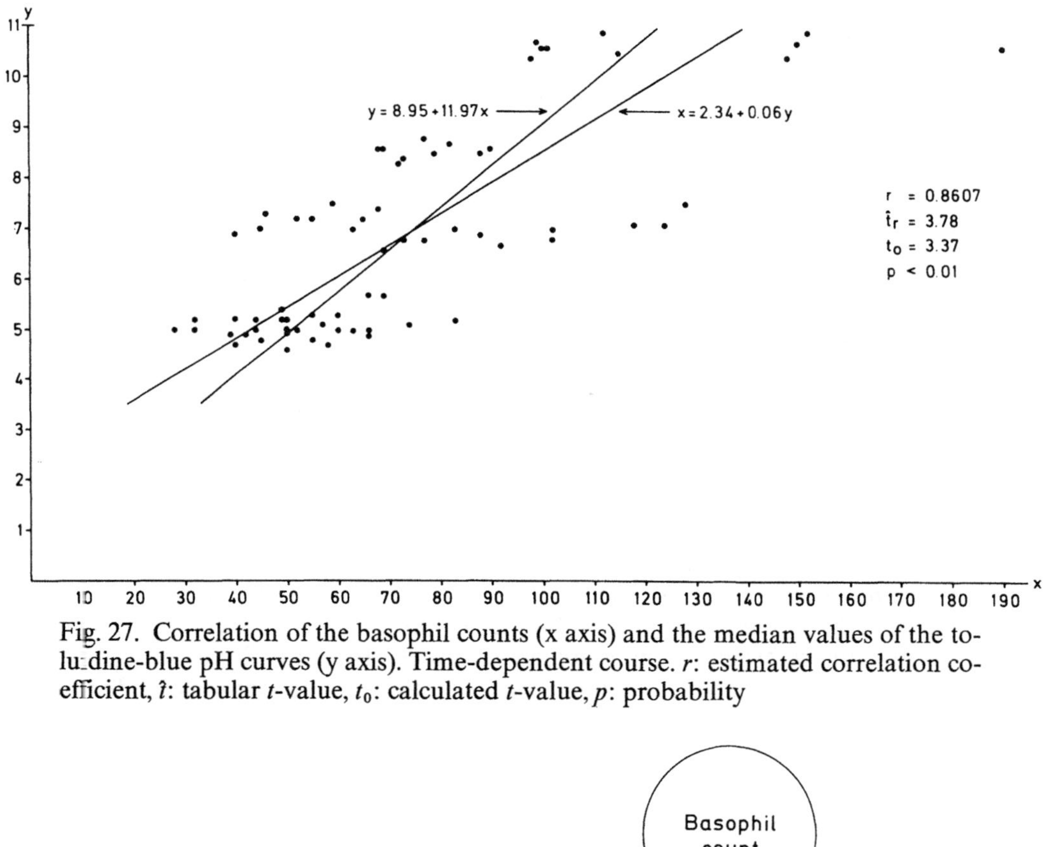

Fig. 27. Correlation of the basophil counts (x axis) and the median values of the toluidine-blue pH curves (y axis). Time-dependent course. r: estimated correlation coefficient, $\hat{t}$: tabular t-value, t_0: calculated t-value, p: probability

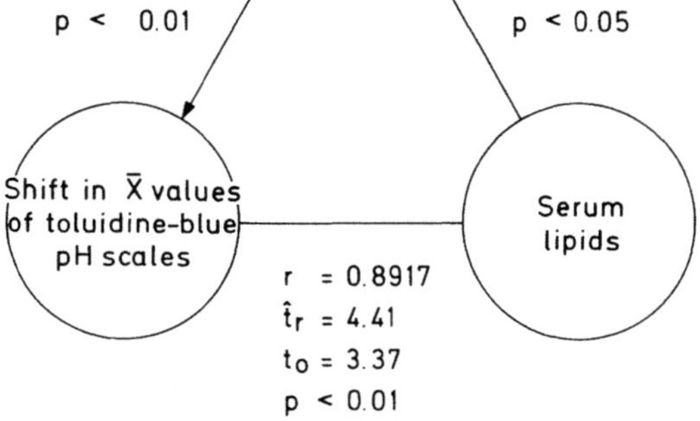

Fig. 28. Illustration of the correlative relationships of the three parameters: serum lipids, blood basophil counts, and extent of the shift of the toluidine-blue pH medians ($\tilde{x}$). *Arrows* indicate the primary dependences.

it usually is no longer possible to detect a difference between the curves obtained from fasting subjects and the curves obtained 5.5 h postprandially.

The increase in the serum lipids is accompanied by an alteration in the histochemical properties of the acidic glycosaminoglycans in the basophil granules. This alteration, which is apparent in a shift of the staining maxima on the toluidine-blue pH scale, can be explained theoretically by two mechanisms. In first hyperlipidemia leads either directly or indirectly to a partial "degranulation" of the basophils. The granule portions left would then contain less polymer and less sulfated glycosaminoglycans and would then only become stained at higher pH levels. We are however, of the opinion that the loss of granules, whether partial or complete, initiates cell death. Necrobiotic cells are rapidly withdrawn from the circulation. The results of our kinetic studies (Chapter C III) support this view. Furthermore, if we accept the theory of partial degranullation, we must produce proof of the occurrence in the circulation of cytologically intact basophils with a lower granule content than the blood basophils in the pre-experimental state. In addition, it must also be shown that the number of 'partially degranulated' cells is high enough both to effect the strong shift in the toluidine-blue pH series and to maintain sufficient heparin for lipolysis.

We cannot on the basis of our findings agree with this hypothesis. In the smears prepared from leukocyte concentrates, we could not detect by light microscopy differences in the granule content of intact blood basophils obtained at different observation times. Ultrastructural results were in good agreement with these findings. Over 50 basophils were studied in each sample. Basophils from the fasting state or even 1.5 h after fat intake showed no significant difference in the number, size, and shape of their granules. The number of basophils present 3 and 4 h after fat intake was found to be significant with reference to myelinized granules (Fig. 29). Some basophils showed large cytoplasmic vacuoles, pyknotic nuclei, and obvious evidence of necrobiosis. The basophils circulating in the blood contain differing amounts of granules even when the subject is fasting (Fig. 30). This difference is at least partly artificial and should not be regarded as the morphological correlate of 'partial degranulation' or of a shift of the toluidine-blue pH maxima. The finding that in hyperlipidemia the necrobiotic basophil count increases (Fig. 31) supports our view and refutes the degranulation theory.

A second possible explanation for the toluidine-blue pH shift is provided by the finding that the circulating blood basophil count simultaneously increases. The strong peripheral consumption apparently proceeds with a massive output of less mature basophils. This not only explains the quantitative basophil increase, but also the shift on the toluidine-blue pH scale. Blood basophils with less mature granules cannot be cytologically differentiated from the fully matured cells but on the toluidine-blue pH scale they can. This is also true of the cytologically mature basophils in normal human bone marrow as they can be stained at significantly higher pH levels than the mature circulating basophils (Parwaresch and Sadighi, 1970). It seems obvious that, in the course of maturation, the basophil content of

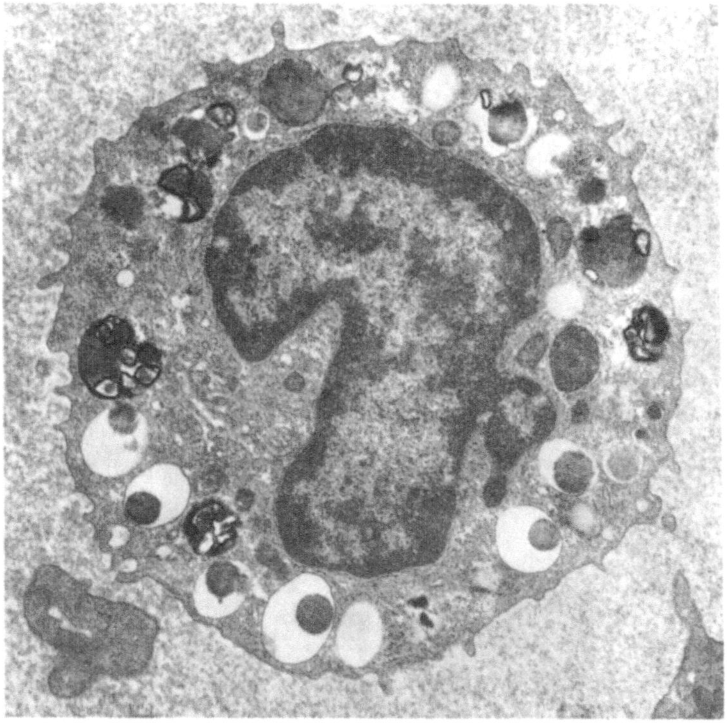

Fig. 29. Typical mild ultrastructural alterations in human basophils after induced hyperlipidemia: Note the abundance of myelin figures and discharged granules. Buffy coat, peripheral blood, 3 h after fat intake (2 g/kg body weight). × 12,000

acidic glycosaminoglycans swiftly increases only in the maturation stages corresponding to the band forms and polymorphonuclear granulocytes. The accumulation of highly polymerized and highly sulfated glycosaminoglycans within the granule matrix occurs not gradualy but quite rapidly in the last phase of maturation. This implies that the maturation process of basophil granules continues for at least part of the circulation time. We made a similar observation with tissue mast cells , which contain considerably more heparin than blood basophils. It appears that the complete maturation process of the granules takes only a few hours (PARWARESCH *et al.,* 1971; DESAGA *et al.,* 1971).

On the basis of the results obtained so far, we believe that the evidence concerning the role of blood basophils in serum lipolysis is convincing. Hyperlipidemia appears to lead to blood basophil cytolysis and thus to the liberation of polyanions. The elevated peripheral consumption stimulates massive flooding of these cells out of their reservoirs, e.g. bone marrow. There has been speculation about the importance of blood basophils in atherosclerosis: In old age as well as in advanced arteriosclerosis, clearing factor activity has been found to decline (BLOCK *et al.,* 1951; OLIVER and BOYD, 1953; DAY *et al.,* 1957; HARTMANN, 1963; ZEMPLENYI, 1964). The

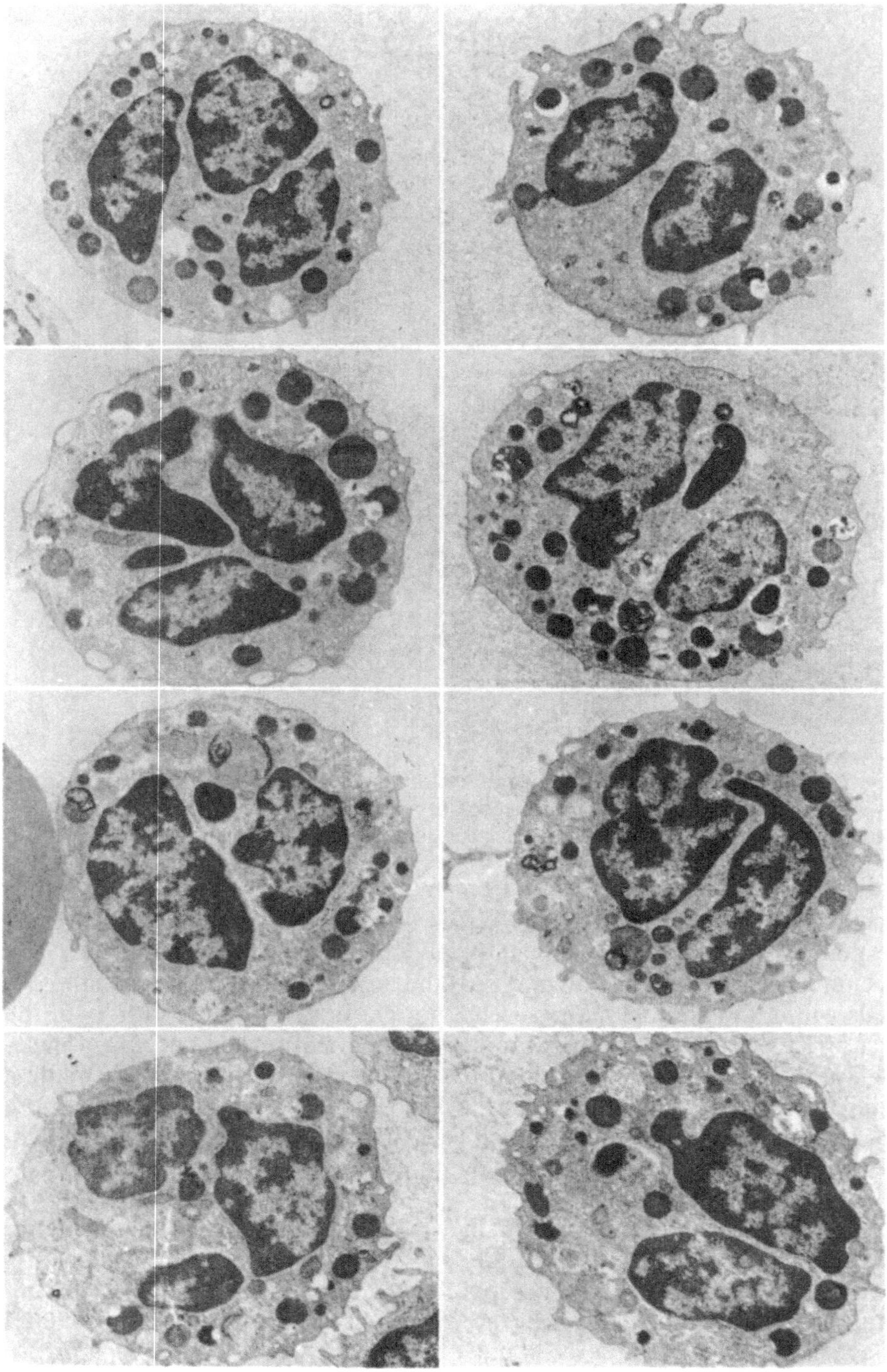

Fig. 30. Blood basophils of fasting normal subjects. The cells show well-preserved granules of varying electron density. Single granules show myelin figures. The granule size varies considerably. The nuclei in all cells possess a coarse chromatin structure with wide condensation zones in the marginal areas. ×4,500

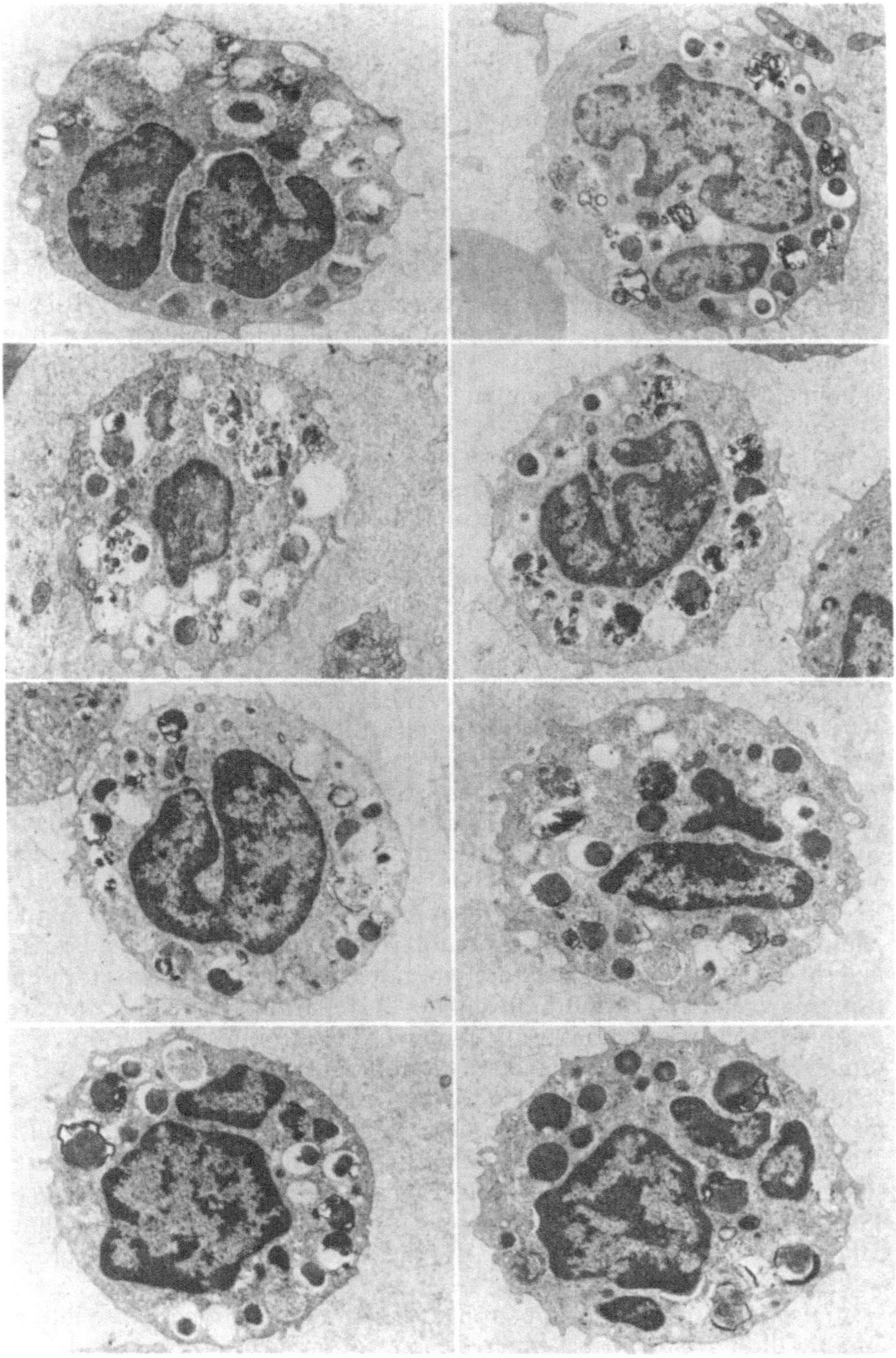

Fig. 31. Blood basophils 3 h after oral fat intake (2 g per kg body weight). Basophils in hyperlipidemic blood show disrupted or coarsely vacuolated granules. Myelin figures are found frequently within the specific granules. The cytoplasm is often hydrated and shows a loose electron-microscopic structure and membrane fragmentation. ×4,500

decline in clearing factor activity and the subsequent slowing of serum lipolysis could be due to various causes. First, there could be a disturbance in the synthesis of lipoprotein lipase in the sense of an absolute or relative enzyme-deficiency syndrome. However, exogenous heparin induces normal serum lipolysis in arteriosclerosis (HOOD *et al.*, 1954; ANGERVALL and HOOD, 1957) so that it seems improbable that enzyme deficiency is the cause of the impaired lipolysis (BAKER, 1957). Impaired serum lipolysis in old age and in arteriosclerosis could also be due to the presence of inhibitors in the serum of such patients (ANGERVALL and HOOD, 1957; HOLLETT and MENG, 1957; DAY and WILKINSON, 1958). The chemical nature of these inhibiting substances is not clear. Their inhibiting action can be completely eliminated by repeated freezing and thawing and by exposure to temperatures over 60° C. The activity of the lipolytic inhibitors in serum is extremely low. Such inhibiting substances also appear in the serum of healthy people, although in much more limited amounts. It is therefore improbable that these substances alone can account for the difference in clearing activity found in the sera of arteriosclerotic and normal individuals (ANGERVALL and HOOD, 1957; DAY and WILKINSON, 1958).

In certain apes (*Saimirishiorea*) that are susceptible to fat-induced arteriosclerosis arterial lesions were prevented by simultaneous administration of heparin (MIDDLETON *et al.*, 1964; PORTMAN and ANDRUS, 1965) or heparin-like glycosaminoglycans (OSHIMA and MURATA, 1960; 1962; MORRISON *et al.*, 1966). Such findings have been taken by a considerable body of authors to suggest that heparin deficiency could be the cause of impaired lypolysis in old age and in atherosclerosis. Some authors hold the view that a critical relationship exists between the physiological amount of circulating endogenous heparin and daily fat consumption (ENGELBERG *et al.*, 1955; MARTIRANI *et al.*, 1962).

The anatomic texture and permeability of the vessel walls are important pathogenetic factors determining the development of arteriosclerosis. The main components of the interstitial ground substance of the vessel wall are hyaluronic acid and chondroitin sulfate-C. Heparitin sulfate and chondroitin sulfate-B are present in small amounts. Chondroitin sulfate-C and hyaluronic acid can both be split by hyaluronidase. Lytic enzymes like hyaluronidase and such physicochemical factors as radiation and thermal and mechanical injuries can lead to severe damage of vessel-wall metabolism. The impaired arterial wall accumulates macromolecular substances during serum perfusion (FELD *et al.*, 1960; BÖTTCHER, 1963; 1968; DAVIS *et al.*, 1963; DUNCAN *et al.*, 1963; WATTS, 1963; CHRISTENSEN, 1964). The significant role of the glycosaminoglycans of the intercellular space of the arterial wall in transport mechanisms has been well elucidated by KLYNSTRA *et al.* (1967). These authors noted a stronger penetration of trypan blue into the aortic wall of swine *in vitro* when the incubation medium contained testicular hyaluronidase, and drew attention to the fact that the infiltrated areas were formally and topically very similar to atherosclerotic lesions. KRUT and WILKENS (1968) found that the permeability of the aortic wall as visualized by ^{32}P-labeling and autoradiography agreed topically very well with the findings of KLYNSTRA *et al.* (1967). On the other hand, histamine has been found to increase the activity of tissue hyaluronidase, whereas heparin exerts a depressive effect on this enzyme (RYVKINA, 1957; KAZNACHEEV and LOZOVOI, 1958; KASATKINA, 1963). These observations agreed with those of WEGELIUS and ASBOE-HANSEN (1957), and RIKHTER (1960).

In summary: The hyperlipidemia subsequent to lipid intake induces lysis of blood basophils, liberating histamine and heparin. The endhanced peripheral utilization stimulates an intense emergence of less mature basophils from the bone marrow.

References

ADAMS, S. S., HEATHCOTE, B. V., MACEY, P. E.: A note on irradiated heparin: some biological and chemical properties. J. Phar. Pharmacol. **13,** 240 – 243 (1961).

ALBRINK, M. J., GLENN, W. W. L., PETERS J. P., MAN, E. B.: Transport of lipids in chyle. J. clin. Invest. **34,** 1467 – 1475 (1955).

AMANN, R.: Über das Verhalten von Heparinen und anderen sulfathaltigen Mucopolysacchariden bei der Papierchromatographie, pp. 547 – 551. Verh. 6. Kongr. europ. Ges. Haemat., Kopenhagen 1957. Basel-New York: Karger 1958.

AMANN, R., WERLE, E.: Über Komplexe von Heparin und Histamin und anderen Di- und Polyaminen. Klin. Wschr. **34,** 207 – 209 (1956).

AMANN, R., MARTIN, H.: see page 56.

ANDERSON, N. G., FAWCETT, B.: An antichylomicronemic substance produced by heparin injection. Proc. Soc. exp. Biol. (N. Y.) **74,** 768 – 771 (1950).

ANDERSON, B., HOFFMAN, P., MEYER, K.: The O-serine linkage in peptides of chondroitin-4- or -6-sulfate. J. biol. Chem. **240,** 156 – 167 (1965).

ANGERVALL, G., HOOD, B.: Studies on heparin and lipemia clearing factor. Acta med. scand. **157,** 407 – 415 (1957).

ASBOE-HANSEN, G.: Autoradiography of mast cells in experimental skin tumors of mice injected with radioactive sulfur (^{35}S). Cancer Res. **13,** 587 – 589 (1953).

ASHWELL, G.: Carbohydrate metabolism. Ann. Rev. Biochem. **33,** 101 – 138 (1964).

ASTALDI, G., RONDANELLI, E. G., BERNADELLI, B.: see page 56.

BAKER, S. P.: Heparin-activated clearing factor. Standardized test, agewise application and clinical observation. Circulation **15,** 889 – 896 (1957).

BARLOW, G. H., SANDERSON, N. D., MCNEILL, P.: Macromolecular properties and biological activity of heparin. Arch. Biochem. Biophys. **94,** 518 – 525 (1961).

BEHRENS, M., TAUBERT, M.: see page 57.

BENNETT, H. S., LUFT, J. H., HAMPTON, J. C.: Morphological classification of vertebrate blood capillaries. Amer. J. Physiol. **196,** 381 – 390 (1959).

BIGGS, R., DOUGLAS, A. S., MAC FARLANE, R. G.: The action of thromboplastic substances. J. Physiol. (Lond.) **122,** 554 – 569 (1953).

BIGGS, R., MAC FARLANE, R. G.: Human Blood Coagulation and Its Disorders. 3rd edition. Philadelphia: Davis 1962.

BLOCK, W. J., BARKER, N. W., MANN, F. D.: Effect of small doses of heparin in increasing the translucence of plasma during alimentary lipemia. Studies in normal persons and patients having atherosclerosis. Circulation **4,** 674 – 678 (1951).

BÖTTCHER, C. J. F.: Phospholipids of atherosclerotic human aorta. In: Jones (Ed.): Evolution of Atherosclerotic Plaques, pp. 109 – 116. Chicago: University of Chicago Press 1963.

Böttcher, C. J. F.: Origin and development of atherosclerotic lesions. Progr. biochem. Pharmacol. **4,** 231 – 234. Basel-New York: Karger 1968.

Borgström, B., Jordan, P.: Metabolism of chylomicron glyceride as studied by C^{14}-glycerol-C^{14}-palmitic acid labeled chylomicrons. Acta Soc. Med. upsalien. **64,** 185 – 193 (1959).

Bragdon, J. H., Havel, R. J.: In vivo effect of anti-heparin agents on serum lipids and lipoproteins. Amer. J. Physiol. **117,** 128 – 133 (1954).

Braswell, L. M.: 1963. Cited in: L. W. Harris, L. M. Braswell and J. P. Fleisher: Metabolites of pinacolyl methylphosphono-fluoridate after enzymatic hydrolysis in vitro. Biochem. Pharmacol. **13,** 1129 – 1136 (1964).

Braunsteiner, H., Thumb, N.: see page 22.

Braunsteiner, H., Höfer, R., Thumb, N., Vetter, H.: Untersuchungen über die basophilen Leukocyten bei Schilddrüsenerkrankungen. Klin. Wschr. **37,** 250 – 252 (1959).

Braunsteiner, H., Thumb, N.: In: Lipoproteid lipase. Ed.: H. Braunsteiner, S. Sailer und F. Sandhofer. Basel-New York: Karger 1963.

Braunsteiner, H., Sailer, S., Sandhofer, F.: The relationship between level of triglycerides in plasma and number of basophils in blood. Metabolism **14,** 1071 – 1075 (1965).

Brimacombe, J. S., Webber, J. M.: Mucopolysaccharides. Chemical structure, distribution and isoliation. Amsterdam-London-New York: Elsevier 1964.

Brown, W. D.: Reversible effects of anticoagulants and protamine on alimentary lipemia. Quart. J. exp. Physiol. **37,** 75 – 84 (1952).

Brown, R. K., Boyle, E., Anfinsen, C. B.: The enzymatic transformation of lipoproteins. J. biol. Chem. **204,** 423 – 434 (1953).

Brown, K. D., Cushing, I. B., Evans, S. M., Helbert, J. R.: Lipoprotein lipase and anticoagulant properties of a heparin derivative: N-succinyl heparin (P). Circulation **26,** 647 (1962).

Christensen, S.: Transfer of labeled cholesterol across the aortic intimal surface of normal and cholesterol-fed cockerels. J. Atheroscler. Res. **4,** 151 – 160 (1964).

Cifonelli, J. A.: Reaction of heparitin sulfate with nitrous acid. Carbohyd. Res. **8,** 233 – 242 (1968).

Cifonelli, J. A., Dorfman, A.: The uronic acid of heparin. Biochem. biophys. Res. Commun. **7,** 41 – 45 (1962).

Cooper, J. R., Cruickshank, C. N. D.: see page 22.

Corvilain, J., Loeb, H., Champenois, A., Abramow, M.: Effect of fasting on levels of plasma non-esterified fatty acids in normal children, normal adults and obese adults. Lancet **1961 I,** 534 – 535.

Davies, J. N., Adams, C. W. M., Bayliss, O. B.: Gradient in cholesterol concentration across human aortic wall. **1963 II,** 1254 – 1255.

Day, A. J., Wilkinson, G. K., Gilmore, H. K., Schwartz, C. J.: Effect of protamine on alimentary lipemia. Ciruclation **16,** 72 – 76 (1957).

Day, A. J., Wilkinson, G. K.: Clearing factor inhibitor in human atherosclerosis. Circulation **18,** 76 – 81 (1958).

Desaga, J. F., Parwaresch, M. R., Müller-Hermelink, H. K.: see page 22.

Dole, V. P.: Fat as an energy source. In: K. Rodahl and B. Issekutz (Eds.): Fat as a Tissue. New York: McGraw-Hill 1963.

Dondoroff, M.: In: S. P. Colowick and N. O. Kaplan (Eds.), Methods in Enzymology, Vol. 5. New York: Academic Press Inc. 1962.

Douglas, A. S.: Factor V consumption during blood coagulation. Brit. J. Haemat. **2,** 153 – 159 (1956).

DUNCAN, L. E., BUCK, K., LYNCH, A.: Lipoprotein movement through canine aortic wall. Science **142**, 972 – 973 (1963).

DURANT, G. J., HENDRICKSON, H., MONTGOMERY, R.: Studies on the structure of heparin. Arch. Biochem. Biophys. **99**, 418 – 425 (1962).

EGGE, H., MURAWSKI, U., MÜLLER, J., ZILLIKEN, F.: Mikrolipidanalysen aus Serum mit dem Eppendorf-System 3000. Z. klin. Chem. klin. Biochem. **8**, 488 – 491 (1970).

EHRLICH, P.: Beiträge zur Kenntnis der granulierten Bindegewebszellen und der eosinophilen Leukocyten. Arch. Anat. Physiol. **3**, 166 – 169 (1879).

ENGELBERG, H.: Human endogenous lipemia clearing activity. Studies of lipolysis and effects of inhibitors. J. Biol. Chem. **222**, 601 – 610 (1956).

ENGELBERG, H., DUDLEY, A., FREEMAN, L.: An improved method for the determination of plasma heparin. J. Lab. clin. Med. **46**, 653 – 656 (1955).

FAWCETT, D. W.: Observations on the cytology and electron microscopy of hepatic cells. J. nat. Cancer Inst. **15**, 1475 – 1503 (1955).

FELD, H., SWELL, L., SCHOOLS, P. E., TREADWELL, C. R.: Dynamic aspects of cholesterol metabolism in different areas of the aorta and other tissues in man and their relationship to atherosclerosis. Circulation **22**, 547 – 558 (1960).

FELTS, J. M.: Lipid transport between adipose tissue and blood. In: K. RODAHL and B. ISSEKUTZ: Fat as a Tissue, p. 95. New York: McGraw-Hill 1962.

FITTON JACKSON, S., HARKNESS, R. D., PATRIDGE, S. M., TRISTAM, G. R.: Structure and function of connective and skeletal tissues. London: Butterworths 1965.

FORSTER, A. B., HARRISON, R., INCH, T. D., STACEY, M., WEBBER, J. M.: Periodate oxidation of heparin and related compounds. Biochem. J. **80**, 12 – 13 (1961).

FORSTER, A. B., HARRISON, R., INCH, T. D., STACEY, M., WEBBER, J. M.: Aminosugars and related compounds. IX. Periodate oxidation of heparin and some related substances. J. chem. Soc. **2**, 2279 – 2287 (1963).

FRANSSON, L.-A.: Structure of dermatan sulfate. IV. Glgycopeptides from the carbohydrate-protein linkage region of pig skin dermatan sulfate. Biochim. biophys. Acta (Amst.) **156**, 311 – 316 (1968 a).

FRANSSON, L.-A.: Structure of dermatan sulfate. III. The hybrid structure of dermatan sulfate from umbilical cord. J. biol. Chem. **243**, 1504 – 1510 (1968 b).

FRANSSON, L.-A., RODÉN, L.: Structure of dermatan sulfate. J. biol. Chem. **242**, 4161 – 4175 (1967).

FREDRICKSON, D. F., GORDON, Jr., R. S.: Transport of fatty acids. Physiol. Rev. **38**, 585 – 630 (1958).

FREDRICKSON, D. F., LEVY, R. J., LEES, R. S.: Fat transport in lipoporoteins – an integrated approach to mechanism and disorders. New Engl. J. Med. **276**, 32 – 44 (1967).

GAGE, S. H., FISH, P. A.: Fat digestion, absorption, and assimilation in man and animals as determined by the dark-field microscope, and a fat-soluble dye. Amer. J. anat. **34**, 1 – 85 (1924).

GIBIAN, H., BAROLLIER, J.: Notiz über die Anfärbung von Mucopolysaccharidsäuren auf Papier. Naturwissenschaften **43**, 60 (1956).

GOFMAN, J. W., LALLA, O. F., GLAZIE, F., FREEMAN, N. K., LINDGREN, F. T., NICHOILS, A. V., STRISHOWER, B., TAMPLIN, A. R.: The serum lipoprotein transport system in health, metabolic disorders, atherosclerosis and coronary artery disease. Plasma Ann. *II*, 413 – 484 (1954).

GORDON, Jr., R. S.: Unesterified fatty acid in human blood plasma. II. The transport function of unesterified fatty acids. J. clin. Invest. **36**, 810 – 815 (1957).

GORDON, Jr., R. S., CHERKES, A.: Unesterified fatty acid in human blood plasma. J. clin. Invest. **35,** 206 – 212 (1956).

GOTTSCHALK, A.: Glycoproteins. Amsterdam: Elsevier 1965.

GRABENER, E.: Funktionsanalytische Untersuchungen an Blutbasophilen. Kiel: Habilitationsschrift 1967.

GREGORY, J. D., LAURENT, T. C., RODÉN, L.: Enzymatic degradation of chondromucoprotein. J. biol. Chem. **239,** 3312 – 3320 (1964).

GRETEN, H., LEVY, R. I., FREDRICKSON, D. S.: A further characterization of lipoprotein lipase. Biochim. biophys. acta (Amst.) **164,** 185 (1968).

HAGEN, P.: Bisoynthesis and storage of histamine, heparin and 5-hydroxytryptamine in the mast cell. Canad. J. Biochem. **39,** 639 – 642 (1961).

HAHN, P. F.: Abolishment of alimentary lipemia following injection of heparin. Science **98,** 19 – 20 (1943).

HAMPTON, J. C.: An electron microscope study of the hepatic uptake and excretion of submicroscopic particles injected into the blood stream and into the bile duct. Acta anat. (Basel) **32,** 262 – 291 (1958).

HARTMANN, G.: In: Lipoproteidlipase. H. BRAUNSTEINER, S. SAILER und F. SANDHOFER (Eds.). Basel-New York: Karger 1963.

HAVEL, R. J.: Early effects of fasting and of carbohydrate ingestion on lipids and lipoproteins of serum in man. J. clin. Invest. **36,** 855 – 859 (1975).

HAVEL, R. J., FELTS, J. M., VAN DUYNE, C. M.: Formation and fate of endogenous triglycerides in blood plasma of rabbits. J. Lipid. Res. **3,** 297 – 308 (1962).

HAVEL, R. J., GOLDFIEN, A.: The role of the liver and of extrahepatic tissues in the transport and metabolism of fatty acids and triglycerides in the dog. J. Lipid Res. **2,** 389 – 395 (1961).

HAVEL, R. J., GORDON, Jr., R. S.: Idiopathic hyperlipemia: metabolic studies in an affected family. J. clin Invest. **39,** 1777 – 1790 (1960).

HELTING, T.: Biosynthesis of heparin: solubilization, partial separation and purification of uridine diphosphate-galactose: acceptor galactosyltransferases from mouse mastocytoma. J. biol. Chem. **246,** 815 – 822 (1971).

HERWERDEN, M. A.: see page 60.

HOLLETT, C., MENG, H. C.: Lipemia clearing factor inhibitor in normal plasma. Fed. Proc. **16,** 60 – 61 (1957).

HOOD, B., ANGERVALL, O. G., ISAKSSON, B., WELIN, G.: Studies on heparin and the lipemia clearing factor I. Scand. J. clin. Lab. Invest. **6,** 1 – 7 (1954).

HORWITZ, A. L., DORFMAN, A.: Subcellular sites for synthesis of chondromucoprotein of cartilage. J. Cell Biol. **38,** 358 – 368 (1968).

HOWELL, W. H., HOLT, E.: see page 60.

INAGAKI, S.: see page 24.

JACOBS, S., MUIR, H.: A heparin sulphate-peptide from human aorta. Biochem. J. **87,** 38 (1963).

JAQUES, L. B., WATERS, E. T., CHARLES, A. F.: A comparison of the heparins of various mammalian species. J. biol. Chem. **144,** 229 – 235 (1942).

JAQUES, L. B., BELL, H. J.: Determination of heparin. Meth. biochem. Anal. **7,** 253 – 309 (1959).

JAQUES, L. B., KAVANAGH, L. W., LAVALLÉE, A.: A comparison of biological activities and chemical analyses for various heparin preparations. Arzneimittel-Forsch. **17,** 774 – 777 (1967).

JENSEN, R., SNELLMAN, O., SYLVÉN, B.: On the inhomogeneity of commercial heparin preparations from the physicochemical point of view. J. biol. Chem. **174,** 265 – 271 (1948).

JORPES, J. E.: Heparin – eine Chondroitinschwefelsäure. Naturwissenschaften **23,** 196 – 197 (1935).

JORPES, J. E., HOLMGREN, H., WILANDER, O.: Über das Vorkommen von Heparin in den Gefäßwänden und in den Augen. Ein Beitrag zur Physiologie der Ehrlichschen Mastzzellen. Z. mikr.-anat. Forsch. **42,** 279 – 301 (1937).

JORPES, J. E., GARDELL, S.: On heparin monosulfuric acid. J. biol. Chem. **176,** 267 – 276 (1948).

JORPES, J. E., WERNER, B., ÅBERG, B.: see page 61.

JORPES, J. E., ODEBLAD, E., BOSTRÖM, H.: see page 74.

JÜRGENS, R., STUDER, A.: Zur Wirkung des Thrombins. Helv. physiol. pharmacol. Acta **6,** 130 – 149 (1948).

JULÉN, Chr., SNELLMAN, O., SYLVÉN, B.: Cytological and fractionation studies on the cytoplasmic constituents of tissue mast cells. Acta physiol. scand. **19,** 289 – 303 (1950).

KASATKINA, L. V.: Effect of histamine on development of experimental atherosclerosis. Kardilogiya **3,** 45 – 48 (1963).

KAZNACHEEV, J. P., LOZOVOI, V. P.: In: Proceedings of the second plenary meeting of the Siberian branch of the All-Union Society of Pathophysiologists, p. 153. Chita 1958.

KEHNSCHERPER, M., BLAU, H.: see page 24.

KELLNER, A., CORRELL J. W., LADD, A. T.: Sustained hyperlipaemia induced in rabbits by means of intravenously injected surface-active agents. J. exp. Med. **93,** 373 – 383 (1951).

KLEINE, O. T., HILZ, H.: Charakterisierung der Protein-Polysaccharide aus Kälberrippenknorpel und ihre in-vitro-Markierung mit $^{35}SO_4$. Hoppe-Seylers Z. physiol. Chem. **349,** 1027 – 1036 (1968).

KLEINE, O. T., KISIG, H. J., HILZ, H.: Über die Koordinierung von Protein-Polysaccharid- und Sulfatester-Synthese im Rippenknorpel von Kälbern. Hoppe-Seylers Z. physiol. Chem. **349,** 1037 – 1048 (1968).

KLYNSTRA, F. B., BOELSMA-VAN HOUTE, E. BÖTTCHER, C. J. F.: Acid mucopolysaccharides and atherosclerosis. Lancet **1967 II,** 1150 – 1151.

KLYNSTRA, F. B., BÖTTCHER, C. J. F., VAN MELSEN, J. A., VAN DER LAAN, E. J.: Distribution and composition of acid mucopolysaccharides in normal and atherosclerotic human aortas. J. Atheroscler. Res. **7,** 301 – 309 (1967).

KOBAYASHI, Y.: Histamine binding by heparin. Arch. Biochem. Biophys. **96,** 20 – 27 (1962).

KORN, E. D., QUIGLEY, T. W.: Studies on lipoprotein lipase of rat heart and adipose tissue. Biochem. biophys. Acta (Amst.) **18,** 143 – 145 (1955).

KORN, E. D., QUIGLEY, T. W.: Lipoprotein lipase of chicken adipose tissue. J. biol. Chem. **226,** 833 – 839 (1957).

KORN, E. D.: In. I. H. PAGE (Ed.): Chemistry of Lipids as Related to Atherosclerosis. Springfield, Ill.: Charles C. Thomas 1958.

KORN, E. D.: A chromatographic and spectrophotometric study of the products of the reaction of osmium tetroxide with unsaturated lipids. J. Cell. Biol. **34,** 627 – 638 (1967).

KRAUP, O.: In. Lipoproteidlipase. H. BRAUNSTEINER, S. SAILER und F. SANDHOFER, (Eds.). Basel-New York: Karger 1963.

LALLA, O. F., GOFMAN, J. W.: Ultracentrifugal analysis of serum lipoprotein. In: D. GLICK (Ed.): Methods of Biochemical analysis. New York: Interscience 1954.

LAURELL, S.: Recycling of intravenously injected palmic acid-I-C^{14} as esterified fatty acid in the plasma of rats and turnover rate of plasma triglycerides. Acta physiol. scand. **47,** 218 – 232 (1950).

LAURENT, T. C.: Studies on fractionated heparin. Arch. Biochem. Biophys. **92,** 224 – 231 (1961).

LAVES, W., THOMA, K.: see page 61.

LENNERT, K., SCHUBERT, J. F. C.: see page 62.

LENNERT, K., SCHUBERT, J. F. C.: see page 24.

LENNERT, K., PARWARESCH, M. R.: Löslichkeit und Fixierungsmöglichkeiten der Blutbasophilen-Granula des Menschen. Z. Zellforsch. **83,** 279 – 287 (1968).

LENNERT, K., PARWARESCH, M. R.: see page 24.

LINDAHL, U.: The structures of xylosylserine and galactosylxylosylserine from heparin. Biochim. biophys. Acta. (Amst.) **130,** 361 – 367 (1966 a).

LINDAHL, U.: Further characterization of the heparin-protein linkage region. Biochim. biophys. Acta. (Amst.) **130,** 368 – 382 (1966 b).

LINDAHL, U.: Structure of the heparin-protein linkage region. Arkiv Kemi **26,** 101 – 110 (1966 c).

LINDAHL, U.: see page 24.

LINDAHL, U., RODÉN, L.: The role of galactose and xylose in the linkage of heparin to protein. J. biol. Chem. **240,** 2821 – 2826 (1965).

LINDBERG, B., SILVANDER, B.-G.: Synthesis of o-β-D-xylopyranosyl-L-Serine. Acta chem. scand. **19,** 530 – 531 (1965).

LINKER, A., HOVINGH, P.: The enzymatic degradation of heparin and heparitin sulfate. I. The fractionation of a crude heparinase from flavobacteria. J. biol. Chem. **240,** 3724 – 3728 (1965).

MARTIN, H., ROKA, L.: see page 63.

MARTIRANI, I., MELO, E. H. L., HÖXTER, G., WAICHENBERG, B. L., CINSTRA, A. B. U.: Heparin-included clearing factor: comparative studies between normal and patients with electrocardiographic singns of a past myocardinal infarction (coronary heart disease). Metabolism **11,** 1210 – 1220 (1962).

MARQUARD, F., WALZMAN, P.: Untersuchungen über den Mechanismus der Antithrombinwirkung des Heparins. Hoppe-Seylers Z. physiol. Chem. **317,** 64 – 77 (1959).

MATHEWS, M. B., LOZAITYTE, I.: Sodium chondrotin sulfate-protein complexes of cartilage. I. Molecular wight and shape. Arch. Biochem. Biophys. **74,** 158 – 174 (1958).

MAXIMOW, A.: Bindegewebe und blutbildendes Gewebe. In: Handbuch der mikroskopischen Anatomie des Menschen, Vol. II, 1. Berlin: Springer 1927.

MCLEAN, J.: The thromboplastic action of cephalin. Amer. J. Physiol. **41,** 250 – 257 (1916).

MEYER, K.: Biochemistry and biology of mucopolysaccharides. Amer. J. Med. **47,** 664– 672 (1969).

MIDDELTON, C. C., CLARKSON, T. B., LOFLAND, H. B., PRICHARD, R. W.: Atherosclerosis in the squirrel monkey. Arch. Path. **78,** 16 – 23 (1964).

MORRISON, L. M., MURATA, K., QUILLIGAN, J. J., SCHJEIDE, O. A., FREEMAN, L.: Prevention of atherosclerosis in subhuman primates by chondroitin sulfate A. Circulation **19,** 358 – 363 (1966).

MUIR, H.: The nature of the link between protein and carbohydrate of a chondroitin sulphate complex from hyaline cartilage. Biochem. J. **69,** 195 – 204 (1958).

MUIR, H.: Chemistry and metabolism of connective tissue glycosaminoglycans (mucopolysaccharides). Intern. Rev. connective tissue Res. **2,** 101 – 154 (1964).

MUIR, H.: The structure and metabolism of mucopolysaccharides (glycosaminoglycans) and the problem of the mucopolysaccharidoses. Amer. J. Med. **47**, 673 – 690 (1969).

NAGAYO, M.: see page 64.

NESTEL, P. J.: Relationship between plasma trilycerides and removal of chylomicrons. J. clin. Invest. **43**, 943 – 949 (1964).

NEUFELD, E. F., GINSBURG V.: Carbohydrate metabolism. Ann. Rev. Biochem. **34**, 297 – 312 (1965).

NINNI, M., BELLONI, F.: Sulla transformazione della leucemia mieloide cronica in leucemia basfilia subacuta. Haematologica (Pavia) **37**, 1455 – 1467 (1953).

NOMINÉ, G., BUCOURT, R., BERTIN, D.: Recherches sur l'héparine et la N-desulfohéparine. Etudes de structure. Bull. Soc. Chim. biol. (Paris) 561 – 567 (1961).

O'BRIEN, J. R.: The effect of heparin on the early stages of blood coagulation. J. clin. Path. **13**, 93 – 98 (1960).

OLIVER, M. F., BOYD, G. S.: The clearing by heparin of alimentary lipemia in coronary artery disease. Clin. Sci. **12**, 293 – 298 (1953).

OSHIMA, Y., MURATA, K.: Atherosclerosis from a viewpoint of abnormal polysaccharide metabolism. Clinics **9**, 115 (1960).

OSHIMA, Y., YOKOHARI, R., ODOI, S., MURATA, K., MURATA, K., WASP, K., OTSUKI, A., NODA, M., MIYAMOTO, T.: Clinical and experimental studies on mucopolysaccharides. Mucopolysaccharides and atherosclerosis, pp. 259 – 272. In: F. EGAM and Y. OSHIMA: Biochemistry and Medicine of Mucopolysaccharides. Tokyo: University Press 1962.

PAPPENHEIM, A.: Allgemeine Zytologie der Entzündung. Theoretische Vorbemerkungen. Folia haemat. (Lpz) **3**, 564 – 569 (1906).

PARWARESCH, M. R.: see page 25.

PARWARESCH, M. R., LENNERT, K.: see page 25.

PARWARESCH, M. R., LENNERT, K.: see page 64.

PARWARESCH, M. R., PETERSEN, A.: Der Einfluß von Histamin und fettreicher Diät auf die Anzahl der Gewebsmastzellen der Ratte. Virchows Arch. Abt. B Zellpath. **4**, 137 – 147 (1969).

PARWARESCH, M. R., SADIGHI, R.: see page 98.

PARWARESCH, M. R., MÜLLER-HERMELINK, H. K., DESAGA, J. F., ZAKARI, V., LENNERT, K.: Die Herkunft der Gewebsmastzellen bei der Ratte, zugleich ein Beitrag zur quantitativen Cytologie der sterilen Peritonitis. Virchows Arch. Abt. B Zellpath. **8**, 20 – 35 (1971).

PATAT, F., ELIAS, H.-G.: Molekulargewicht und Aktivität von Heparin. Naturwissenschaften **46**, 322 (1959).

PORTMAN, O. W., ANDRUS, S. B.: Comparative evaluation of three species of new world monkeys for studies of dietary factors, tissue lipids and atherosclerosis. J. Nutr. **87**, 429 –438 (1965).

QUINTARELLI, G., SCOTT, J. E.: International symposium on the chemical physiology of mucopolysaccharides. Carlo Erba foundation, Milano 1965. Little & Brown, Boston 1966.

RIKHTER, A.: In: Symposium on Connective Tissue, p. 143. Moscow 1960.

ROBINSON, D. S., FRENCH, J. E.: The heparin clearing reaction and fat transport. Quart. J. exp. Physiol. **42**, 151 – 163 (1957).

ROBINSON, E. D., HARRIS, P. M., RICKETTS, C. R.: The production of lipolytic activity in rat plasma after the intravenous injection of dextran sulphate. Biochem. J. **71**, 286 – 292 (1959).

RODÉN, L., ARMAND, G.: Structure of the chondroitin 4-sulfate-protein linkage region. Isolation and charakterization of the disaccharide-3-o-β-D-glucuronosyl-D-galactase. J. biol. Chem. **241,** 65 – 70 (1966).

RODÉN, L., SMITH, R.: Structure of the neutral trisaccharide of the chondroitin-4-sulfate-protein linkage region. J. biol. Chem. **241,** 5949 – 5954 (1966).

ROKA, L., MARTIN, H.: Über ein Antiprothrombin in den Myelocyten. Klin. Wschr. **29,** 468 – 477 (1950).

ROUILLER, C.: Les canalicules biliaires. Acta anat. (Basel) **26,** 94 – 109 (1956).

RYVKINA, D. E.: Effect of histamine on development of experimental atherosclerosis. Usp. sovrem. Biol. **44,** 389 – 395 (1957).

SAILER, S., SANDHOFER, F., BRAUNSTEINER, H.: Untersuchungen über die Lipoproteidlipase. I. Mitteilung: Bestimmung der Postheparin-Lipoproteidlipase beim Menschen durch Messung der Triglycerid-Spaltung. Klin. Wschr. **39,** 585 – 588 (1961).

SAILER, S., SANDHOFER, F.: In: Lipoproteidlipase. H. BRAUNSTEINER, S. SAILER und F. SANDHOFER (Eds.). Basel-New York: Karger 1963.

SCHILLER, S.: Connective and supporting tissues: mucopolysacchrides of connective tissues. Ann. Rev. Physiol. **28,** 137 – 158 (1966).

SCHÖLL, H.: In: Lipoproteidlipase. H. BRAUNSTEINER, S. SAILER und F. SANDHOFER: Basel-New York: Karger 1963.

SCHUBERT, J. F. C.: see page 99.

SCHUBERT, J. F. C.: Histochemische Untersuchungen an Gewebsmastzellen des menschlichen Knochenmarks. Inaugural Disseration, pp. 1 – 47, Frankfurt 1958.

SCHÜRER, W.: Speicherung von Heparin in den Zellen des Retikuloendothels. Helv. med. Acta **13,** 161 – 171 (1946).

SERAFINI-FRACASSINI, A., PETERS, T. J., FLOREANI, L.: The protein-polysaccharide complex of bovine nasal cartilage. Biochem. J. **105,** 569 – 575 (1967).

SERAFINI-FRACASSINI, A., DURWARD, J. J., FLOREANI, L.: The heparin-protein complex of ox-liver capsule. Biochem. J. **112,** 167 – 172 (1968).

SERAFINI-FRACASSINI, A., DURWARD, J. J., CRAWFORD, J.: The morphology of the heparin-protein macromolecule and its organization in the mast cell granule. J. Ultrastruct. Res. **28,** 131 – 140 (1969).

SHAFRIR, E.: Partition of unesterified fatty acids in normal and nephrotic syndrome serum and its effect on serum electrophoretic pattern. J. clin. Invest. **37,** 1775 – 1782 (1958).

SHELLEY, W. B., JUHLIN, L.: Degranulation of the basophil in man induced by alimentary lipemia. Amer. J. med. Sci. **242,** 211 – 222 (1961).

SLEIN, M. W.: In: Methods in Enzymology, Vol. 5 , S. P. COLOWICK and N. O. KAPLAN (Eds.). New York: Academic Press 1962.

SNELLMAN, O., SYLVÉN, B., JULÉN, C.: Analysis of the native heparin-lipoprotein complex including the identification of a heparin complement (heparin co-factor) obtained from extracts of tissue mast cells. Biochim. Biophys. Acta (Amst.) **7,** 98 – 109 (1951).

SPITZER, J. J.: Influence of protamine on alimentary lipemia. Amer. J. Physiol. **147,** 43 – 45 (1953).

SPITZER, J. A., SPITZER, J. J.: Effect of liver on lipolysis by normal and postheparin sera in the rat. Amer. J. Physiol. **185,** 18 – 22 (1956).

STAEMMLER, M.: Untersuchung über Vorkommen und Bedeutung der histiogenen Mastzellen im menschlichen Körper unter normalen und pathologischen Verhältnissen. Frankfurt. Z. Path. **25,** 391 – 435 (1921).

STEIN, Y., SHAPIRO, B.: Uptake and metabolism of triglycerides by the liver. J. Lipid Res. **1,** 326 – 331 (1960).

STIVALA, S. S., HERBST, M., KRATKY, O., PILZ, I.: Physico-chemical studies of fractionated bovine heparin. Arch. Biochem. Biophys. **127,** 795 – 802 (1968).

THOMA, K., WERCINSKI, A.: Untersuchungen über die Funktion der Granula der basophilen Leukocyten. Dtsch. med. Wschr. **75,** 86 – 87 (1950).

TOMINAGA, F., OKA, K., YOSHIDA, H.: The isolation and identification of Oxylosylserine and S-methylcysteine sulfoxide from human urine. J. Biochem. (Tokyo) **57,** 717 – 720 (1965).

TROUT, E. L., ESTES, E. H., FRIEDBERG, S. J.: Titration of free fatty acids of plasma: a study of current methods and a new modification. J. Lipid Res. **1,** 199 – 202 (1960).

TURIN, E.: see page 27.

WALTON, K. W.: Chemistry and mode of action of heparin and related compounds. Brit. med. Bull. **11,** 62 – 69 (1955).

WALTON, P. L., RICKETTS, C. R., BANGHAM, D. R.: Heterogeneity of heparin. Brit. J. Haemat. **12,** 310 – 325 (1966).

WASSERMANN, F.: The concept of the „fat organ“. In: Fat as a Tissue, p. 22. K. RODAHL and B. ISSEKUTZ (Eds.). New York: McGraw-Hill 1963.

WEGELIUS, O., ASBOE-HANSEN, G.: Histamine and connective tissue. Acta chem. scand. **3,** 18 – 21 (1957).

WERLE, E., AMANN, R.: Zur Physiologie der Mastzellen als Träger des Heparins und Histamins. Klin. Wschr. **34,** 624 – 630 (1956).

WERMEL, E., SASSUCHIN, D.: see page 69.

WESTPHAL, O., LÜDERITZ, O., BISTER, F.: Über die Extraktion von Bakterien mit Phenol/Wasser. Z. Naturforsch. **7 b,** 148 – 155 (1952).

WILLS, E. D.: Lipases, pp. 197 – 240. In: Advances in Lipid Research, Vol. 3, R. PAOLETTI and D. KRITCHEVSKY (Eds.). New York-London: Academic Press 1965.

WISLOCKI, G. B., DEMPSEY, E. W.: see page 69.

WOLFROM, M. L., WEISBLAT, D. I., KARABINOS, J. V., MCNELLY, W. H., MCLEAN, J.: Chemical studies on crystalline barium acid heparinate. J. Amer. chem. Soc. **65,** 2077 – 2085 (1943).

WOLFROM, M. L., MCNEELY, W. H.: The relation between the structure of heparin and the anticoagulant activity. J. Amer. chem. Soc. **67,** 748 – 753 (1945).

WOLFROM, M. L., SHEN, T. M., SUMMERS, G. G.: 1953. Cited in: J. S. BRIMACOMBE and J. M. WEBBER: Mucopolysaccharides, Vol. 6, Amsterdam-Lond-New York: Elsevier 1964.

WOLFROM, M. L., VERCELLOTTI, J. R., HORTON, D.: A disaccharide from carboxylreduced heparin. J. org. Chem. **27,** 705 – 706 (1962).

WOLFROM, M. L., VERCELLOTTI, J. R., HORTON, D.: The linkage in the disaccharide from carboxyl-reduced heparin. J. org. Chem. **28,** 278 – 279 (1963).

WOLFROM, M. L., VERCELLOTTI, J. R., HORTON, D.: Two disaccharides from carboxyl-reduced heparin. The linkage sequence in heparin. J. org. Chem. **29,** 540 – 547 (1964).

YOSHIZAWA, Z.: Heparin. Protein (Tokyo) **14,** 595 – 603 (1969).

ZEMPLÉNYI, T.: The lipolytic and esterolytic activity of blood and tissue and problems of atherosclerosis, p. 235. In: Advances in Lipid Research, Vol. 2, R. PAOLETTI and D. KRITCHEVSKY (Eds.). New York-London: Academic Press 1964.

ZÖLLNER, N.: In: Lipoproteidlipase. H. BRAUNSTEINER, S. SAILER and F. SANDHOFER (Eds.). Basel-New York: Karger 1963.

ZÖLLNER, N., SCHENCK, R., MANNMEUSEL, L.: Veränderungen des Dispersionsgrades der Plasmalipoide durch Heparin. Naturwissenschaften **39**, 111 – 114 (1952).
ZÖLLNER, N., SEITZ, W., KÖNIG, E.: Die Hemmung der Lipaemie-Klärungsreaktion durch Heparin. Hoppe Seylers Z. physiol. Chem. **314**, 177 – 182 (1959).
ZÖLLNER, N., KIRSCH, K.: In: Untersuchungen und Bestimmungen der Lipide im Serum. N. ZÖLLNER und D. EBERHAGEN (Eds.). Berlin-Heidelberg-New York: Springer 1965.
ZOLLINGER, H. U.: Gewebsmastzellen und Heparin (phasenmikroskopische Untersuchung) Experientia (Basel) **6**, 384 – 386 (1950).

II. Histamine in Blood Basophils

1. Detection of Histamine in Basophils

CODE (1937) was the first to find histamine in leukocyte concentrates obtained from various species and he believed the eosinophils to be carriers of blood histamine (CODE and MITCHELL, 1957). CODE and MACDONALD (1937) pointed out that the histamine concentration in serum is greatly increased in myeloproliferative diseases. In chronic myeloid leukemias, the activity of serum histaminase was also found to be increased (THIERSCH, 1947 a, b). In addition, a positive correlation could be found between the leukocyte count and the serum histamine level.

Further studies carried out on thrombocyte concentrates, isolated lymphocytes from lymph nodes, and ascites monocytes yielded no significant amounts of histamine (CODE, 1952; GRAHAM *et al.*, 1955). The hypothesis that serum histamine derives from granulocytes was supported by the observation of a considerable hyperhistaminemia in chronic myeloid leukemias but not in chronic lymphatic leukemias. SHIMKIN and BIERMAN (1950) found the histamine level in patients with chronic myeloid leukemia to be about 2300 µg/100 ml, hence very much higher than in healthy subjects (2 – 8.5 µg/100 ml). The blood histamine level in cases of reactive leukocytosis, however, showed normal values. At first, this finding appeared to speak against the relationship of granulocytes to histamine. The exact localization of histamine in the blood remained uncertain until 1952.

A relationship between blood basophil count and the histamine concentration of serum was discussed by VALENTINE *et al.* (1950). In 1952, GRAHAM *et al.* were able to demonstrate the presence of histamine in blood basophils. This study showed that blood basophils contain about 50 times more histamine than any other blood cell; fractionation of the blood cells was carried out with fibrinogen and albumin gradients at 12° C and pH 7. The histamine was determined by transferring it into basic mono-dinitrofluorobenzol after extraction in methylene-N-hexylketone, followed by treatment with concentrated hydrochloric acid. The thrombocyte fraction obtained by this technique contained 0.009 µg/10^9 platelets. Further platelet samples with a leukocyte: thrombocyte ratio of 1 : 200 showed double this histamine concentration. On the other hand, leukocyte concentrates with an average basophil count of 6/mm³ showed a histamine concentration of 49×10^6 μg and those with 104/mm³ a concentration of 222×10^6 μg. This shows that more than half the blood histamine is derived from the basophils. Other studies showed that the histamine concentration in the total leukocyte population is almost equal to that in the total granulocyte fraction. VALENTINE *et al.* (1955) calculated for granulocytes an average histamine content of 25 μg/10^9 cells. A similar study by GRAHAM *et al.* (1955) yielded a histamine content of 27 μg/10^9 granulocytes. For total leukocytes the value was, of course, somewhat lower. For example, HUMPHREY and JAQUES (1954) found 15 μg/10^9 cells, and GRAHAM *et al.* (1955) 13 μg/10^9 leukocytes. According to the last-mentioned authors, the histamine concentration in blood basophils amounted to 20,000 times that in platelets and 1,000,000 times that in serum. Blood basophils contain about 1 pg of histamine per cell, i.e. more than 1/20 that found in tissue mast cells.

The investigations of VALENTINE *et al.* (1955) on 14 cases of chronic myeloid leukemias yielded similar results and revealed a positive correlation between the histamine level of the leukocyte concentrates and the blood basophil count. These authors found that the histamine content was 1.9 to 3.3 g/10^8 myeloid leukocytes when the blood basophil count was 1.7 to 5.1% of the total leukocytes, and when the basophil count was 6.1 to 37.1%, the histamine content was 3.4 to 76.7 μg/10^8 leukocytes. The amount of non-basophil myeloid cells found during these investigations was between 76.2 and 90.4% of leukocytes. The findings of GRAHAM and VALENTINE were later confirmed by several other workers.

The sharp decrease in basophil count observed by CODE and MITCHELL (1957) subsequent to cortisone administration was found to be accompanied by a swift fall in the blood histamine concentration.

Direct evidence for the occurrence of histamine in blood basophils was produced on the basis of new concentration procedures for these cells. SAMPSON and ARCHER (1967), for instance, were able to increase the proportion of blood basophils up to 17.5% of total leukocytes by fractional centrifugation of leukocyte concentrates. According to these authors, the histamine content of normal blood basophils amounts to 2.4 ± 0.6 μg/10^6 basophils. Similar investigations in cases of chronic myeloid leukemias yielded an average histamine content of 1.8 ± 1.4 μg/10^6 basophils.

The blood histamine concentration has been well investigated in cases of chronic myeloid leukemias and in so-called basophil leukemias. As early as 1936, MARCU *et al.* found that the normal blood histamine concentration (10 – 30 μg/100 ml) was significantly elevated in cases of chronic myeloid leukemia and could be up to 100 times the normal values. In further communications, MARCU *et al.* (1937) pointed out that blood histamine concentrations were elevated in all his 6 cases of myeloid leukemia, especially after X-ray treatment. Further evidences have been maintained by other authors (CODE, 1937; 1953; CACCIAVILLANI and GIBERTINI, 1942; THIERSCH, 1947; ASTALDI and ALLEGRI, 1951; VALENTINE *et al.*, 1952; KELEMAN *et al.*, 1953; RILEY, 1954; VALENTINE *et al.*, 1957; GINGOLD and TEITEL, 1959; 1966; NORDEN *et al.*, 1967).

The elevation of the blood histamine concentration in cases of myeloid leukemia appears to be a fairly constant phenomenon. GINGOLD and his coworkers attempted to use the blood histamine level as a differential-diagnostic criterion for distinguishing myeloid leukocytes from leukemoid reactions (GINGOLD, 1939 a, b, c). These authors consider the blood histamine determination to be much more reliable in the differential diagnosis of chronic myeloid leukemia than the determination of alkaline leukocyte phosphatase or evidence of the Philadelphia chromosome.

The high histamine level in chronic myeloid leukemia, myelofibrosis with myeloid metaplasia, and polycythemia rubra vera is attributed to an increase in the basophil count. GINGOLD (1968) took the view that leukemic blood basophils have a higher histamine content than normal cells. This is contrary to the direct analytical studies of SAMPSON and ARCHER (1967), who found a lower histamine content in myeloid blood basophils. The blood basophil count is often elevated in myeloproliferative disorders. Hence, the increased blood histamine concentration in these cases is solely due to an increase in the blood basophil count; the individual blood basophils, in fact, contain less histamine than normal basophils.

There is still no unanimous agreement concerning the ability of the human orgnism to synthesize histamine. GADDUM (1956) believed histamine to be a substance similar to vitamins, possibly formed by the bacterial flora in the intestine and absorbed. This idea had its origin in the findings of WATON (1956), who could not detect any histidine-decarboxylating enzymes in human tissue. GADDUM's hypothesis was based upon the idea that some bacteria of the intestinal flora can decarboxylate histidine to histamine. Oral administration of L-histidine produces an increase in both free and conjugated histamine in the urine; this effect is inhibited by pretreatment with succinyl sulfate thiazol (IRVINE *et al.*, 1959). However, after a dose of 14 mg ^{14}C-labeled L-histidine (10 μCi), these authors could not detect ^{14}C-labeled histamine or its metabolites in the urine of either healthy persons or patients with urticaria pigmentosa.

The hypothesis on the vitamin nature of histamine was contradicted by DUNÉR *et al.* (1961), who could find no increase in the urine histamine after oral administration of 5 mg L-histidine in 4 healthy persons. Moreover high doses of histamine (133 mg) provoked no increase in the urine histamine concentration (ADAM, 1950). Orally administered histamine, according to these investigations, appears to be almost completely destroyed. LINDELL and WESTLING (1966) believe that the question whether or not histamine can be synthesized out of elementary metabolites in the human organism has not yet been settled. So long as this question remains open, it cannot be accepted that the only pathway of histamine synthesis is through decarboxylation of histidine.

The ability of tissue mast cells to transform histidine into histamine directly has been adequately demonstrated. LILJA *et al.* (1960) demonstrated the transformation of L-histidine labeled on the imidazole ring intohistamine in sterile lung specimens. DEMIS and BROWN (1961) and LINDELL *et al.* (1961 a) showed that histidine is converted into histamine in human tissue mast cells in urticaria pigmentosa. The studies of HARTMANN *et al.* (1960) showed that human blood basophils are able to synthesize histamine through decarboxylation of ^{14}C-L-histidine. Their findings were supported by other authors (LINDELL *et al.*, 1961; LINDELL and VISKE, 1961). The ability of the leukocyte concentrates to form histamine correlated with the blood basophil count.

It is now confirmed that the specific enzyme histidine-decarboxylase occurs in measurable amounts in histamine-synthesizing cells (SCHAYER, 1966). Since then, numerous methods for measuring the activity of this enzyme have been developed (review by SCHAYER, 1966).

2. Biochemical-Functional Significance of Histamine

It is not the purpose of this monograph to review the current state of knowledge concerning histamine. We refer here only to works which, directly or indirectly, contribute to our understanding of the functional potencies of basophils as 'histaminocytes' (WERLE and AMANN, 1955). This section deals briefly with the chemical properties of histamine as they affect its role in the cytochemistry of blood basophils. In addition, we give selected data on the biological activity and its pathogenetic significance. The structure-action relationship can be only marginally covered. For detailed information on histamine, we recommend the reviews and monographs by ROCHA E SILVA (1955; 1966) and SCHAYER (1956).

Histamine is a low-molecular-weight organic base. Depending upon its structural configuration, the free base occurs in two tautomeric forms, 4-(2-aminoethyl)-imidazole and 5-(2-aminoethyl)-imidazole. The steady equilibrum can be arrested by substitution at position 1 of the imidazole ring. The free base and many of its salts are readily soluble in water, alcohol, and chloroform, and slightly soluble in ether. Histamine is extremely heat-stable in acidic media. Through titration, two basic elements can be detected on the histamine molecules at pH 5.94 and 9.80 (HOLMES and JONES, 1960).

Among the physicochemical properties of histamine, the solubility of its salt is important for the cytochemistry of blood basophils for, through certain reactions, stabilization of the otherwise extremely water-soluble basophil granules can be achieved. As early as the turn of the century, researchers knew that a water-insoluble histamine precipitate occurs after the addition of mercuric chloride and potassium hydroxide. In histamine-containing solutions, a gelatinous precipitate of the complex salts $(Ag(C_5H_9N_3)NO_3 \cdot XH_2O$ can be obtained after addition of silver nitrate at pH 7.5 (HATEM, 1955). Contrary to earlier ideas, complex compounds with zinc are not water-soluble. The insolubility of the zinc-histamine complex salts has been successfuly employed for histamine determinations (ACKERMAN and FUCHS, 1939; KAPELLER-ALDER, 1941). The complex salt is strongly water-soluble in acidic media (WEITZEL and FRETZDORFF, 1956). The chelate-like complex salts of histamine with copper, cobalt, and nickel are moderately water-soluble.

Histamine, being a primary amine, possesses some chemical properties typical of this group, such as the ability to react with carbohydrates (aryl and alkyl) and aromatic aldehydes.

By heating an acidic aqueous histamine solution with formaldehyde, a bicyclic compound can be obtained (Hoffman *et al.*, 1951). The reaction with diazotized aromatic amines represents a typical property of imidazoles and leads to the formation of azo-dyes which can be applied for analytical purposes.

a) Structure-Activity Relationship of Histamine

The varied biological activities of histamine make an exact analysis of its structure-activity relationship problematical. Over 200 different compounds with a histamine-like activity have been developed. Histamine is said to induce three basic biological effects: contraction of the smooth muscle fibers, lowering of the arterial blood pressure, and stimulation of stomach secretion. Many other effects are also ascribed to histamine. Schayer (1960) believes that the promotion of the microcirculation on the capillary level is the most important physiological function of this biogenic amine. Histamine has been found to be liberated in abundance by muscle action, producing tissue hyperemia (Dunér and Pernow, 1958; Schayer 1964). The increase in capillary permeability brought on by the action of histamine also leads to better perfusion of the extravasal space (Majno and Palade, 1961). An increase has been observed in the phagocytic activity of leukocytes under the influence of histamine (Fernex, 1968).

When used in appropriate experimental procedures, histamine can strongly increase hyaluronidase activity (Kasatkina, 1963). Ryvkina (1957) reported a singnificant increase in hyaluronidase activity after application of low doses of histamine. The findings of Rikhter (1960) support this observation. In addition, Wegelius and Asboe-Hansen (1957) found that after addition of histamine, a strong depolymerization of the tissue acid glycosaminoglycans occurs, accompanied by increased permeability of the tissue ground substance and an increase of glycoproteins in serum.

There does not seem to be any clear connection between a particular molecular site and one or more of these biological properties. The situation is further complicated by the observation that the various histamine equivalents exert very different effects in various animals.

According to Walker *et al.* (1941), the molecule fragment $=N{>}C-C-C-N{<}$ presents the structural requirements for a histamine-like activity. Lee and Jones (1949) and Jones *et al.* (1954), however, could not support this view. Pyrazole compounds substituted at position 1 by $-CH_2-CH_2NH_2$ have a histamine-like activity but do not demonstrate an atomic configuration of the type mentioned above. Furthermore, numerous substances are known to possess the postulated 'histamine specific group' (Walter *et al.*, 1941) but do not biologically develop a histamine-like effect.

According to JONES (1966), histamine and histamine equivalents possess relatively small nitrogen-containing heterocyclic rings with a 2-aminoethyl side chain. He divided the histamine equivalents into imidazole, pyrazole, and triazole derivatives and distinguished them from another group of substances which are not chemically uniform.

An intramolecular hydrogen bond between the side chain and the ring was also deemed responsible for the development of a histamine-like activity (LEE and JONES, 1949). The activity of histamine is not impaired by methylation at position 2, but the introduction of methyl groups at position 5 of the ring leads to a strong decrease in biological activity. According to ROCHA E SILVA (1944), histamine possesses two active groups which are responsible for reacting with the cellular receptors. The imine group of the imidazole ring performs the haptophore function and the amino groups of the side chain the toxophore function. At the pH found in tissue, histamine may act as a proton donor. A linkage develops between the imine group of the imidazole ring and the free amino groups (ROCHA E SILVA, 1961). Such a mode of linkage, which would explain the bonding character of the receptors of the organ and of the tissue storage sites, is compatible with the action of numerous histamine liberators. If this hypothesis is accepted, it becomes possible to explain the histamine-liberating action of many different groups of substances, such as organic solvents, proteolytic enzymes (trypsin, chymotrypsin), amines, tubocurarine, strychnine, atropine, and such synthetic polymers as compound 48/80. The factor common to histamine liberation, in spite of the different mechanisms underlying it, would be that practically all of the substances cited lead to a breaking off of such hydrogen bonds. The energy-requiring processes that occur with phosphorylation of the corresponding receptor groups (imidazole or arginine) would then lead to a histamine release. Evidence for such a mechanism has been suggested in connection with immuno-reactions of the immediate type and the action of compound 48/80 (MOUSSATCHÉ and PROUVOST-DANON, 1958; ROTHSCHILD *et al.*, 1961).

Histamine is interesting because of its manifold biological actions. The pharmacological importance of histamine – the biological mechanisms of its liberation and the substructural configuration of its local concentration – have been the subject of numerous papers and provoked much lively speculation. A local accumulation of very water-soluble and biologically highly active substances in certain circumscribed areas of a cell is only conceivable if their action is in some way restrained by appropriate blockade of the active sites. A very special structural cell equipment would be necessary to stabilize and bind biogenic amines in such high concentrations.

The development of suitable experimental models, such as concentrates of blood basophils and tissue mast cells resuspended in certain media, has made it possible to gain an insight into the finer mechanisms underlying histamine accumulation and release. A review of the results so far obtained on tissue mast cells is required for a better understanding of the problems at hand.

The special structures which allow a local concentration of histamine to exist in a stabilized form must possess certain physicochemical properties:

1. They must show a high affinity for histamine.
2. The resulting complex must be very stable and as far as possible water-insoluble.
3. The bound histamine must be stored in a biologically inactive form.
4. The receptor must be able to release the amine when necessary.

If the substances present in blood basophils and tissue mast cells are examined under these aspects, heparin is seen to be an ideal compound. While histamine is able to form labile bonds with peptides by means of hydrogen bonding, the acid valences of heparin offer an appropriate matrix for binding cationic substances like histamine. WERLE and AMANN (1955) investigated the bonding capacity of heparin for histamine by using appropriate test models. With an optimum pH of 2.8, the reaction showed a strong dependency upon the hydrogen ion concentration *in vitro*. According to the results of these authors, the amino group of histamine and the sulfo groups of heparin are involved in such bondings. Assuming a molecular weight of 16,000 for heparin, they calculated a heparin: histamine molar ratio of 1 : 29. PATON (1955; 1957) also ascribed the granular accumulation of histamine to its basic affinity for the strongly acidic heparin.

We attempted to check this question on human blood basophils. The test was carried out on a case of chronic myeloid leukemia with a total leukocyte count of $230{,}000/mm^3$. The blood basophil count amounted to $188{,}600/mm^3$, or 82% of the total leukocytes. To settle such questions, heparin and histamine must, for methodological reasons, be present in sufficient amounts. As normal blood basophils cannot easily be obtained in such large amounts, we were forced to use leukemic cells. If we consider the results obtained with purified compounds, this does not seem to have any bearing on the results of the experiment. Using the experimental procedures described below, we isolated the leukocytes and studied them in dialysis chambers.

60 ml of blood was collected from the cubital vein in siliconized glass containers previously moistened with a 2.5% Na_2 EDTA solution and dried in a heating chamber at 50° C. The total leukocyte count was determined by the usual method in Thoma-Neu chambers, and the blood basophil count by the technique of COOPER and CRUICKSHANK (1966) in Fuchs-Rosenthal chambers. Finally, the blood sample was centrifuged for 10 min at 150 to 200 g, and the leukocyte layer carefully isolated. Only a few leukocytes could be detected in the remaining plasma and erythrocyte fraction; the leukocyte yield always amounted to over 95%, so that possible errors resulting from this could be neglected. The leukocytes obtained in this manner were then resuspended in a slightly modified buffer solution as described by UVNÄS and THON (1961) and GILLESPIE and LEVINE (1969) to give a final volume of 18 ml. The buffer solution contained 154 mM NaCl, 2,7 mM KCl, 4 mM Na_2HPO_4, 2.7 mM KH_2PO_4 and 100 mg/1 disodium

EDTA. The pH of the solution was adjusted with 1N HCL to 5.0. The entire procedure was conducted at room temperature.

Three chamber systems were utilized (Nos. 1 – 3) which, in a total volume of 6 ml per chamber, contained an average of $3{,}661.26 \times 10^6$ blood basophils (610.21×10^6 per ml). After resuspension, the basopil portion amounted to about 97% of the initial value. The chamber system was composed of a funnel-shaped inner chamber (liquid volume 6 ml) which, after cytolysis, was brought into the outer chamber (liquid volume 54 ml). The bottom of the funnel-shaped inner chamber was closed with dialysis foil. The whole system contained a liquid volume of 60 ml. The histamine concentration was measured in the cell-free inner chamber, 15 min after the start of the test by the fluorometric method of SHORE *et al.* (1959). For this purpose we used a spectral fluorometer (SF-1-Flurispec from BAIRD-Atomic). Finally, the contents of the three inner chambers were frozen, thawed and ultra-sonicated for 5 sec three times at short intervals, and the histamine concentration was once again determined (Table. 15). After cytolysis, we added 1 mg/ml of protamine sulfate to inner chamber No. 2; 0.025 mg/ml of compound 48/80 to No. 3. The inner chambers were then inserted into the outer chambers and the histamine concentration in the outer chambers was measured at intervals for the first then again after 8, 9 and 10 h (Table 16).

Table 15. Basophil count and histamine concentration in three inner dialysis chambers (V = 6 ml) prior to and after cytolysis. For details, refer to text

Inner chamber No.	Basophil count $\times 10^6$ per ml	Total histamine µg/ml Prior to Cytolysis	After Cytolysis
1	611.46	2,266	10,493
2	609.80	3,124	12,110
3	609.36	2,662	10,200

We found that even a careful suspension of blood basophils in buffer solutions leads to a liberation of histamine, which in our investigations amounted to about 25% of the total histamine content. The liberation of this so-called labile portion of histamine proceeds without light-optically detectable cell alterations. Suspended tissue mast cells also liberate part of their histamine content without any obvious structural alterations. Some findings support the assumption that heparin is not set free by the liberation of this labile histamine. At any rate, our results show a swift equilibration of the concentration in both chambers, which makes this assumption probable. It is possible that the histamine portion that is released is bonded to the peptide chain by weak secondary bonds (hydrogen bonds).

Cytolysis led to a rapid increase in the histamine concentration in the inner chambers. The values (Table 15) were approximately equal and aver-

Table 16. Histamine concentration in three outer dialysis chambers (V = 54 ml). Samples were taken at intervals after cytolytic destruction of the suspended basophils in inner chambers. Compounds administered additionally are given in brackets

Sampling intervals after cytolysis h	Histamine concentration (μg/ml) in outer chambers Chamber No. 1	2 (+Protamine)	3 (+C 48/80)
0.5	1,794	6,048	4,876
1	1,917	7,563	4,988
1.5	1,922	8,078	6,385
2	2,052	9,477	7,036
8	2,496	9,704	7,801
9	2,878	10,200	8,138
10	4,439	10,465	8,802

aged 2010.29 μg/ml of the incubation solution and 2.9 μg/10^6 blood basophils. In spite of the high histamine level in the inner chambers, the concentration in the outer dialysates remained very low. This is especially clear from the values for outer chamber No. 1. Here, the histamine concentration 2 h after cytolysis was 2,052 μg/ml. Even eight hours later, only a low histamine concentration was determined (2,496 μg/ml). In contrast, a swift concentration equilibrium between the chamber spaces occurred in the other two chamber systems (Nos. 2 and 3). The values for all three outer chambers are given in Table 16. This procedure showed that protamine sulfate and compound 48/80, whose high affinity for heparin has long been known, liberate histamine from its bonding onto heparin. The unbound histamine can, following the concentration gradient, pass through the semipermeable membrane, whereas the complex of heparin and histamine cannot be dialysed by this procedure.

The affinity of histamine for heparin has also been demonstrated in other studies. WERLE and AMANN (1955), for instance, showed that heparin can easily be precipitated out of an alcohol solution by adding histamine. After addition of histamine or serotonin, metachromatic heparin-toluidine blue solutions lose their metachromasia (KELLER, 1958).

KELLER (1958) calculated a molecular ratio of 1 : 16 for the heparin-histamine complex. He further pointed out that the imidazole ring of histamine takes part in the bonding onto heparin. Similar findings have also been reported by SANYAL and WEST (1956).

Even if none of these findings alone can be accepted as absolute proof, when they are taken together it can hardly be doubted that heparin forms a salt-type bonding with biogenic amines. The resulting complex is extremely stable, which shows the high affinity of its reacting partners. As the example of protamine sulfate in our investigations shows, it is possible, under certain conditions, to displace histamine from the complex.

Numerous papers on the degranulation mechanism of blood basophils and particularly tissue mast cells support the assumption that an intragranular heparin-histamine complex is formed. According to WALTON (1955) and HIGGINBOTHAM (1959; 1966), many cations are able to liberate histamine from its bonds with heparin. As the concentration of liberated histamine increases in the incubation solution, so cationic substances accumulate in the granules. Toluidine blue, for example, can be traced through the metachromasia and stilbamidine by its strong fluorescence. Compound 48/80, a low polymer of p-methoxy-N-methylphenethylamine, which effects a strong degranulation of the mast cells, like protamine also forms a bonding with heparin, according to the investigations of MOTA *et al.* (1953). The histamine portion, which has been thus displaced and liberated, leads in sufficiently high dosage to a lethal circulatory collapse in experimental animals (PAPACOSTAS *et al.*, 1959). Pretreatment of the animals with heparin prevents a lethal outcome. Similar observations have also been made with snake venom (HIGGINBOTHAM, 1959 a, b; 1962 a, b). Also typical is the finding that the toxic effect of compound 48/80 is increased by the simultaneous administration of toluidine blue or protamine sulfate.

ACTH, which forms a complex bond with heparin, also increases the toxic effect of otherwise sublethal doses of the histamine liberator polymyxin B (HIGGINBOTHAM and DOUGHERTY, 1956 a, b). We are not in a position to judge whether the observation that heparin inhibits the suppressive action of glucocorticoids upon eosinophils and decreases the production of aldosterone, thereby causing an increase of the sodium diuresis (WEISBECKER and SCHRÖTER, 1954; BRAUNSTEINER *et al.*, 1959; CEJKA *et al.*, 1960; SCHLATMANN *et al.*, 1960; WILSON and GOETZ, 1964), is in fact connected with mechanism discussed above. MACINTOSH and PATON (1949) and PATON (1955; 1957) have shown that histamine can be displaced in the complex by stronger organic bases. The ability of many organic bases to liberate histamine is based upon their strong affinity for heparin.

DABNEY and STANLEY (1960) studied the affinity of heparin for the known histamine liberators and established three criteria for estimating this affinity:

1. Loss of metachromasia of a heparin-toluidine blue solution.
2. The inhibiting effect of histamine liberators upon heparin-activated serum lipoylsis.
3. The effect of heparin upon the toxicity of histamine liberators.

In this investigation, compound 48/80 showed the highest affinity in a concentration of 100 µg/ml and displaced 34 µg of toluidine blue. To displace the same amount of toluidine blue, 10 times as much reserpine and more than 1000 µg of polyvinylpyrrolidone were found to be necessary.

In agreement with other results, histamine liberators were found to be potent inhibitors of serum lipolysis. Serum to which 0.025 mg/ml of compound 48/80 was added showed a densitometric clearing of 0.002 after 15 and 30 min, and a decrease of 0.004 in optical density after 60 min. The control group showed a much higher lipolytic activity of 0.018 after 15 min, 0.028 after 30 min, and 0.036 after 60 min. Similar results were obtained in investigations of the effect of heparin upon toxic doses of tubocurarine and strychnine in C57 BL mice. Out of 73 mice treated with 0.55 mg of tubocurarine per kg body weight, 35 died. The mortality rate among 72 mice treated with the same dose of tubocurarine and 2.85 mg of heparin per kg body weight was 11; a considerable reduction. Similar results were obtained with strychnine sulfate.

In summary, it can be stated that intragranular heparin is bound onto certain cellular structures composed of lipid-protein complexes. Histamine forms a salt-type complex with heparin; this complex is relatively stable and very insoluble. Some 20 to 25% of the total histamine appears to be bound in a labile form, probably through hydrogen bonding, to the intragranular protein structures. The bound histamine exists in a biologically inactive form, and can be competitively displaced from its complexes by numerous substances with an affinity for heparin. Under *in-vitro* conditions, this process appears to be the primary mechanism of action of the histamine liberators. It is not yet definitely known whether, under *in-vivo* conditions, similar processes also play a decisive role in histamine liberation. It is highly suggestive that under *in-vivo* conditions certain transmitters or mediators take part in basophil granulolysis. At any rate, numerous findings support the assumption that histamine liberation *in vivo* is an energy-consuming process linked with phosphorolysis and not a simple ion-exchange mechanism. The last step in histamine liberation, the release of histamine from the excorporated histamine complex, may involve an ion-exchange mechanism.

b) Immunological Significance of Blood Basophils

Qualitative and quantitative alterations in the blood basophils have been repeatedly reported in connection with hypersensitivity reactions. Although it is now generally accepted that these cells and their tissue counterparts are involved in certain immune reactions, the question still remains open as to whether these changes have a significant bearing on human diseases. Experiments with rats, rabbits and guinea pigs and therapeutic and prophylactic administration of sera to humans have suggested a connection between blood basophils and allergic reactions. Observations made on patients with bronchial asthma, urticaria, and anaphylactic reactions brought further insights into the relationship of blood basophils to the immune response. Especially interesting findings were obtained by morphological studies of immune reactions of the delayed type.

Generally, allergic edema is traced back to a histamine-induced increase in vascular permeability (Majno and Palade, 1961). The fact that blood basophils are rich in histamine is therefore considered to be of importance in this context. In order to analyse the numerous individual observations and the results of systematic investigations in the light of a generally accepted nosological classification, we distinguish with ZINSSER (1921) immune reactions of the immediate type and those of the delayed type. The next section covers immune reactions of the immediate type, after which the delayed type of immune response is discussed, including the closely related JONES-MOTE reaction.

α) Blood Basophils in Immune Reactions of the Immediate Type. In 1902, LEVADITI succeeded.in producing selective eosinophil and basophil leukocytosis in rabbits and guinea pigs by repeated intrapertitoneal injections of bacterial toxin. He determined in further experiments that a single subcutaneous injection of staphylococcal toxin induced basophil leukocytosis. Similar results were reported by PRÖSCHER (1909), who applied smallpox viruses to rabbits, and by SCHLECHT (1918) after administration of heterologous sera to guinea pigs. RINGOEN (1923) took advantage of the fact that repeated treatment with ovalbumin causes an increase in the basophil granulocytes in bone marrow in order to study the origin of these cells. CARVAHLO (1922) detected basophil leukocytosis in patients treated with antirabies serum. At first, these observations could not be clearly explained, and RINGOEN (1923) assumed a positive chemotactic response of blood basophils to the applied sera.

Since then similar observations have been made on tissue mast cells. Degranulation in immune reactions of the immediate type has been described by ASBOE-HANSEN (1950), DRENNAN (1951), HUMPHREY and MOTA (1959), and BOREUS (1961). It has been shown that the antigen-antibody reaction induces granulolysis of the tissue mast cells with liberation of histamine, which causes the local edema and is supposedly partly responsible for the inflammatory symptoms.

Various observations have been reported on the participation of basophil granulocytes in anaphylactic reactions. A significant decrease in the blood histamine was regularly observed in patients with acute urticarial manifestations (ROSE, 1941; NILZEN, 1947). This finding supports the involvement of blood basophils in immune reactions, as it is not seen in nonallergic skin diseases (TEDESCHI *et al.*, 1957; RORSMAN, 1958; BERSANI, 1959; SCHULZ *et al.*, 1959; BBRAUNSTEINER *et al.*, 1960). Patients with urticaria have been found to have significantly ($p < 0.001$) lower basophil counts ($8.1 \pm 2.7/mm^3$) compared with normal values ($44.8 \pm 2.4/mm^3$ recorded in 97 normal subjects) (RORSMAN, 1957).

The anaphylactic basophil fall can be explained in four different ways. (a) the emergence of basophils from the marrow pool may be selectively blocked; (b) the discharge of secretory granules may render the basophils unrecognizable; (c) basopenia may occur due to intravascular cytolysis; (d) the basophils may migrate into various organs and revert to cytolysis. The organs predominantly involved, the so-called shock organs, vary from species to species.

The first possibility is easily excluded: the fall in the basophil count in the peripheral blood is so rapid, taking at most a few minutes, that it cannot be due to a mechanism of this kind. Many authors believe that degranulation of blood basophils is associated with an anaphylactic reaction (FRICK and FRICK, 1966). Some secretory activity of the merocrine type is ascribed to blood basophils. According to this degranulation theory, the blood basophils secrete their biologically active substances in the manner of gland cells and are believed to be restored after degranulation by regranulation of the same cells. The observation that during anaphylaxis blood basophils reach such a low level that they can no longer be detected with the usual methods does not seem to be consistent with the theory of a secretory degranulation of these cells. We believe the fall in the basophil count of the peripheral blood and the swift drop in the blood histamine level to be due to basophils migrating into the so-called shock organs. The fact that the symptoms in the 'shock organs' closely resemble those observed in a local histamine accumulation supports this view. It is, therefore, very probable that the antigen-antibody complex, or agents liberated as a result of antigen fixation onto the lymphocyte surface, exert a positive chemotactic effect upon the blood basophils. The migration of the basophil granulocytes into the so-called shock organs would account for both the fall in blood histamine and the low basophil count. The assumption that granule resynthesis occurs subsequent to granule discharge implies recirculation of these cells, which, however, is inconsistent with the general biological behavior of the granulocytic cells.

Numerous findings support the view that basophils migrate into shock organs. Reference should first be made to the results of kinetic studies with ^{3}H-thymidine (Chapter C III). The average survival time of basophils in the blood under steady-state conditions in humans and in rabbits amounts to about 12 h, a finding that demonstrates the brisk kinetic activity of bloodbasophils. Our quantitative studies of bone marrow supply further evidence that the kinetic behavior of basophil granulocytes is very similar to that of neutrophils (Chapter B II). Repeated efforts to detect quantitative changes in the granule content in the course of an experimentally induced basophil fall in serial preparations of blood smears also failed (Chapter C III). Since the first papers by JUHLIN and SHELLEY (1961 a, b) and SHELLEY and JUHLIN (1962), there have been many studies of the qualitative, cytologically identifiable alterations in blood basophils during allergic reactions of the immediate type. In order to study the morphological alterations of blood basophils in immunologic reactions, JUHLIN and SHELLEY (1961 a) developed a method of basophil assay from the peripheral blood. Blood basophils were classified according to granule content into 18 different groups. The authors found an exceedingly wide variation in the number of granules in normal people, and large variations within their defined groups in allergic reactions of the immediate type, as well as in *in-vitro* experiments in which basophils were incubated with known allergens (JUHLIN and SHELLEY, 1961 b; SHELLEY and JUHLIN, 1962). Although most of the recent authors speak of degranulation (fired cells) on observing basophils with a low granule content, JUHLIN (1963) in his *in-vivo* experiments did not exclude the possibility that these cells could also be young blood basophils. He also suggested that such alterations might represent artifacts.

Anaphylactic sensitivity could be detected by means of this technique in cases of drug and food hypersensitivity (penicillin and milk allergy) without administration of the allergen (JUHLIN and WESTPHAL, 1962; SHELLEY, 1963). SHELLEY and CARO (1962) sensitized 26 4-week-old albino rabbits with intraperitoneally administered albumin solutions (5 injections, each of 2 ml of 3% albumin in physiologic saline, every 2nd day). After sufficient sensitization, heparinized blood samples were incubated at room temperature for 15 min with albumin (0.25 ml of blood and 0.025 ml of albumin solutions of different concentrations). The basophil exposure test *in vitro* with an antigen titer of 1 : 100 showed strong degranulation of the cells in all cases. In a dilution of antigen at 1 : 1000, positive results were obtained in 12 out of 15 animals. Further dilution of the antigen to 1 : 10,000 decreased the number of positively reacting animals to 3 out of 15. A parallel study of basophils in the peripheral blood showed that as early as 5 to 30 min after the albumin injection no blood basophils at all could be detected in 13 out of 14 sensitized animals. This observation was made in both smears and cell filtrates. The basophil count in the peripheral blood did not regain its initial value until 5 days post-injection (p.i.). This finding clearly shows that blood basophils are destroyed in the course of immune reactions of the immediate type.

It seems probable that during immune reactions of the immediate type blood basophils migrate into the organs concerned and are destroyed. The mode of basophil participation seems to be independent of the type of immune reaction. The alterations reported in blood basophils are similar in cases of hay fever, bronchial asthma, and their equivalents (BRECHTER and RORSMAN, 1965; DOLEN and AAS, 1966; PARRA *et al.*, 1966; KIMURA *et al.*, 1968; KAWAI, 1969; LICHTENSTEIN and NORMAN, 1969), as well as in consequence of a food allergy (fish).

Basophil alterations resulting from a drug allergy are clinically of more importance. Thrombocytopenic purpura, allergic skin manifestations, spastic bronchitis, true asthma, and catarrhal inflammations of the upper respiratory tract have all been observed in connection with drug allergies (aspirin, menthol, t-chlorobenzol and penicillin) (NALBANDIAN and PEARCE, 1965; RESNIK and SHELLEY, 1965; VIALLIER and SEDALLIAN, 1965; CHARPIN *et al.*, 1966; DREYFUSS *et al.*, 1966; GORDON, 1966; MACGOWAN, 1966; BOWSZYC and BOWSZYC, 1967; COHEN, 1967; GUDOWSKI and DIECKHOFF, 1967; KIRSCHBAUM *et al.*, 1967; LEVIN, 1967 a, b; REYNOLDS and SMITH, 1967; SOFTIC, 1967; CONSTANZI and COLTMAN, 1967; CRUICKSHANK and HAYE, 1968; GIRALDO *et al.*, 1969). Most of these studies were carried out with SHELLEY's basophil degranulation test. CHARPIN *et al.* (1966), in their *in-vitro* studies on humans pointed out the significance of this test for the recognition of penicillin allergy. The SHELLEY test may be useful not only for recognizing the allergenic and sensitizing properties of recently developed drugs, but also for the diagnosis of hypersensitivity to drugs already in use. This test has also proved useful in distinguishing allergic skin diseases from nonallergic dermatoses (MACGOWAN, 1966; CONSTANZI and COLTMAN, 1967; FEINBERG *et al.*, 1967).

Animal experiments have been of great help in devising sero-diagnostic tests involving animal basophils, the antigen in question, and serum from the patient under observation. Rapid cytolysis of blood basophils indicates hypersensitivity (VIALLIER and TOURAINE, 1966; ZIMMER *et al.*, 1966; FEIZI, 1967; SCHUPPLI, 1969). Similar experimental models using guinea pigs have been developed by ALBANUS and WINQVIST (1961) and RORSMAN (1962), GIERTZ *et al.* (1964), FRIEDBERG and BAUER (1965), BERNAUER *et al.* (1966), GREAVES and BURDIS (1968), HAHN *et al.* (1970) and STARR (1970). The results of these investigations agree fully with the results achieved in humans and rabbits. GREAVES and BURDIS (1968) and GREAVES and MONGAR (1968) were able to produce anaphylactic shock in guinea pigs through repeated applications of ovalbumin. They detected a massive degranulation of blood basophils, which was accompanied by histamine release.

The basic immunochemical mechanisms of basophil degranulation during allergic reactions, especially at the cellular or subcellular level, have only recently been systematically studied. The results obtained so far indicate that the antigen-antibody reaction proceeds directly upon the cell surface and initiates granulolysis through activation of the membrane ATPases. There is as yet no unanimous agreement over the preferentially participating immunoglobulin classes. By means of immuno-electrophoresis and gel diffusion in cases of cold urticaria, CONSTANZI and COLTMAN (1967) claimed to have found some cold-precipitable immunoglobulins belonging to the IgG class. HUBSCHER and GOODFRIEND (1969) studied the significance of reagins with sedimentation constants of 7 S and 19 S for basophil degranulation in allergic reactions of the immediate type. They pointed out the significance of these antibodies for a positive outcome of the indirect basophil test. The investigations of MIDDLETON *et al.* (1960), LICHTENSTEIN and OSSLER (1964, 1966 a, b), BERGQVIST and NILZEN (1966; 1969), LICHTENSTEIN *et al.* (1968) and VAN METRE *et al.* (1969) have provided further evidence for the participation of blood basophils in the immuno-reactions mediated by humoral factors.

Experiments devised by HASTIE (1971) have shed new light upon the cellular mechanisms of the allergic degranulation of blood basophils. He examined patients suffering from bronchial asthma and hay fever who showed a marked allergic reaction to certain plant extracts. As controls, he used normal persons and patients with bronchial asthma without detectable hypersensitivity to a certain antigen. Freshly obtained blood samples were centrifuged for 5 min at 150 to 200 g, and the leukocyte layer was removed and resuspended in a buffer solution (8 g NaCl; 0.2 g KCl; 1.15 g $Na_2HPO_4 \cdot 2H_2O$; 0.2 g KH_2PO_4 in 1000 ml distilled water). After repeated washings, the cells were centrifuged and collected in another solution (6.87 g NaCl; 0.43 g KCl; 0.184 g $CaCl_2 \cdot 2H_2O$; 0.29 g $MgSO_4 \cdot 7H_2O$; 0.18 g $NaH_2PO_4 \cdot 2H_2O$; 2.1 g Na_2HPO_3 and 1 g glucose in 1000 ml distilled water). The final molarity was for sodium 0.143, potassium 0.58, and calcium and magnesium 0.0012. The samples were injected into specially prepared chambers and studied under the phase-contrast microscope. No alterations in basophil morphology were observed when plant extracts were added to the basophil suspensions from control subjects. Basophils from 'atopic' persons showed a broadening of the cytoplasm on antigen contact. The alteration in cellular adhesiveness indicated altered membrane properties. Many basophils stopped their movements. In some cases, obvious degranulation of the blood basophils could be observed. Degranulation was accompanied by the appearance of optically empty vacuoles, which underwent fusion and occasionally formed lacunae up to 5μm in diameter. This phenomenon has also been described in the degranulation of tissue mast cells. Repeated washings of the cells strongly reduced their reactivity to allergen contact. Reincubation of the cells with autologous plasma or with the solution used for washing led to the reinstatement of their reactivity. On the basis of these investigations, HASTIE declared that antigen-induced granulolysis does not lead to cell death. He reached this conclusion, even though experiments on the same cells were only carried out for a short time, and those cells that were exposed to antigen were not observed over a longer period. He also failed to take into consideration the observation that granulolysis was accompanied by the formation of large vacuolar lacunae of up to 5 μm in diameter. This last finding, which is also known from degranulated tissue mast cells, is a clear indication of beginning cytolysis. On this point HASTIE's conclusion from his experimental results deviates from that of LICHTENSTEIN and OSSLER (1964; 1966 a, b) as well our own.

In summary, it can be concluded that blood basophils are involved in immune reactions of the immediate type, especially in drug and food allergies and atopic reactions. The antigen-antibody reaction proceeds on the surface of the cell. The resulting alteration in the membrane leads to basophil cytolysis, and degranulation proceeds with the liberation of histamine and heparin.

β) Blood Basophils in Immune Reactions of the Delayed Type. (Histopathology of the JONES-MOTE *Reaction)*

Histological visualization of blood basophils in tissue sections still presents a major technical problem. KLAUSNER und KREIBICH (1909, 1913) reported the occurrence of basophils (exudative mast cells) in local skin efflorescences in cases of scabies infestation, miliaria crystallina, eczema, erythema exudativum multiforme, herpes zoster, and herpes simplex. Later authors reported the presence of blood basophils in the lesions of contact dermatitis (WOLF-JÜRGENSEN, 1962; ASPEGREN *et al.*, 1963 a, b) and in areas of skin tests with staphylococcal extracts in patients with repeated staphylococcal infections (HU *et al.*, 1963). These observations gave rise to the hypothesis that basophils are also involved in allergic reactions of the delayed type. FREGERT and RORSMAN (1963) described basophil accumulations in local exudates in sensitized patients after intradermal injection of certain metal salts. ASPEGREN *et al.* (1964) detected numerous blood basophils in skin infiltrates after tuberculin sensitization. JUHLIN (1964) achieved selective inhibition of basophil migration in cantharidin-induced blisters of the skin through premedication with the glucocorticoid fluocinolone.

Investigations of this sort can be carried out either on skin-window preparations according to REBUCK u. CROWLY (1955) or on skin specimens treated prior to a surgical operation. For this purpose skin areas lying in the incision region of a previously planned surgical operation are suitable. The skin-window technique has been widely used because of its simplicity, but diffuculties arise when statements on the size and distribution of the inflammatory infiltrates are required. Furthermore, the quantity of the various cells present on skin-window preparations cannot be regarded as randomly representative due to the different speeds of cell migration during epidermis passage. Also, the excoriation required may induce an unspecific suppurative inflammation, which accounts for the high percentage of neutrophils found in this technique. The occurrence of blood basophils in the foci of allergic reactions of delayed type has been demonstrated by many authors by means of the skin window method (BARTH, 1958; WOLF-JÜRGENSEN, 1962; ASPEGREN *et al.,* 1963 a, b; HU *et al.,* 1963; JUHLIN, 1964; FREGERT and RORSMAN, 1964; FULTON and DERBES, 1964; WOLF- JÜRGENSEN, 1968).

Studies on successive skin excisates have only been occasionally reported. In their survey on local histological findings during immune reactions of ARTHUS, JONES-MOTE and tuberculin type, MARTINS and RAFFEL (1964) did not mention the presence of blood basophils. In skin specimens from corresponding foci, blood basophils were first reproted in guinea pigs by RICHERSON *et al.* (1969), DVORAK *et al.* (1970), RICHERSON *et al.* (1970), and DESAGA *et al.* (1970). Further evidence of the general participation of blood basophils in local allergic reactions is their occurrence in foci of the Arthus phenomenon, as observed by LUPOVITCH *et al.* (1968). Nevertheless, the number of basophils in the inflammatory foci seems to be fairly specific for the different forms of hypersensitivity reactions. In tuberculin reactions, as well as in other inflammatory reactions in which blood basophils have been observed, the percentage of blood basophils has never been found to exceed 1 to 2%. The JONES-MOTE reaction, however, seems to be exceptional in that blood basophils are the predominant cells in such lesions. Systematic investigations by RICHERSON *et al.* (1969; 1970) and DVORAK *et al.* (1970) have shown that this type of reaction can be differentiated from the usual forms of immediate and delayed types of immune reactions on the basis of clear differences in the genesis and quantitative cellular composition of its infiltrates. A proposal has been made by RICHERSON *et al.* (1970) and DVORAK *et al.* (1970) to term this special type of immune reaction *cutaneous basophil hypersensitivity* (CBH) and to regard it as synonymous with the JONES-MOTE reaction (JONES and MOTE, 1934), which can be also induced by incomplete FREUND's adjuvant and soluble proteins. Whereas the symptoms of acute inflammation in the classic tuberculin reaction are apparent between the 18th and 24 th h, the JONES-MOTE reaction shows only a moderate reddening. The inflammatory induration is also less than that of the classic tuberculin reaction within this time span; the central necrosis that sometimes occurs is never seen in the JONES-MOTE reaction. The neutrophil granulocytes regularly detectable in small numbers in the cellular infiltrates of the beginning phase of tuberculin reactions are not present in the foci of the

JONES-MOTE reaction. In contrast to the tuberculin reaction, eosinophil granulocytes are somewhat more often observed. The strong tissue infiltration with blood basophils represents the most striking finding and is highly characteristic for the JONES-MOTE reaction. DVORAK *et al.* (1970) found that a minimum of 23±7.1% and a maximum of 44±8.9% of the total exudate cells consisted of blood basophils. The corresponding values in classic tuberculin reactions are significantly lower. The lymphocyte count, on the other hand, predominates in the tuberculin reaction. The monocytes and monocytogenic macrophages are almost twice as numerous in the JONES-MOTE reaction as in the tuberculin reaction. According to some investigations, there is some involvement of regional lymph nodes in the JONES-MOTE reaction, a marked increase in the immunoblast content of the paracortical regions of the lymph nodes being observed 4 days after antigen contact.

The blood basophil count in the immediate subepidermal layers of the skin has been found to be markedly increased. According to DVORAK *et al.* (1970), the blood basophils in the upper layers of the epidermis amounted to 70% of the exudate cells. In typical tuberculin reactions, the basophil count was found to be higher (6.5±2.8) in the subepidermal areas than in the deeper epidermis layers. The authors attribute the high basophil count observed with the classic tuberculin reactions in the skin window slides to this phenomenon (WOLF-JÜRGENSEN, 1968). DESAGA *et al.*(1970) studied the histology of the classic tuberculin reaction and also found a strong participation of blood basophils. Between 12 and 36 h p.i. blood basophils made up about 2% of the total inflammatory cells; 36 h p.i. the absolute basophil count was several times more than the neutrophil count. Lymphocytes and monocytes, which made up 15 to 20% of the total inflammatory cells 3 h p. i., increased to over 50% 24 h p. i. Within 48 h, the percentage of neutrophils fell from 60% to less than 1%.

Lymph node involvement with development of tertiary follicles and increase of immunoblasts is also found in classic tuberculin reactions and other immune reactions of delayed type. LENNERT and ELSCHNER (1954) detected a raised basophil content in the regional lymph nodes in cases of dermatopathic lymphadenitis in man.

The induction of an immune reaction of delayed type is mainly done through application of antigen with complete FREUND's adjuvant, but the JONES-MOTE reaction is specifically induced with incomplete FREUND's adjuvant. Further, the JONES-MOTE reaction is induced through application of soluble proteins, antigen-antibody complexes with antigen surplus, or repeated application of minimal antigen concentrations. Other immunological peculiarities also distinguish the JONES-MOTE reaction from the classic tuberculin reaction. With the tuberculin reaction, about 3 weeks is required for sensitization, which then lasts for a long time. Induction time for the JONES-MOTE reaction is only 5 to 11 days, and the reaction is only detectable during this period. It is thus a 'temporary' mode of reaction or a transitional reagibility. Both the tuberculin reaction and the JONES-MOTE reaction have their maximum between the 24th and 48th h and are thereby distinguished from the rapid course (2 – 3 h) of the Arthus reaction. The Arthus reaction can be transferred with serum, whereas the tuberculin and Jones-Mote reactions can only be transferred by cells or cell fractions. The termination of local alterations is also characteristic. Whereas the tuberculin reaction with its typical morphology persists for a long time, the Jones-Mote reaction

Table 17. Skin lesions associated with different types of immune reactions

Specifications	Type of hypersensitivity reaction Tuberculin	Jones-Mote	Arthus
Inducible by	complete Freund's adjuvant and antigen	– incomplete Freund's adjuvant – soluble proteins * – antigen-antibody complex with antigen surplus * – minimal antigen concentrations: contact allergens * – viral components * – allografts * * without Freund's adjuvant	intravenous antigen apllication and successive s.c. antigen administration
Site of application	s.c.	s.c.	i.v. and s.c.
Time span between antigen application and reactivity on readministration	about 3 weeks	5 – 11 days	about 2 weeks
Time span between reapplication and appearance of inflammatory skin reaction	24 – 48 hours	24 – 48 hours	2 – 3 hours
Skin response inducible	for a long time	for 5 – 11 days (transitional)	antibody titer dependent
Transferable by	lymphocytes or lymphocyte lysates	lymphocytes	serum
	±	+ + +	+ + +
Duration of skin inflammatory lesion	long lasting	subsides with appearance of circulating antibodies	normal wound healing

heals with the appearance of circulating antibodies. The outcome of the Arthus phenomenon corresponds largely to normal wound healing. The main features of these three types of immune reponse are shown in Tables 17 and 18.

Table 18. Histological specification of skin foci of different hypersensitivity reactions

Histological Details	Type of Hypersensitivity Reaction Tuberculin	Jones-Mote	Arthus
Necrosis	+	–	+ + +
Intensity of inflammation	+ +	+	+ + +
Lymph node participation in inflammatory process	+	+ +	±
Neutrophils	+ +	+	+ + +
Eosinophils	±	+ +	±
Basophils	+	+ + +	±
Lymphocytes	+ + +	+ +	±
Monocytes	+ +	+ + +	+

Histamine liberation from mast cells and blood basophils might appear to be an epiphenomenon of the immediate and delayed type of immune response. In the Jones-Mote reaction, however, the involvement of these cells attains a significant importance. Recent results indicate that the antigen-antibody reaction proceeding on the surface membrane of blood basophils is the main mechanism underlying basophil or mast cell discharge in certain cases of hypersensitivity. This is in good agreement with the observation that repeated washings reduce the reagibility of blood basophils (Hastie, 1971).

There have been many attempts to determine which of the different immunoglobulins is responsible for triggering basophil granulolysis. Hubscher and Goodfriend (1969) ascribed the main granulocytic activity to immunoglobulins of the G class. From their findings that anti-IgE antibodies attach to human basophils resulting in histamine release in certain cases of hypersensitivity, Ishizaka *et al.* (1969) claimed that IgE was responsible for atopic basophil discharge. This new aspect proved fairly consistent with earlier results. Juhlin and Öhmann (1964) could find no significant relationship between the basophils and immunoglobulin classes G, A, and M.

In the past few years the significance of reaginin-like immunoglobulins in atopic reactions has increasingly been accepted. The investigations of Johnsson and Bennich (1967) and of Iishizaka and Ishizaka (1968) have shown that this type of immunoglobulin corresponds fully with the heat-labile immunoglobulins of the E type. IgE from atopic patients gives a positive PRAUSNITZ-KÜSTNER test and, *in vitro,* is able to passively sensitize isolated human or rabbit blood basophils. *In vitro* it initiates granulolysis on allergen contact. Both the PRAUSNITZ-KÜSTNER reaction and the leukocyte sensitizing effect *in vitro* can be reduced to a minimum of 20% after heating at 50° C for 30 min. Further heating leads to a complete loss of activity (STANWORTH and KUHNS, 1963). There appears to be a certain parallel here with the findings of MORSE *et al.* (1969), in that these authors identified two types of the so-called homocytotropic antibodies (IgE and IgG) in rats, IgE triggering histamine liberation from the tissue mast cells and IgG being responsible for the liberation of slow-reacting substance A (SRS-A). Today there is hardly any doubt that the immediate type of hypersensitivity is mediated through the so-called cytotropic antibodies of the IgE type. The absorption of the IgE molecule is generally believed to take place onto certain receptors of the basophil surface by means of the Fc fragment of the Ig molecule. Supporting this is the finding that Fc fragments obtained after pepsination could prevent the sensitization of the cells through the entire antibody molecule (STANWORTH *et al.* 1968; 1970). This correlates well with the findings of ISHIZAKA and ISHIZAKA (1968). They found that the histamine-liberating cytotropic effect of IgE occurs both after addition of specific antigens to the immunoglobulins, and through an unspecific aggregation of the IgE molecules by means of bis-diazotized benzidine. STANWORTH (1970) achieved the same results. In their studies with monomers and molecule aggregates of IgE, a cytotropic effect could only be verified after intradermal injection of IgE aggregates. This was expressed in terms of histamine liberation. In this relation, IgG and IgE display a similar behaviour (HENNEY and STANWORTH, 1966).

The experiments mentioned appear to confirm to a large extent the mode of the antigen-antibody reaction proposed by STANWORTH *et al.* (1969). According to this, several antibody molecules of the E type react with the corresponding basophil membrane receptors. Blood basophils laden with IgE possess at this stage the specific receptors for fixing of the corresponding antigen. The flexibility of the heavy chains permits the localization of an antigen molecule between the two light chains of the neighbouring IgE molecules. The side chains, with their reactible groups, can then initiate the chain reaction for histamine liberation. According to STANWORTH *et al.* (1969), the enzymatically controlled histamine liberation can be initiated by a similar mechanism through the sulfhydryl groups of the antibody side chains, and also through other groups which are able to react. The reaction has its optimum at 37° C and in the presence of sufficient quantities of calcium and magnesium ions. It takes about 5 min at this temperature for the absorption on the cell surface of sufficient antibodies to liberate 50% of the total histamine. The corresponding times necessary at 20° and 4° C, based on the same testing procedure, were 40 and 100 min, respectively (OSSLER *et al.*, 1968; OSSLER, 1970). According to LICHTENSTEIN (1968), histamine liberation can be completely repressed by inhibitors of glycolysis. In contrast, respiratory enzyme inhibitors show no such effect. LICHTENSTEIN and MARGOLIS (1968) have shown that, for example, theophylline, a phosphodiesterase inhibitor, can inhibit immunological histamine liberation. Phosphodiesterase mediates the hydrolysis of cyclic AMP (adenosine 3′,5′-monophosphate). The catecholamines, which also increase the intracellular AMP content, show a similar effect and inhibit antigen-induced histamine liberation (LEVY and CARLTON, 1969).

IgE antibodies are proteins with an average molecular weight of 200,000. Electrophoretically, they are localized in the region of gamma-1 and have a sedimentation constant of 8.2. Their carbohydrate component amounts to 10.7% (review by ISHIZAKA and ISHIZAKA, 1970). Direct detection of the IgE on the cell surface of basophils, for example with the immunofluorescence method, has not yet been achieved. On the other hand, ISHIZAKA and ISHIZAKA (1970) found label in 1 to 2% of the leukocytes after incubation of leukocyte suspensions with iodine-125-labeled IgE and subsequent radioautography. The identification of blood basophils in the preparations is reported in this paper to have been substantiated by toluidine-blue metachromasia. SULLIVAN *et al.* (1971) succeeded in demonstrating IgE on the surface of human basophils by means of electron microscopy.

In summary, human blood basophils have been shown to participate in immune responses of immediate and delayed type. Both circulating immunoglobulins (humoral) and some cell mediated (cellular) factors may induce a detectable histamine release.

Extensive basophil infiltration has been reported to occur in the lesions of the JONES-MOTE reaction. This type of delayed-onset cell-mediated immune response is preferentially observed when hypersensitivity has been induced by minimal antigen doses (contact allergens) proteins, viral components, or allografts without the use of FREUND's adjuvant. The humoral reaginin-like factor triggering histamine release in atopic cases has found to be identical with the immunoglobulin E.

Radio-iodine-labeled IgE was found to accumulate on human blood basophils, as detected by autoradiography. Ferritin-labeled IgE could also be traced on the surface membrane of basophils.

In-vitro sensitization of blood basohils has been effected through incubation with IgE. Passively sensitized basophils and those obtained from atopic subjects react with massive histamine liberation on allergen contact.

References

ACKERMANN, D., FUCHS, H. G.: Zur Frage des Vorkommens von Histamin im normalen Harn. Hoppe-Seylers Z. physiol. Chem. **259**, 32 – 34 (1939).

ADAM, H. M.: Excretion of histamine in human urine Quart. J. exp. Physiol. **35**, 281 – 293 (1950).

ALBANUS, L., WINQVIST, G.: Basophils, eosinophils and histamine in the bone marrow of the guinea pig. Acta haemat. (Basel) **26**, 365 – 371 (1961).

ASBOE-HANSEN, G. A.: Origin of synovial mucin: Ehrlich's mast cell secretory element of connective tissue. Ann. rheum. Dis. **9**, 149 – 157 (1950).

ASPEGREN, N., FREGERT, S., RORSMAN, H.: Basophil leukocytes in allergie eczematous contact dermatitis. Int. Arch. Allergy **23**, 150 – 156 (1963 a).

ASPEGREN, N., FREGERT, S., RORSMAN, H.: Basophil leukocytes in non-vascular allergic patch-test reactions. J. invest. Derm. **41**, 107 – 108 (1963 b).

ASPEGREN, H., FREGERT, S., RORSMAN, H.: Basophil leukocytes at sites of intracutaneous tuberculin test reactions. Int. Arch. Allergy **24**, 35 – 38 (1964).

ASTALDI, G., ALLEGRI, A.: Sul tasso istaminico ematico e midollare nella norma e in diverse emopatie. Haematologica (Pavia) **34**, 851 – 868 (1951).

BARTH, H.: Über die Zellelemente des entzündlichen Exsudates, ihre quantitativen Änderungen im Entzündungsablauf und ihre Herkunft. Frankfurt: Inaugural-Dissertation 1958.

BERGQVIST, G., NILZÉN, A.: 1966. Cited in: G. BERGQVIST and A. NILZÉN: The release of histamine from blood corpuscles by antigen-antibody reactions. I. A method for detecting allergy in vitro in atopic persons. Acta allerg. (Kbh.) **23**, 263 – 273 (1969).

BERGQVIST, G., NILZÉN, A.: The release of histamine from blood corpuscles by antigen-antibody reactions. I. A method for detecting allergy in vitro in atopic persons. Acta allerg. (Kbh.) **23**, 263 – 273 (1969).

BERNAUER, W., SESEKE, G., HAHN, F., SCHMUTZLER, W., GIERTZ, H.: Über die anaphylaktische Histaminfreisetzung am Herzlungenpräparat des Meerschweinchens. Arch. int. Pharmacodyn. **162**, 319 (1966).

BERSANI, R. B.: see page 21.

BOREUS, L. B.: Anafylaksi og Mastceller, pp. 14 – 17. Uppsala: Almqvist & Wiksells 1961.

BOWSZYC, J., BOWSZYC, J.: The importance of the 1967 basophil degranulation test for the detection of allergy to penicillin. Pol. med. J. (Eng.) **6**, 130 – 136 (1967).

BRAUNSTEINER, H., POTUZHEK, O., THUMB, N.: Über die Beeinflussung der Eosinophilenzahl durch Heparin. Acta haemat. (Basel) **22**, 153 – 157 (1959).

BRAUNSTEINER, H., POTUZHEK, O., THUMB, N.: Variations observées dans le nombre des leucocytes basophiles chez l'homme. Rev. Hémat. **15**, 241 – 249 (1960).

BRECHTER, C., RORSMAN, H.: Basophil leukocytes in hypersensitization. Int. Arch. Allergy **28**, 35 – 40 (1965).

CACCIAVILLANI, B., GIBERTINI, G.: 1942. Cited in: GIBERTINI, G.: La istidina non spiega effeto antiistaminico sull'intestino isolato. Boll. Soc. ital. Biol. sper. **17**, 234 (1942).

CARVAHLO, M. G.: Sur la labrocytose (mastzellose) chez les individus soumis au traitment antirabique. C. R. Soc. Biol. (Paris) **87**, 701 – 723 (1922).

CEJKA, V., de VRIES, L. A., SMORENBERG-SCHOORL, M. E., VAN DAATSELAAR, J. J., VORST, J. G. G., MAJOOR, G. L. H.: Effect of heparinoid and spirolactone on the renal excretion of sodium and aldosterone. Lancet **1960 I**, 317 – 319.

CHARPIN, J., AUBERT, J., OHRESSER, P., BOUTIN, C., FRANCAL, P.: Comparison of the basophil test with penicillin and the clinical data. Acta allerg. (Kbh.) **21**, 1 – 8 (1966).

CODE, C. F.: The histamine-like activity of white blood cells. J. Physiol (Lond.) **90**, 485 – 510 (1937 a).

CODE, C. F.: The quantitative estimation of histamine in the blood. J. Physiol. (Lond.) **89**, 257 – 268 (1937 b).

CODE, C. F.: Histamine in blood. Physiol. Rev. **32**, 47 – 65 (1952).

CODE, C. F.: The histamine content of white blood cells. In: J. TULLIS (ed.): Blood Cells and Plasma Proteins, Their State in Nature. New York: Harvard University-Academic Press. 1953.

CODE, C. F., MACDONALD, A. D.: see page 57.
CODE, C. F., MITSCHELL, R. G.: see page 22.
COHEN, H. A.: The role of hetero- and isohemagglutinins in the indirect basophil reaction. Arch. Derm. Syph. (Chic.) **95**, 313 – 318 (1967).
CONSTANZI, J. J., COLTMAN, C. A. Jr.: Kappa chain cold-precipitable immunoglobulin G (IGG) associated with cold urticaria. Clinical observations. Clin. exp. Immun. **2**, 167 – 178 (1967).
COOPER, F. K., CRUICKSHANK, C. N. D.: see page 22.
CRUICKSHANK, C. N. D., HAYE, K. R.: The responses of the basophil leukocyte. J. invest. Derm. **51**, 324 – 329 (1968).
DABNEY, J. M., STANLEY, A. J.: The affinity of heparin for certain liberators of histamine. Tex. Rep. Biol. Med. **18**, 194 – 201 (1960).
DEMIS, J. D., BROWN, D. D.: Histidine metabolism in urticaria pigmentosa. J. invest. Derm. **36**, 253 – 272 (1961).
DESAGA, J. F., TIETZ, G., LENNERT, K.: Zur Cytologie der Tuberkulinreaktion. Verh. dtsch. Ges. Path. **54**, 265 – 267 (1970).
DOLEN, T., AAS, K.: Studies of hypersensitivity to fish. An evaluation of the indirect basophil degranulation test for the in vitro demonstration of hypersensitivity to fish. Int. Arch. Allergy **30**, 405 – 415 (1966).
DRENNAN, J. M.: The mast cells in urticaria pigmentosa. J. Path. Bact. **63**, 513 – 520 (1951).
DREYFUSS, F., HELLMAN, M., KLOPSTOCK, A., SCHWARTZ, J., VARDINON, N.: The basophil degranulation test in patients hypersensitive to drugs. Acta allerg. (Kbh.) **21**, 17 – 24 (1966).
DUNÉR, H., PERNOW, B.: see page 23.
DUNÉR, H., LILJEDAHL, S. O., PERNOW, B.: Does the urinary excretion of imidazole acetic acid reflect the endogenous histamine metabolism in man? Acta physiol. scand. **51**, 41 – 46 (1961).
DVORAK, H. F., DVORAK, A. M., SIMPSON, B. A., RICHERSON, H. B., LESKOWITZ, S., KARNOVSKY, M. J.: Cutaneous basophil hypersensitivity. II. A light and electron microscopic description. J. exp. Med. **132**, 558 – 582 (1970).
EHRICH, W. E.: Histamine in mast cells. Science **118**, 603 (1953).
FEINBERG, A. R., FEINBERG, S. M., LEE, F.: Leukocytes and hypersensitivity reactions. I. Eosinophil response in skin window to ragweed extract, histamine, and compound 48/80 in atopic and nonatopic individuals. J. Allergy **40**, 73 – 87 (1967).
FEIZI, T.: The indirect basophil degranulation test for allergy to penicillin. Trans. St. John's Hosp. derm. Soc. (Lond.) **53**, 162 – 164 (1967).
FERNEX, M.: The mast cell-system, its relationship to atherosclerosis, fibrosis and eosinophils. Basel-New York: S. Karger 1968.
FREGERT, S., RORSMAN, H.: Basophil leukocytes in intracutaneous test reactions to metals. J. invest. Derm. **41**, 361 – 362 (1963).
FREGERT, S., RORSMAN, H.: Allergens in epoxy resins. Acta allerg. (Kbh.) **19**, 296 – 299 (1964).
FRICK, G., FRICK, U.: Zur Rolle der basophilen Leukozyten und Mastzellen in Fibrinolyse und Allergie. I. Wirkung von Fibrinolytica und Antifibrinolytica auf den Degranulationsgrad von basophilen Leukocyten. Folia haemat. (Lpz.) **86**, 389 – 403 (1966 a).
FRICK, G., FRICK, U.: Zur Rolle der basophilen Leukozyten und Mastzellen in Fibrinolyse und Allergie. II. Wirkung eines Antihistaminicums und einer allergi-

schen Sofortreaktion auf Zahl und Degranulierung basophiler Leukozyten. Folia haemat. (Lpz.) **87,** 178 – 189 (1966 b).

FRIEDBERG, K. D., BAUER, U.: Anaphylaktischer Schock nach passiver Sensibilisierung am anaphylatoxinvorbehandelten Meerschweinchen. Arch. exp. Path. Pharmacol. **250,** 171 – 172 (1965).

FULTON, J. E., DERBES, V. J.: Basophil leukocyte infiltration in the positive tuberculin skin test in man. J. invest. Derm. **43,** 125 – 128 (1964).

GADDUM, J. H.: The origin of histamine in the body, p. 285. Ciba Foundation Symposium on Histamine. London: J. & A. Churchill Ltd. 1956.

GIERTZ, H., HAHN, F., SCHMUTZLER, W., KOLLMEIER, J.: Plasma- und Bluthistamin bei verschiedenen Schockformen des Meerschweinchens. Int. Arch. Allergy **25,** 26 – 45 (1964).

GILLESPIE, E., LEVINE, R. J.: Histamine release by reserpine from rat peritoneal mast cells in vitro. Biochem. Pharmacol. **18,** 934 – 935 (1969).

GINGOLD, N.: Un élément dans le diagnostic différential de la leucémie myéloide chronique. Bull. Acad. Méd. Roum. **4,** 382 – 384 (1939 a).

GINGOLD, N.: Zur Differentialdiagnose zwischen chronischer Leukaemie und myeloisch-leukaemoiden Blutbildern. Klin. Wschr. **18,** 1217 – 1218 (1939 b).

GINGOLD, N.: Un nouveau moyen de diagnostic différential des leucémies et des réactions leucémoides. Sang **13,** 920 – 923 (1939 c).

GINGOLD, N.: Der Bluthistaminspiegel in der Differential- und Frühdiagnose der chronischen myeloischen Leukaemie. Wien. Z. inn. Med. **49,** 180 – 186 (1968).

GINGOLD, N., TEITEL, P.: Differentialdiagnose zwischen chronischer Myelose und leukaemoider Reaktion. Probl. Gemat. **4,** 28 – 29 (1959).

GINGOLD, N., TEITEL, P.: Bluthistaminmenge in der Differentialdiagnose der chronischen Myeloleukose. Stud. Cercet. Med. intern. **7,** 163 – 172 (1966).

GIRALDO, B., BLUMENTHAL, M. N., SPINK, W. W.: Aspirin intolerance and asthma. A clinical and immunological study. Ann. intern. Med. **71,** 479 – 496 (1969).

GORDON, V. H.: The indirect basophil test and drug hypersensitivity. Ann. Allergy **24,** 171 – 178 (1966).

GRAHAM, H. T., WHEELWRIGHT, F., PARISH, H. H., MARKS, A. R., LOWRY, O. H.: Distribution of histamine among blood elements. Fed. Proc. **11,** 350 (1952).

GRAHAM, H. T., LOWRY, O. H., WHEELWRIGHT, F., LENZ, M. A., PARISH, H. H.: Distribution of histamine among leukocytes and platelets. Blood **10,** 467 – 481 (1955).

GREAVES, M. W., BURDIS, B. D.: Anaphylactic histamine release from guinea pig basophil leukocytes. Int. Arch. Allergy **34,** 313 – 323 (1968).

GREAVES, M. W., MONGAR, J. L.: The histamine content of rabbit leukocytes and its release during in vitro anaphylaxis. Immunology **15,** 733 – 742 (1968).

GUDOWSKI, G., DIECKHOFF, J.: Basophil leukocytes and histamine in blood in childhood diseases caused by allergic reactions. Allergie u. Asthma **13,** 1 – 5 (1967).

HAHN, F., MAACK, T., MÜLLER, G., MITZE, R., EBNER, C.: Anaphylatoxin tachyphylaxis and anaphylactic histamine release. Int. Arch. Allergy **37,** 596 – 606 (1970).

HARTMAN, W. J., CLARK, W. G., CYR, S. D.: see page 60.

HASTIE, R.: The antigen-induced degranulation of basophil leukocytes from atopic subjects studied by phase-contrast microscopy. Clin. exp. Immunol. **8,** 45 – 61 (1971).

HATEM, S.: 1955. Cited in: C. CHAMPY and S. HATEM. Une réaction argentique de l'histamine. C. R. Soc. Biol. (Paris) **150,** 1325 – 1326 (1956).

HENNEY, C. S., STANWORTH, K.: Effect of antigen on the structural configuration of homologous antibody following antigen-antibody combination. Nature (Lond.) **210,** 1071 – 1972 (1966).

HIGGINBOTHAM, R. D., DOUGHERTY, T. F.: Micellophagosis and detoxification. RES Bull. **2,** 27 – 31 (1956 a).

HIGGINBOTHAM, R. D., DOUGHERTY, T. F.: Mechanism of heparin protection against a histamine releaser (48/80). PSEM **92,** 493 – 498 (1956 b).

HIGGINBOTHAM, R. D.: On the participation of micellophagosis in the resistance of tissues to injurious agents. Int. Arch. Allergy **15,** 195 – 222 (1959 a).

HIGGINBOTHAM, R. D.: Effect of compound 48/80 on toxicity of histamine and of serotonin in mice. Proc. Soc. exp. Biol. (N. Y.) **102,** 4 – 8 (1959 b).

HIGGINBOTHAM, R. D.: Mast cells and local resistance to RUSSEL's viper venom. Fed. Proc. **21,** 279 (1962 a).

HIGGINBOTHAM, R. D.: Sulfated polysaccharides and resistance to RUSSEL's viper venom. Proc. Soc. exp. Biol. (N. Y.) **110,** 135 – 138 (1962 b).

HIGGINBOTHAM, R. D.: Interaction of mast cells with cationic histamine releasers. In: Histamine and Antihistaminics. M. ROCHA E SILVA (Ed.). Berlin-Heidelberg-New York: Springer 1066.

HOFFMAN, J. B., SCHWARTZ, J.: Tropical eosinophilia versus LOEFFLER's syndrome. New York med. J. **51,** 2261 – 2263 (1951).

HOLMES, W. N., JONES, I. C.: 1960. Cited in: W. N. HOLMES, J. G. PHILLIPS and I. C. JONES: Adrenocortical factors associated with adaptation of vertebrates to marine environments. Recent Progr. Hormone Res. **19,** 619 – 672 (1963).

HU, F., FOSNAUGH, R. P., LIVINGOOD, C. S.: Human skin window to Staphylococcus in controls and in patients with cutaneous bacterial infections. J. invest. Derm. **41,** 325 – 334 (1963).

HUBSCHER, T., GOODFRIEND, L.: Role of human reaginic and hemagglutinating antibodies in the indirect rabbit basophil degranulation reaction. Int. Arch. Allergy **35,** 298 – 307 (1969).

HUMPHREY, J. H., JAQUES, R.: The histamine and serotonin content of the platelets and the polymorphonuclear leukocytes of various species. J. Physiol. (Lond) **124,** 305 – 310 (1954).

HUMPHREY, J. H., MOTA, I.: The mechanism of anaphylaxis: specificity of antigen-induced mast cell damage in anaphylaxis in the guinea pig. Immunology **2,** 31 – 43 (1959).

IRVINE, W. T., DUTHIE, H. L., WATON, N. G.: Urinary output of free histamine after a meat meal. Lancet **1959 I,** 1061 – 1064.

ISHIZAKA, K., ISHIZAKA, T.: Human reaginic antibodies and immunoglobulin E. J. Allergy **42,** 330 – 363 (1968 a).

ISHIZAKA, K., ISHIZAKA, T.: Reversed type allergic skin reactions by anti-γE globulin antibodies in humans and monkeys. J. Immunol. **100,** 554 – 562 (1968 b).

ISHIZAKA, T., ISHIZAKA, K., JOHNSSON, S. G. O., BENNICH, H.: Histamin release from human leukocytes by anti-γE antibodies. J. Immunol. **102,** 884 – 892 (1969).

ISHIZAKA, K., ISHIZAKA, T.: Biological function of γE antibodies and mechanisms of reaginic hypersensitivity. Clin. exp. Immunol. **6,** 25 – 42 (1970).

JOHNSSON, S. G. O., BENNICH, H.: Studies on a new class of human immunoglobulins. I. Immunological properties. Nobel Symposium 3. Stockholm: Almqvist & Wiksell 1967.

JONES, R. G.: Chemistry of histamine and analogs. Relationship between structure and pharmacological activity. In: Histamine and Antihistaminics. M. ROCHA E SILVA (Ed.). Berlin-Heidelberg-New York: Springer 1966.

JONES, T. D., MOTE, J. R.: Phases of foreign protein sensitization in human beings. New Engl. J. Med. **210,** 120 – 123 (1934).

JONES, R. G., MANN, M. J., MCLAUGHLIN, K. C.: Substituted β-aminoethylpyrazoles. J. org. Chem. **19,** 1428 – 1434 (1954).

JUHLIN, L., SHELLEY, W. B.: Plastic tube technic of centrifugal separation of leukocytes from human blood. Blood **18,** 477 – 480 (1961 a).

JUHLIN, L., SHELLEY, W. B.: A new test for detecting anaphylactic sensitivity: The basophil reaction. Nature (Lond.) **191,** 1056 – 1058 (1961 b).

JUHLIN, L., WESTPHAL, O.: Degranulation of basophil leukocytes in a case of milk allergy. Acta derm.-venereol. (Stockh) **42,** 273 – 279 (1962).

JUHLIN, L.: Basophil leukocyte differential in blood and bone marrow. Acta haemat. (Basel) **29,** 89 – 95 (1963).

JUHLIN, L.: Effect of fluocinolone on basophil and eosinophil leukocytes in inflammatory exudates. Acta derm.-venereol. (Stockh.) **44,** 327 – 329 (1964).

JUHLIN, L., ÖHMAN, S.: Basophil and eosinophil leukocytes in cantharidin blisters of patients with various dermatoses. Acta derm.-venereol. (Stockh.) **44,** 303 – 414 (1964).

KAPELLER-ALDER, R.: Histidine metabolism in toxemia of pregnancy. Isolation of histamine from urine of patients with toxemia of pregnancy. Biochem. J. **35,** 213 – 218 (1941).

KASATKINA, L. V.: see page 129.

KAWAI, T.: Studies on bronchial asthma, concerning histamine release reaction. Keio J. Med. **18,** 129 – 145 (1969).

KELEMAN, E., BIKICH, G., BORBALA, J., TANOS, B.: Clinical investigation on the histamine of leukemic granulocytes. Acta haemat. (Basel) **9,** 171 – 184 (1953).

KELLER, R.: Zur Bindung von Histamin und Serotonin in den Mastzellen. Arzneimittel-Forschung **8,** 390 – 394 (1958).

KIMURA, J., MORITANI, Y., NISHIZAKI, Y., TANIZAKI, Y.: see page 24.

KIRSHBAUM, B. A., COHEN, H. B., BEERMAN, H., PASTRAS, T.: The basophil degranulation test. A review of the literature. Amer. J. med. Sci. **253,** 473 – 492 (1967).

KLAUSNER, E., KREIBICH, C.: Über exsudative Mastzellen. Arch. Derm. Syph. (Chic.) **96,** 235 – 241 (1909).

KLAUSNER, E., KREIBICH, C.: Über den Mastzellengehalt vesiculöser Hauteffluorescenzen. Folia haemat. (Lpz.) **15,** 347 – 350 (1913).

LEE, H. M., JONES, R. G.: The histamine activity of some β-aminoethylheterocyclic nitrogen compounds. J. Pharmacol. exp. Ther. **95,** 71 – 78 (1949).

LENNERT, K., ELSCHNER, H.: Zur Kenntnis der lipomelanotischen Retikulo(cyto)se. Frankfurt: Z. Path. **65,** 559 – 577 (1954).

LEVADITI, C.: see page 97.

LEVIN, R. A.: An indirect basophil degranulation slide test for detection of immediate type hypersensitivity reactions. Amer. J. clin. Path. **48,** 150 – 152 (1967 a).

LEVIN, R. A.: An indirect basophil degranulation slide test for detection of immediate type hypersensitivity reactions. Tech. Bull. Reg. med. Technol. **37,** 168 – 170 (1967 b).

LEVY, D. A., CARLTON, J. A.: Influence of temperature on the inhibition by colchicine of allergic histamine release. Proc. Soc. exp. Biol. (N. Y.) **130,** 1333 – 1336 (1969).

LICHTENSTEIN, L. M.: Characteristics of leukocytic histamine release by antigen and by anti-immunoglobulin and anticellular antibodies. Int. Symp. canad. Soc. Immunol. Toronto 1968.

LICHTENSTEIN, L. M., OSLER, A. G.: Studies on the mechanisms of hypersensitivity phenomena. Histamine release from human leukocytes by ragweed pollen antigen. J. exp. Med. **120**, 507 – 530 (1964).

LICHTENSTEIN, L. M., OSLER, A. G.: Studies on the mechanism of hypersensitivity phenomena. XI. The effect of human serum on the release of histamine from human leukocytes by ragweed pollen antigen. J. Immunol. **96**, 159 – 168 (1966 a).

LICHTENSTEIN, L. M., OSLER, A. G.: Studies on the mechanisms of hypersensitivity phenomena. XII. An in vitro study of the reaction between ragweed pollen antigen, allergic human serum, and ragweed-sensitive human leukocytes. J. Immunol. **96**, 169 – 179 (1966 b).

LICHTENSTEIN, L. M., MARGOLIS, S.: Histamine release in vitro: inhibition by catecholamines and methylxanthines. Science **161**, 902 – 903 (1968).

LICHTENSTEIN, L. M., NORMAN, P. S.: Human allergic reactions. Amer. J. Med. **46**, 163 – 173 (1969).

LILJA, B., LINDELL, S.-E., SALDEEN, T.: Formation and destruction of ^{14}C-histamine in human lung tissue in vitro. J. Allergy **31**, 492 – 496 (1960).

LINDELL, S.-E., VISKE, K.: A note on the distribution of ^{14}C-histamine added to blood. Brit. J. Pharmacol. **17**, 131 – 136 (1961).

LINDELL, S.-E., RORSMAN, H., WESTLING, H.: Histamine formation in urticaria pigmentosa. Acta derm.-venereol. (Stockh.) **41**, 277 – 280 (1961 a).

LINDELL, S.-E., RORSMANN, H., WESTLING, H.: Histamine formation in human blood. Acta allerg. (Kbh.) **16**, 216 – 227 (1961 b).

LINDELL, S.-E., WESTLING, H.: Histamine metabolism in man. In: Histamine and Antihistaminics. M. ROCHA e SILVA (Ed.). Berlin-Heidelberg-New York: Springer 1966.

LUPOVITCH, A., GREKIN, T., KRAEGER, C.: A localized Arthus-type hypersensitivity reaction to penicillin. Ann. Allergy **26**, 206 – 210 (1968).

MACGOWAN, E. M.: Menthol urticaria. Arch. Derm. **94**, 62 – 63 (1966).

MACINTOSH, F. C., PATON, W. D.: The liberation of histamine by certain organic bases. J. Physiol. (Lond.) **109**, 190 – 211 (1949).

MAJNO, G., PALADE, G. E.: Studies on inflammation. I. The effect of histamine and serotonin on vascular permeability: An electron microscopic study. J. Biophys. biochem. Cytol. **11**, 571 – 601 (1961).

MARCU, I., PARHON, C. C., COMSA, Gh.: La teneur en histamine du sang normal et pathologique. Bull. Soc. méd. Hôp. (Bucarest) **18**, 246 – 251 (1936).

MARCU, I., GINGOLD, N., PARHON, C. C.: L'histamine dans les maladies du sang. Bull. Acad. Méd. Roum. **3**, 3 – 9 (1937).

MARTINS, A. B., RAFFEL, S.: Cellular activities in hypersensitive reactions. I. Comparative cytology of delayed "Jones-Mote" and Arthus reactions. J. Immunol. **93**, 937 – 947 (1964).

MIDDELTON, E., SHERMAN, W. B., FLEMING, W., VAN ARSDEN, P. P.: Some biochemical characteristics of allergic histamine release from leukocytes of ragweed-sensitive subjects. J. Allerg. (Kbh.) 448 – 454 (1960).

MORSE, H. C., AUSTEN, K. F., BLOCK, K. J.: Biologic properties of rat antibodies. III. Histamine release mediated by two classes of antibodies. J. Immunol. **102**, 327 – 337 (1969).

Moussatché, H., Prouvost-Danon, A.: Influence of oxidative phosphorylation inhibitors on the histamine release in the anaphylactic reaction in vitro. Experientia (Basel) **14,** 414 – 415 (1958).

Mota, I., Beraldo, W. T., Junqueira, L. C. U.: Protamine-like property of compound 48/80 and stilbamidine and their action on mast cells. Proc. Soc. exp. Biol. (N. Y.) **83,** 455 – 457 (1953).

Nalbandian, R. M., Pearce, J. F.: Allergic purpura induced by exposure to p-dichlorobenzene. Confirmation by indirect basophil degranulation test. J. amer. Med. Ass. **194,** 828 – 829 (1965).

Nilzén, A.: Studies in histamine (h-substance) with special reference to the conditions obtaining in urticaria and related skin changes. Acta derm.-venereol. (Stockh.) **27,** 225 – 230 (1947) Suppl. 17.

Norden, A., Brandt, L., Stählberg, K. G., Tryding, N.: Blood histamine and serum vitamin B12 in polycythaemia vera, chronic myeloid leukemia and other myeloproliferative disorders. X. Congr. Soc. Europ. Haematol. Strassburg 1965. Basel: S. Karger 1967.

Osler, A. G., Lichtenstein, L. M., Levy, D. A.: In vitro studies of human reaginic allergy. Advanc. Immunol. **8,** 183 – 231 (1968).

Osler, A. G.: Immunology of reaginic allergy: in vitro studies. Clin. exp. Immunol. **6,** 13 – 23 (1970).

Papacostas, C. A., Loew, E. R., West, G. B.: Studies on the toxicology of a histamine liberator, compound 48/80. Arch. int. Pharmacodyn. **120,** 353 – 362 (1959).

Parra, C. A., Alvarez, M. A., Laciar, T.: On the basophil degranulation test in spastic bronchitis. Allergie u. Asthma **12,** 295 – 298 (1966).

Paton, W. D. M.: The mechanism of histamine release. Ciba Foundation Symposium on Histamine **1,** 59 – 73 (1955).

Paton, W. D. M.: see page 64.

Pröscher, F.: see page 98.

Rebuck, J. W., Crowly, J. H.: A method of studying leukocytic functions in vivo. Ann. N. Y. Acad. Sci. **59,** 757 – 805 (1955).

Resnik, S. S., Shelley, W. B.: Penicillin hypersensitivity detection by basophil response to challenge. J. invest. Derm. **45,** 269 – 274 (1965).

Reynolds, R. D., Smith, R. E.: The indirect basophil degranulation test. Ann. Allergy **25,** 318 – 323 (1967).

Richerson, H. B., Dvorak, H. F., Leskowitz, S.: Cutaneous basophilic hypersensitivity: A new interpretation of the Jones-Mote reaction. J. Immunol. **103,** 1431 – 1434 (1969).

Richerson, H. B., Dvorak, H. F., Leskowitz, S.: Cutaneous basophil hypersensitivity. I. A new look at the Jones-Mote-reaction; general characteristics. J. exp. Med. **132,** 546 – 557 (1970).

Rikhter, A.: see page 131.

Riley, J. F.: The riddle of the mast cells. A tribute to Paul Ehrlich. Lancet **1954 I,** 841 – 843.

Ringoen, A. R.: see page 26.

Rocha e Silva, H.: Inhibition of histamine effects by compounds of histamine, histidine and arginine. J. pharmacol. exp. Ther. **80,** 399 – 408 (1944).

Rocha e Silva, M.: Histamine. Its Role in Anaphylaxis and Allergy. Springfield: Charles C. Thomas 1955.

Rocha e Silva, M.: On the nature of the receptors for histamine. Chemoterapia **3,** 544 – 559 (1961).

ROCHA E SILVA, M.: Histamine und Antihistaminics. In: Handbuch der exp. Pharmakol. Berlin-Heidelberg-New York: Springer 1966.

RORSMAN, H.: Basophil leukocytes in asthma, atopic dermatitis and psoriasis. Acta derm.-venereol. (Stockh.) **38,** 175 – 179 (1958).

RORSMAN, H.: Basophils and other leukocytes in allergic reactions in guinea pigs. Acta allerg. (Kbh.) **17,** 36 – 48 (1962).

ROTHSCHILD, A. M., VUGMANU, I., ROCHA E SILVA, M.: Metabolic studies on the release of histamine by compound 48/80 in the rat diaphragm. Biochem. Pharmacol. **7,** 248 – 255 (1961).

RYVKINA, D. E.: see page 132.

SAMPSON, D., ARCHER, G. T.: see page 26.

SCHAYER, R. W.: Histamine. Ciba Foundation Symposium I. London: Churchill 1956.

SCHAYER, R. W.: Histamine formation as a control of circulating hemostasis. Amer. J. Physiol. **198,** 1187 – 1190 (1960).

SCHAYER, R. W.: Histamine and hyperemia of muscular exercise. Nature (Lond.) **201,** 195 (1964).

SCHAYER, R. W.: Enzymatic formation of histamine from histidine. In: Histamine and antihistaminics. M. ROCHA E SILVA (Ed.). Berlin-Heidelberg-New York: Springer 1966.

SCHLATMANN, R. J. A. F. M., JANSEN, A. P., PENEN, H., MAJOOR, C. L. H.: The natriuretic action of heparin and some related substances. Lancet **1960 I,** 314 – 317.

SCHLECHT, W.: Über experimentelle Eosinophilie und basophile Leukocytose. Verh. Kongr. inn. Med. **27,** 483 – 487 (1918).

SCHULTZ, H. J., CODE, C. F., BRUNSTING, L. A.: Blood histamine and basophil-eosinophil counts in skin diseases. AMA Arch. Dermat. **80,** 44 – 52 (1959).

SCHUPPLI, R.: Experimental studies on SHELLEY's indirect basophil degranulation test. Dermatologica (Basel) **138,** 124 – 127 (1969).

SHELLEY, W. B., CARO, W. A.: Detection of anaphylactic sensitivity by the basophil degranulation response. J. Amer. med. Ass. **172,** 170 – 176 (1962).

SHELLEY, W. B., JUHLIN, L.: Functional cytology of the human basophil in allergic and physiologic reactions. Technic and Atlas. Blood **19,** 208 – 216 (1962).

SHELLEY, W. B.: Indirect basophil degranulation test for allergy to penicillin and other durgs. J. Amer. med. Assoc. **184,** 171 – 178 (1963).

SHIMKIN, M. B., BIERMAN, H. R.: Blood histamine in leukemia. Amer. J. Med. **8,** 542 – 543 (1950).

SHORE, P. A., BURKHALTER, A., COHN, V. H.: see page 67.

SOFTIC, N.: The normal absolute numerical values, the number and role of basophilic granulocytes in allergic diseases and in some other pathological states. Acta Allerg. (Kbh.) **22,** 360 – 372 (1967).

STANWORTH, D. R.: Immunochemical mechanisms of immediate-type hypersensitivity reactions. Clin. exp. Immunol. **6,** 1 – 12 (1970).

STANWORTH, D. R., KUHNS, W. J.: 1963. Cited in: D. R. STANWORTH and W. J. KUHNS: Quantitative studies on the assay of human skin-sensiziting antibodies (reagins). I. An examination of factors affecting the accuracy of the Prausnitz-Küstner (P-K)-test. Immunology **8,** 323 – 344 (1965).

STANWORTH, D. R., HUMPHREY, J. H., BENNICH, H., JOHANSSON, S. G. O.: Inhibition of Prausnitz-Küstner reaction by proteolytic-cleavage fragments of a human myeloma protein of immunoglobulin class E. Lancet **1968 II,** 17 – 18.

STANWORTH, D. R., HOUSLEY, J., BENNICH, H., JOHANSSON, S. G. O.: Effect of reduction upon the PCA-blocking activity of immunoglobulin E. Immunochemistry **7**, 321 – 325 (1970).

STANWORTH, D. R., HOUSLEY, J., BENNICH, H., JOHANSSON, S. G. O.: Inhibition of reagin-induced passive anaphylaxis in baboons by myeloma IgE and certain of its proteolytic cleavage fragments. Zitiert nach: D. R. STANWORTH: Clin. exp. Immunol. **6**, 1 – 12 (1970).

STARR, M. S.: Further studies on the process of histamine release from sensitized guinea-pig bone marrow basophils by antigen. Int. Arch. Allergy **37**, 376 – 384 (1970).

TEDESCHI, G., CAVAZZUTI, F., ANGELI, G.: 1957. Cited in: G. TEDESCHI, F. CAVAZZUTI, G. ANGELI: Variazioni quantitative dei granulociti basofili del sangue periferico in diverse condizione patologiche. Min. med. **50**, 1535 – 1538 (1959).

THIERSCH, J. B.: Histamine and histaminase in the blood of cases of lymphoid and monocytic leukemia. Aust. J. exp. Biol. med. Sci. **25**, 73 – 78 (1947 a).

THIERSCH, J. B.: Histamine and histaminase in chronic myeloid leukemia of man. Aust. J. exp. Biol. med. Sci. **25**, 79 (1947 b).

UVNÄS, B., THON, I. L.: Evidence for enzymatic histamine release from isolated rat mast cells. Exp. Cell Res. **23**, 45 – 57 (1961).

VALENTINE, W. N., PEARCE, M. L., LAWRENCE, J. S.: Studies on the histamine content of blood with special reference to leukemia, leukemoid reactions and leukocytoses. Blood **5**, 623 – 647 (1950).

VALENTINE, W. N., BECK, W. S., FOLLETTE, J. M., MILLS, H., LAWRENCE, J. S.: Biochemical studies in chronic myelocytic leukemia, polycythemia vera and other idiopathic myeloproliferative disorders. Blood **7**, 959 – 977 (1952).

VALENTINE, W. N., LAWRENCE, J. S., PEARCE, M. L., BECK, W. S.: The relationship of the basophil to blood histamine in man. Blood **10**, 154 – 159 (1955).

VALENTINE, W. N., FOLLETTE, J. H., SOLOMON, D. H., REYNOLDS, J.: Biochemical and enzymatic characteristics of normal and leukemic leukocytes. In: Leukemias. New York: Academic Press 1957.

VAN METRE, E., LICHTENSTEIN, L. M., TURK, S.: 1969. Cited in: A. G. OSLER: Immunology of reaginic allergy: in vitro studies. Clin. exp. Immunol. **6**, 13 – 23 (1970).

VIALLIER, J., SEDALLIAN, A.: The Shelley test. A serological test in allergology. Its diagnostic value. Critic of results obtained. Ann. Biol. clin. **23**, 993 – 1006 (1965).

VIALLIER, J., TOURAINE, R.: Degranulationstest of polynuclear basophils in rabbits – Shelley test. Clinical and experimental data. Acta Allerg. (Kbh.) **21**, 9 – 16 (1966).

WALTER, L. A., HUNT, W. H., FOSBINDER, R. J.: β-(2- and 4-pyridylalkyl)amines. J. Amer. chem. Soc. **63**, 2771 – 2796 (1941).

WALTON, K. W.: see page 133.

WATON, N. G.: Studies on mammalian histidine decarboxylase. Brit. J. Pharmacol. **11**, 119 – 127 (1956).

WEGELIUS, O., ASBOE-HANSEN, G.: see page 133.

WEISBECKER, L., SCHRÖTER, A.: Untersuchungen über die Beeinflussung der ACTH-Cortison- und Adrenalinwirkung durch Heparin. Acta endocr. (Kbh.) **15**, 66 – 70 (1954).

WEITZEL, G., FRETZDORFF, A. F.: 1956. Cited in: G. WEITZEL, F. SCHNEIDER and A. M. FRETZDORFF: Zink-Komplexe von Histidylpeptiden (Zinc complexes of histidyl peptides). Hoppe Seylers Z. physiol. Chem. **307**, 23 – 35 (1957).

WERLE, E., AMANN, R.: Über eine Bindung des Histamins an Heparin. Klin. Wschr. **42,** 583 (1955).
WILSON, D., GOETZ, F. C.: Selective hypaldosteronism after prolonged heparin administration. A case report with post-mortem findings. Amer. J. Med. **36,** 635 – 640 (1964).
WOLF-JÜRGENSEN, P.: Cytological examination of experimental contact allergy using the skin window technique. Acta allerg. (Kbh.) **17,** 547 – 557 (1962).
WOLF-JÜRGENSEN, P.: The inflammatory exudate in delayed hypersensitivity. Biochem. Pharmacol. Suppl. 87 – 98 (1968).
ZIMMER, J., BERGOEND, H., BASSET, A.: Technic of the in vitro Shelley test. Bull. Soc. franç. Derm. Syph. **73,** 252 – 255 (1966).
ZINSSER, H.: Studies on the tuberculin reaction and on specific hypersensitiveness in bacterial infection. J. exp. Med. **34,** 495 – 524 (1921).

III. Granulolysis and Kinetic Properties of Blood Basophils

1. The Degranulation Mechanism of Blood Basophils

The findings on tissue mast cells have largely determined the direction of research on the degranulation mechanisms of blood basophils. The important experimental advances have mainly been derived from studies on tissue mast cells, and it has so far been impossible to discover more than a few aspects of the mechanisms involved in the degranulation of blood basophils. This is primarily due to the extreme fragility and water-solubility of blood basophils. A major additional difficulty arises from the extreme rarity of these cells.

An attempt has been made here to assess what is known of the mechanisms involved in basophil degranulation. Comparisons with tissue mast cells may help to bridge the gaps. Analogous conclusions will only be drawn from findings supported by justifiable experimental evidence.

The methods available for studying the action of endogenous and exogenous factors upon blood basophils are limited to two. Information about the quantitative fluctuations can be obtained by direct determination of the basophil count at various time intervals. Cytomorphologic examinations at regular time intervals give some insight into the condition of the basophil granules and therefore the pharmacodynamic behavior of their biologically active substances. Special observation chambers have recently been developed in which blood basophils can be exposed to various agents and their behavior observed directly with a phase-contrast microscope. Artifacts of various kinds are to be expected with practically all such techniques, and it is necessary to recognize these artifacts and take them into consideration when evaluating the results.

Quantitative alterations of blood basophils were described by MORELL as early as 1931. After intravenous application of 1% mercuric sulfide solution, MORELL observed a strong fall in the basophil count. He spoke of a selective basophil loss. He did not, in this experiment, go into the functional origins of the observed basopenia. However, he pointed out that the blood basophil count can in theory decrease independently of either the total leukocyte count or the neutrophil count.

BOSEILA (1958) made some of the first systematic investigations of the mode of degranulation of blood basophils. Considering the results on the tissue mast cells, he studied the effect of the widely used histamine liberator, compound 48/80, upon the blood basophil count. After intravenous injection in rabbits of 1 mg/kg body weight of compound 48/80, he determined the blood basophil count using a modified technique from MOORE and JAMES (1953). There was a significant decrease in the basophil count (2.88% of the leukocytes as opposed to the control groups of 5.05%; $p < 0.01$). The determinations were carried out 2, 4, 6 and 24 h p.i., with the lowest values observed about 6 h p.i. After 24 h the basophil count was only slightly below the normal values. On the basis of these results, BOSEILA assumed that degranulated basophils were still present in the peripheral blood but could no longer be stained. Similar investigations were carried out independently by MARKS *et al.* (1959), who also observed basophil degranulation following compound 48/80 in rabbits. They termed the morphological alterations of the blood basophils under *in-vivo* conditions basophil 'destruction'. The same findings *in vitro* were interpreted as 'decoloration phenomenon'.

With reference to the findings of HÖGBERG and UVNÄS (1957; 1960) on tissue mast cells, the opinion was expressed that the degranulation of blood basophils, as with tissue mast cells, might be an enzymatically controlled process. The degranulation of tissue mast cells by compound 48/80 and the subsequent reduction in tissue histamine (RILEY and WEST, 1953 a, b; FELDBERG and TALESNIK, 1953; FAWCETT, 1955) led HUNT and HUNT (1957; 1958) to study the behavior of blood basophils too. After intravenous injection of 0.25 mg of compound 48/80, they found that the circulating blood basophil count in roosters fell to 9% of the initial value within 10 min. Blood smears prepared at the same time showed only a few blood basophils with small and weakly stained granules. HUNT and HUNT believed that the swift fall in blood basophils resulted from both degranulation and selective destruction. However, no destroyed blood basophils were observed in either smears or counting chambers. The hypothesis that damaged basophils might be withdrawn from the circulation by spleen or liver could not be substantiated in further investigations by the same authors (HUNT and HUNT, 1959).

Compound 48/80 leads to a clear basophil damage and histamine release in guinea pigs (GRAEVES and BURDIS, 1968). The reaction of human blood basophils to compound 48/80 has not yet been completely clarified. In laboratory animals, intravenous injection of compound 48/80 regularly leads to a manifest circulatory collapse and, according to the majority of authors, the blood basophil count is strongly decreased. NORDLANDER (1957) reported clinical observations after intravenous injection of 48/80 in humans. He pointed out that the mode of reaction varies greatly from individual to individual. In parallel tests with lecithinase A the so-called histamine effect was observed only in a few testsubjects. LEVI and MENEGHINI (1959) also reported there were major differences in the response of humans to a single intravenous injection of 3 mg of compound 48/80. The blood basophil count showed no significant alteration in these investigations. Here, too, it seems that there is a certain 'individual susceptibility' (SHELLEY and JUHLIN, 1962) in the response of human blood basophils to histamine liberators. SHELLEY and JUHLIN (1962) observed in their *in-vitro* investigations a massive disintegration of human blood basophils after addition of compound 48/80. The results of these authors, however, are contrary to those of others (HAYE and SCHNEIDER, 1966).

SAMPSON and ARCHER (1967) observed no clear histamine liberation after addition of 100 µg/ml of compound 48/80 to human blood basophil concentrates. They incubated human blood basophil concentrates (41×10^1 to 28×10^6 basophils/0.1 mm^3) for 15 min at 37° C and observed a spontaneous histamine liberation of $3.2 \pm 2.6\%$ of the total amine content. In identical trials, after addition of increasing concentrations of compound 48/80, a maximum histamine liberation of $4.3 \pm 1.0\%$ was measured. The difference was not statistically significant. Although, according to some authors, degranulation of blood basophils in humans occurs under the influence of histamine liberators, it still appears, allowing for individual variations and comparing results with animal blood basophils and tissue mast cells, that blood basophils possess a certain resistance to compound 48/80 and protamine sulfate. These varying results are difficult to reconcile. Until this question is settled, compound 48/80 cannot be regarded a universial histamine liberator (largely independent of species and the cell type). The few authors who have directly studied this subject do not come to any definite conclusion. SAMPSON and ARCHER (1967) used physiological saline as the incubation solution. Such a medium alone causes a decrease in basophil granules (PARWARESCH and LENNERT, 1967). The absence of histamine liberation in the control tests could be explained by the procedures used to produce basophil concentrations, which included repeated washings. On the basis of these experimental variations, it cannot be determined whether the action of compound 48/80 on human blood basophils is to release histamine as it does from tissue mast cells and the blood basophils of rabbits and guinea pigs, or not.

In spite of the contradictions in the literature it has been possible to find many parallels between the mechanisms of granule discharge in blood basophils and tissue mast cells. The granulolytic effect of biological extracts and animal venoms upon tissue mast cells has repeatedly been demonstrated. Phospholipase A or lecithinase A are thought to be responsible for the action of these extracts. This connection has also been tested in blood basophils. The venom of *Crotalus atrox* contains a high activity of lecithinase, and it is possible to obtain fractions which contain most of the lecithinase activity. The investigations of HÖGBERG and UVNÄS (1957; 1960) on tissue mast cells were applied to rabbit blood basophils in 1962 by MARKS and OBERER. They found that a single injection of *Crotalus atrox* venom (1 mg/kg body weight) causes a considerable 'basophil fall' (from 757 to 331 per mm^3). During the first hour after the injection and following the massive basophil fall, the mean basophil count rose again to normal values. After that the blood basophil count steadily decreased and 3 h p.i. was 223 per

mm^3; 6 h p.i. the basophil count in the peripheral blood amounted to 267 per mm^3, and 12 h p.i. it had reached 90% of the initial value. After 24 h it corresponded to the normal value. Similar results were obtained *in vitro*. After incubation of 0.005 mg/ml of the same venom fraction with blood, the basophil count fell over 34 h to 1% of the initial value. The total leukocyte count showed no significant alteration.

The strong granulolytic effect of the lecithinase-rich fraction in *Crotalus atrox* venom is not observed with other fractions with a low enzyme content. The granulocytic effect of the lecithinase-rich fraction showed a marked dose dependency within certain concentration ranges; MARKS and OBERER (1962) found a linear correlation between activity and dose in the range 1 to 3 mg/kg. Their investigations provided the first experimental evidence of a similarity between the mode of degranulation of tissue mast cells and blood basophils, and caused them to retract their earlier statement (MARKS *et al.*, 1959) that blood basophils were capable of 'merocrine' secretion. They believed that the discharged granules were resynthetized.

The granulolytic action of compound 48/80 upon blood basophils is said to be largely similar to the effect of lecithinase A. In accordance with the findings on tissue mast cells, this is not thought to be due to unspecific impairment of cell membrane, as it is with proteases and unspecific lipases (SHELLEY and JUHLIN, 1962). As with tissue mast cells, the extent of degranulation was found to depend directly on incubation temperature, substance concentration, and incubation time.

A massive granulolysis of blood basophils was observed in the course of an antigen-antibody reaction. This finding in particular underlines their close functional relationship with tissue mast cells. Basophil participation in immune reactions of immediate and delayed types has been dealt with in detail in Section C II b; here we review findings that contribute to an understanding of degranulation mechanisms.

Recent work has shown that numerous allergic diseases in humans, such as drug allergies, serum disease, contact dermatitis, bronchial asthma, hay fever, and colitis ulcerosa, are accompanied in their acute phases by a massive disintegration of blood basophils and, to some extent, by a so-called basophil fall (SHELLEY and CARO, 1962; SHELLEY, 1963; FRIEDLAENDER and FRIEDLAENDER, 1964; HUBSCHER and GOODFRIEND, 1969).

The liberation of histamine during immune reactions showed a marked dose dependency and was found to require the presence of calcium ions (MONGAR and SCHILD, 1962; LICHTENSTEIN and OSSLER, 1964). The reaction intensity can be influenced by the incubation temperature (HAYE *et al.*, 1968): room temperature inhibits the reaction and at 0° C granulolysis is halted. The action of heterologous protein upon the blood basophils of sensitized guinea pigs was demonstrated by STARR and WEINSTOCK, (1970). With increasing antigen concentration (0.01, 0.05, 0.1, 0.5 and 1 μg/ml) they observed the dose dependence of histamine liberation. In agreement with the results of HAYE *et al.* (1968), they also found that histamine liberation depends upon the calcium ion concentration, the optimum concentration being 12×10^{-7} M. Lower and higher concentrations led to suppression of basophil degranulation. Extensive withdrawal of the calcium ions by disodium-EDTA instantly halted the reaction process. This phenomenon was used for determining the reaction velocity. Only 30 sec after the addition of calcium, over 50% of the total histamine content was released. After 2 min the reaction came to an end. Hence, basophil degranulation also occur quickly and explosively, as repeatedly described for tissue mast cells. Under *in-vitro* conditions it was possible to increase the antigen-induced histamine liberation found in sensitized animals by the addition of either fresh or stored serum (HAYE *et al.*, 1968). Such findings suggest that certain serum factors act upon termination of basophil granulolysis as mediators or biocatalysts with enzyme-like properties. As with tissue mast cells, the participation of certain components of complement cannot be excluded (LICHTENSTEIN and OSSLER, 1966 a; STARR and WEINSTOCK, 1970).

Immunoglobulin E with its clear 'basophil affinity' plays a special role in immunologically induced basophil alterations. It is therefore necessary to distinguish the action of such immunoglobulins and of complement components from basophil-specific mediators and enzyme-like factors. The strong dependence of basophil granulolysis on pH and temperature also supports the existence of such factors, also the fact that certain physicochemical conditions have been found necessary for the process of granulolysis in nonimmunologically induced basophil degranulation. The physiological pH range (pH 7.0 to 7.4 at 37° C) was found to be optimal. Basophil granulolysis also required a critical electrolyte concentration. On this point, as well, there exists a good aggreement with the corresponding findings on tissue mast cells.

According to SAMPSON and ARCHER (1967), the heat-labile complement components play an important role in immunological basophil granulolysis. Basophil suspensions of blood group 0 were incubated with an anti-A hemolysin-containing serum of group 0. After addition to 5% of erythrocytes of group A, immediate liberation of 83% of the total histamine content was observed. The observation that granulolysis occurred only in the presence of fresh serum and not after addition of heat-inactivated serum has been taken as further evidence for the participation of complement.

Numerous other substances have been reported to lead to the degranulation or disintegration of blood basophils. FRICK and KONRAD (1963; 1964) reported on the degranulation effect of glucocorticoids; some fibrinolytics show a similar action (FRICK and FRICK, 1966 a, b). Fibrinolytic-induced basophil degranulation has been reported to be inhibited by the addition of 500 mg beta-amino-caproic acid (1.25 ml of a 40% solution), or 10 mg para-aminomethylbenzoic acid (FRICK nd FRICK, 1968). The action of antihistaminics on tissue mast cells has already been discussed. Related studies on blood basophils showed that these cells, too, revert to granulolysis under the influence of antihistaminics (FRICK and FRICK, 1967). Many authors have used the SHELLEY test for studying basophil degranulation and the action of various substances upon these cells. SHELLEY and JUHLIN (1961) developed a scheme of classifying human blood basophils to enable standardized statements to be made on the granule content of basophils.

This technique has been used extensively in connection with different problems (JUHLIN and SHELLEY, 1961 a, b; SHELLEY and JUHLIN, 1961; 1962; JUHLIN and WESTPHAL, 1962; JUHLIN, 1963; SHELLEY, 1963; SCHÖNHERR and HERMANN, 1964; LANGNER and STEIGLEDER, 1966; FRICK and FRICK, 1968; HAYE *et al.*, 1968; HUBSCHER and GOODFRIEND, 1969). In this technique, fresh blood samples are mixed with a surplus of fixing solution, which serves at the same time to hemolyse the erythrocytes, and then filtered through a membrane. For the selective demonstration of blood basophils, a 0.33% aqueous solution of toluidine blue (pH 5) is used. Filters are stained in this solution for 30 sec. Blood basophils are classified into 3 groups (A, B, and C) according to the size of their metachromatic granulation, and each group is subdivided into 6 types according to the distribution pattern of the granules. The authors distinguish in this way 18 different stages of basophil degranulation.

SHELLEY (1963) introduced a modification of this technique for the early recognition of penicillin allergy. He used a mixture of penicillin and diluted patient serum and added to it rabbit leukocytes (buffy coat containing test basophils). In positive cases, basophil degranulation ensues. The SHELLEY test is used to detect allergic reactions of the immediate type, in particular, drug and food allergies. Its increasing use is perhaps also due to the fact that the reliability of skin tests is no longer beyond all doubt (SHELLEY, 1962, 1963; SHELLEY and JUHLIN, 1962; SHELLEY and CARO, 1962; KATZ *et al.*, 1964; BOBITT *et al.*, 1964; FRIEDLAENDER and FRIEDLAENDER, 1964; SCHWARTZ *et al.*, 1965; KRAVIS *et al.*, 1965; REYNOLDS and SMITH, 1967).

SHELLEY and JUHLIN (1962) also applied this exploratory procedure wherever the functional participation of basophil granulocytes was expected. Arguing that these cells, because of their heparin content, should be important for the activation or liberation of serum lipoprotein lipase, they also attempted to study the lipid-induced alterations of metachromatic basophil granules. They observed an increase of degranulated cells in man from 20 to 50% to 80 to 90 % of the total basophils in the third hour after oral administration of lipids.

A positive SHELLEY test was also obtained on blood basophils treated with compound 48/80 or lecithinase A. In contrast, unspecific proteases, for example, papain, did not lead to morphological alterations of the granular basophil structures (SHELLEY and JUHLIN, 1962).

SHELLEY's technique is very valuable for covering a sufficiently large number of blood basophils from small blood samples. Under suitable *in-vitro* conditions, the explosive course of basophil degranulation can be well verified by the morphologically destroyed cells. Marked differences in the distribution patterns of basophil granules can also be shown with this technique. There are also some basophils that contain a few optically dense metachromatic granules (cells of groups A 6 and B, according to the SHELLEY classification). Along with these groups and the normal blood basophils, another group can be distinguished with a faded granule structure. These basophils show metachromatic clouds which cover large areas of the cytoplasm and cell nucleus. Destroyed blood basophils possessing an enlarged, weakly stainable nucleus are also observed. In such cells, cytoplasm is hardly recognizable. The metachromatic material in the cell vicinity is dispersed as a faintly red, cloudy structure (groups C 3 to 6 in the SHELLEY classification).

Under *in-vitro* conditions, destroyed blood basophils can confidently be taken as indication of a degranulation, but it is still not certain whether it is possible to obtain such cells from the peripheral blood after the action of certain drugs or after the termination of an immune reaction. Differentiation of blood basophils according to their content of metachromatic granules affords an insight into the morphodynamics of these cells. The selective staining permits a standardized grading, so that comparable statements can be made about the morphology of blood basophils under various experimental and clinical conditions. However, it does not give any information about the way in which the different contents of the granules in the various cells occur. The investigations carried out to date only allow the descriptive statement that certain drugs or reactions lead to a selective destruction of blood basophils. With the SHELLEY test it has been possible to demonstrate this effect under *in-vitro* conditions; the significance of the SHELLEY test for *in-vivo* experiments is disputable. Blood basophils with varying granule contents do occur in the peripheral blood under normal conditions. On the other hand, it is hard to imagine that destroyed blood basophils would remain in the circulating blood. This brings us again to the question of the mode of degranulation. SHELLEY and JUHLIN have never maintained in any of their papers that blood basophils were capable of genuine secretory activity, but other authors, using the basophil differential evaluation as the basis of their investigations, have assumed that basophil granulocytes are capable, as active secretory cells, of an excorporation of their granules. With the SHELLEY test, then, it should be possible to detect the total of the 'residual granules'. Such an assumption contradicts the results of *in-vitro* experiments, since most of the degranulated cells detected by the Shelley test are destroyed blood basophils incapable of sustaining life. Nor can the secretion theory be reconciled with the findings from *in-vivo* experiments. A rapid drop in the basophil count can be observed under the influence of various exogenous stimuli that give a positive SHELLEY test. However, in a subsequent examination of blood smears by cytochemical and enzyme-cytochemical methods, we were unable to detect intact cells that could correspond to or be regarded as partially or completely degranulated basophils. This clearly shows that what the SHELLEY test indicates is destroyed blood basophils under *in-vitro* conditions and intact cells with a limited granule content under *in-vivo* conditions. The low content of metachromatic substances observed in blood basophils under certain *in-vivo* conditions (for example, after an asthma seizure, in anaphylactic shock, after stress, and in massive hyperlipidemia) can only be attributed to the fresh emergence of immature basophils from the bone marrow. In other words, the sparse metachromatic granulations seen probably do not represent 'residual granules' left by a partial degranulation process, but are more likely less mature granules which appear as a result of accelerated emergence. JUHLIN (1963) compared the so-called basophil index of human bone marrow with that of the peripheral blood and found that about 10% of the mature bone marrow basophils are 'partially degranulated'. This 'degranulation' can only be partly explained by the presence of recirculating peripheral blood cells. While JUHLIN referred to the reduced granules as 'residual' granules, he left open the possibility that they might be less mature basophils with only a few metachromatic granules. Although this possibility is expected for bone marrow, it is not usually considered in relation to the peripheral blood. The differences in content of metachromatic substances are attributed entirely to 'varying degrees of degranulation'.

In summary, it is of decisive importance for an understanding of the physiology of blood basophils to determine whether degranulated blood basophils are capable of resynthesis of their 'fired' granules, or whether degranulation leads to the death of the cells. To look upon the blood basophil as a monocellular endocrine gland capable of merocrine secretion and resynthesis of granules is to grant this element of the granulocytic system an exceptional position. It would mean that blood basophils exhibit a property, i.e. secretion, that is uncommon in myeloid cells but fairly specific to long-lived glandular tissue. This phenomenon can hardly be reconciled with the characteristics of the other granulocytes. Moreover, the basophil count in the peripheral blood is so low that the quantity of heparin and histamine available would not be sufficient to be biochemically effective.

In our opinion, blood basophils are indeed capable of degranulation. This degranulation, however, is not consistent with the criteria for genuine merocrine secretion. It seems more likely that each granule discharge is associated with cytolysis leading to the death of the cell. Only this seems consistent with the majority of the different physiological functions of blood basophils and with the general properties of the granulopoietic cells. All cells of the granulocytic series are distinguished by a particularly short circulation time.

We know of no systematic investigation which explains these matters with any certainty. The situation is further complicated by the complete lack of information on the circulation time and life span of blood basophils. Reliable statements on the mode of degranulation of blood basophils require an exact knowledge of their kinetics. To clarify this point, we first determined the biological half-life (T/2) of blood basophils by injecting tritium-labeled thymidine in rabbits (PARWARESCH *et al.*, 1973) and in man. In parallel experiments, we studied the kinetic behavior of blood basophils under the influence of compound 48/80 both *in vivo* and *in vitro*. We discuss these investigations in detail in the following two sections.

2. Kinetics of Blood Basophils in Rabbits

Kinetic investigations with ^{3}H-thymidine were carried out on 3 noninbred male rabbits (K_1-_3) about 6 months old, weighing 2300 to 2800 g. All animals were examined after a one-week adjustment period in a fully controlled environment on a standard diet (Altromin-K). Each animal received a single intravenous injection of 1 μCi of ^{3}H-thymidine (Radiochemical Centre, Amersham; specific activity 5.0 μCi/mM) per gram body weight. Twenty-four hours later blood samples were taken at 6-h intervals and blood smears were prepared from leukocyte concentrations. Total leukocyte count and blood basophil count were determined directly in FUCHS-ROSENTHAL chambers. The blood basophils were then examined in smear preparations by autoradiography. The extreme water solubility of the basophil granules rendered the usual fixation and staining techniques inappropriate. A special procedure that enabled good preservation and selective demonstration of the blood basophils was therefore developed (DESAGA and PARWARESCH, 1971; PARWARESCH *et al.*, 1973). The slides were than mounted with a tracer emulsion (Eastman Kodak NTB 2) and exposed for 12 days. After developing (Kodak D-19), rinsing, and drying, selective staining of the metachromatic basophil granules was effected by staining with saturated methylene-blue solution in tertiary butanol.

The grain count of 100 basophils was determined for each time period investigated. All data were subjected to a background correction. The random grain count per μm^2 in cell-free areas was determined for each preparation. Further, the average area of cell nucleus of 50 cells was measured. This amounted to 90.5 μm^2 in smears. In our autoradiographic preparations we obtained 0.3 to 1.0 grains in this area. The individual background values were subtracted from the counted grains. After correction, all cells were divided into 4 groups according to their labeling intensity: those with more than 4, more than 9, more than 14 and more than 24 grains over the nucleus. In order to estimate the level of discrimination above which cells may be regarded as really labeled, the probability of the occurrence of background grains on basophil nuclei was computed according to the POISSON distribution:

The probability (p) that the basophil nuclei will be labeled by a certain number of background grains (k) is calculated by the formula:

$$p(k)=\frac{\lambda^{k}\cdot e^{-\lambda}}{k!}. \qquad (1)$$

Hence, the background-induced grains show a random distribution and their mean number per basophil nucleus (λ) is in the range $\lambda=0.3$ to 1.0. Therefore, λ varies within an interval of $\lambda \leqq 3$, a situation in which random distributions are best approximated on the basis of a POISSON frequency pattern. As this distribution is applicable for $\lambda=3$, it can therefore also be used for $\lambda=1$. The probability, even in the most improbable of cases, that more than 4 artifact-induced grains will be counted over one cell is only 0.36‰. Thus, in our investigations, only blood basophils with more than 4 grains per nucleus were considered as really labeled.

The following results were obtained from the determination of the labeling indices of the blood basophils at various periods after ^{3}H-thymidine injection. The 'emergence time' (the time between the end of the last DNA synthesis phase and the first appearance of labeled basophils in the blood) for the individual animals was between the 24th and 36th h. A labeling index of 60% was reached between the 67th and 78th hours p.i. This corresponds to an initial basophil influx of 0.77 to 0.89% per h. The maximum labeling index of 63 to 66% was reached between the 96th and 120th h p.i. After that there was a fall in the count of labeled cells reaching a first minimum of 17 to 23% between the 14th and 192nd h. The first peak was followed by a second peak, which had a labeling index of 28 to 36% between the 198th and 216th h. The second curve maxima are statistically significant. The probability that there is no actual effect is equal to the area immediately to the right in Fig. 32 (hatched) of the ordinate going through 10. It amounts to about 10‰. This is ascertained by the following considerations.

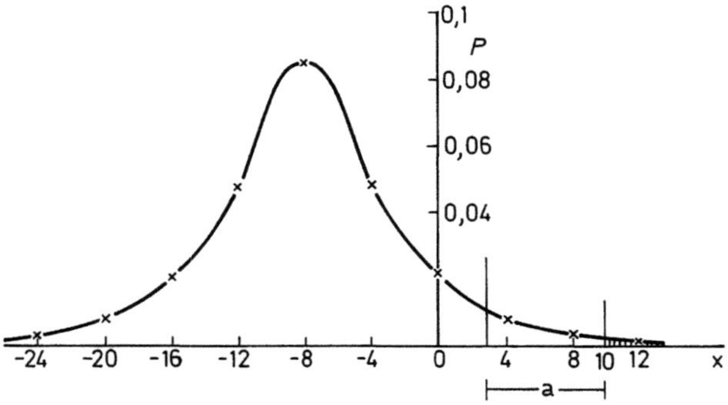

Fig. 32. Illustration of the probability p (x) d (x) by which the peaks of the second curve (see Fig. 33) represent true biologic effects (white curve area) and are not due to counting errors (left hatched area with p=1‰). For this estimation the curve connecting the maximum the first peak with the minimum of the second curve was assumed to bisect the transitional sequents of both peaks

The second curve maximum represents a true second rise in the labeling index curve and is not induced by artifacts or by accidental undulation of the curve due to scattering of the values. An accidental effect could result from random dispersion of the experimentally obtained values around the most probable one, namely the 'real' mean value. This dispersion reveals a binominal pattern of distribution. The dispersion itself (δ) depends upon:

n = the number of basophils considered per slide
p = relative portion of labeled basophils
q = relative portion of unlabeled basophils.

Therefore

$$n = p + q. \tag{2}$$

and the relation can be expressed as:

$$\delta = \sqrt{n \cdot p \cdot q}. \tag{3}$$

Let us assume instead of the experimentally obtained basophil labeling index curve (Fig. 33) with an obvious second peak a constantly falling linear curve as drawn in Fig. 34.

Lines drawn from the intermediate minimum and from the second maximum of the original curve vertically cross this hypothetical prolongation of the curve, and designate the points μ_1 and μ_2 as the assumed means. In Fig. 34 the probability (p) is illustrated for the case that an accidental second rise may occur, exceeding the curve minimum by the height x.

Accordingly

$$p(x)\,dx = \int_{-\infty}^{+\infty} P_1(t) \cdot P_2(t-x)\,dt \tag{4}$$

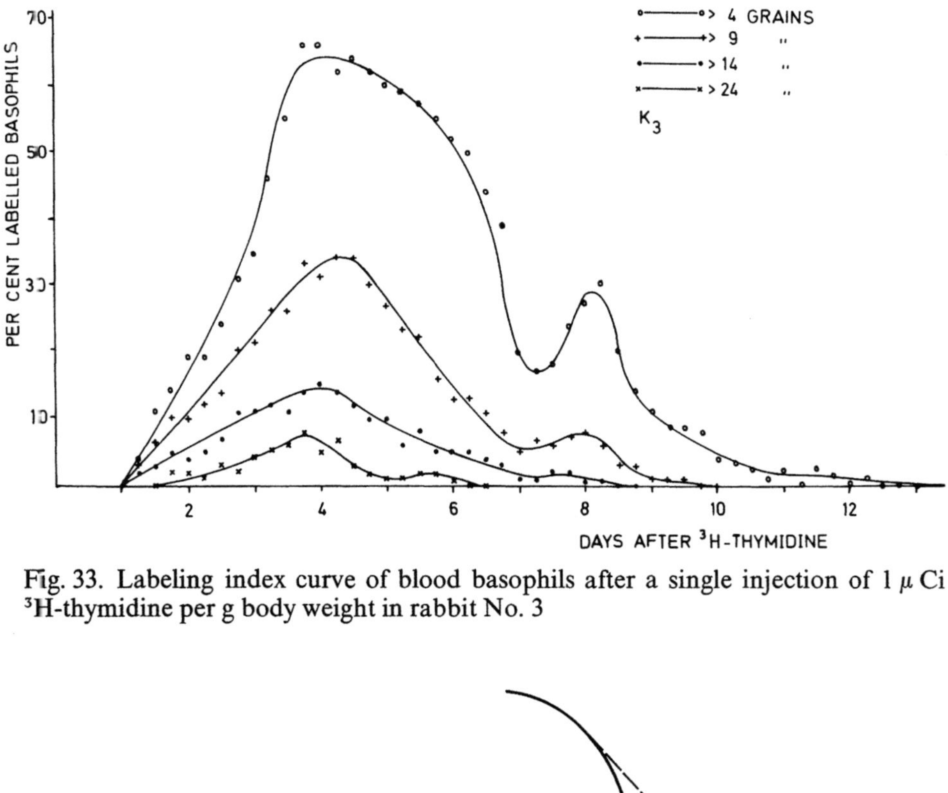

Fig. 33. Labeling index curve of blood basophils after a single injection of 1 μ Ci ^{3}H-thymidine per g body weight in rabbit No. 3

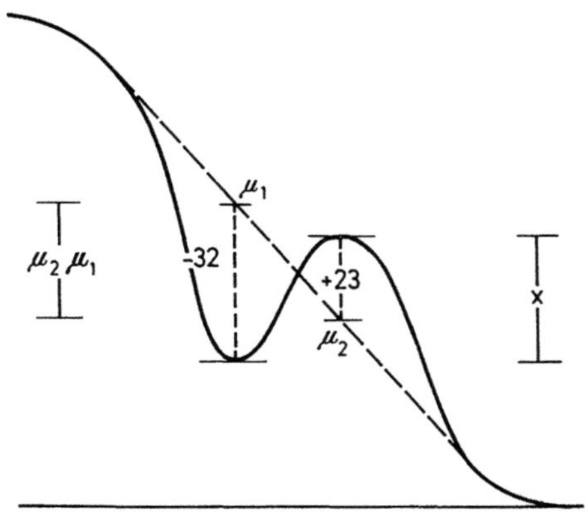

Fig. 34. Assumption of a linearly falling labeling index curve for the computation of the significance of the second peak in fig. 33

P_1 (t) or P_2 (t – x) is the probability of the dispersion from the assumed means by t or by t – x at the intermediate minimum or at the second peak.

On the basis of a normal distribution, the following relation is obtained:

$$P_1(t) = \frac{1}{\sigma_1 \sqrt{2\pi}} \cdot e^{-1/2 \frac{(\mu_1 - t)^2}{\sigma_1}}. \quad (5)$$

The same is valid for P_2 (t – x).

Taking the curve K_3 (Fig. 33) as an example, where

$n = 100$ and $\mu = 23$. This leads to
$P_1 = 0.31$ and $P_2 = 0.23$
$q_1 = 0.69$ and $q_2 = 0.77$.

According to Eq. (3) the dispersion can be estimated yielding

$\delta_1 = 4.6$ and
$\delta_2 = 4.2$.

By entering Eq. (5) in Eq. (4) the value for p (x) can be approximated:

p (+12) = 0.001	p (+8) = 0.005	p (+4) = 0.008
P (0) = 0.021	p (–4) = 0.048	p (–8) = 0.085.

Because the curve is bilaterally symmetrical (Fig. 32) to its maximum at – 8 ($\mu_2 - \mu_1 = -8$), it follows that

p (– 12) = 0.048
p (– 16) = 0.021
p (– 20) = 0.008.

Where x equals + 10, the probability that the second peak represents no actual second rise in the labeling index curve and that it occurs only by chance (no real effect) equals the small hatched area (Fig. 32), or approximately 3‰.

The terminal decrease of the labeling index occurred steeply within 24 to 48 h. Practically no more labeled blood basophils were observed after day 12 p.i. Taking only cells with high labeling intensities, we obtained a somewhat later (6 h) emergence time in the most intensely labeled cell class. The maximum labeling index for cells with more than 9 grains lay at 34%, for cells with more than 14 grains between 13 and 20%, and for cells with more than 24 grains between 5 and 8%. A second peak between day 8 and day 9 was observed for all cells labeled with more than 9 grains and for two animals in which cells with more than 14 grains were found. Cells with more than 9 grains were observed for 10 days, those with more than 14 for 9 days and those with more than 24 for 6 days (Fig. 33).

To determine the intravasal life expectancy (biological half-life T 1/2), the time for which a cell circulates after having been released from the bone marrow, and the mean circulation time, the two cell classes with a labeling intensity of more than 24 or 34 grains per cell, respectively, were evaluated. Figure 35 shows semilogarithmically the falling curve portion of this special basophil population.

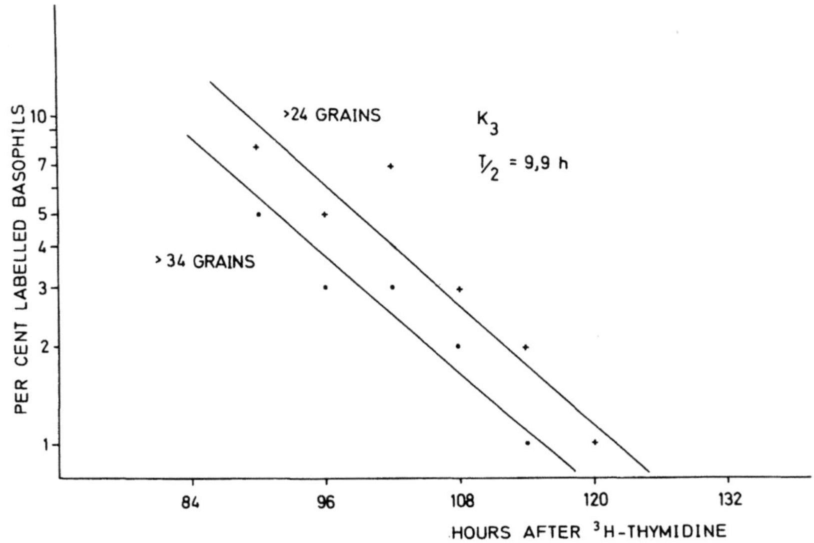

Fig. 35. Semilogarithmic illustration of the descending curve portion for intensely labeled blood basophils (grain number per cell > 24 and > 34) in rabbit No. 3.

Table 19. Kinetic data for all labeled blood basophils in three rabbits ($K_1 - K_3$)

Rabbit No.	K_1	K_2	K_3
Emergence time (h)	30 – 36	24 – 30	24 – 30
Time after application of ^{3}H-thymidine required to reach a labeling index of 60% (h)	103	108	99
Emergence rate per hour	0.89%	0.77%	0.86%
Maximum labeling index	63%	68%	64%
Time after ^{3}H-Thymidine application required to reach maximum labeling index (h)	108	120	108
First minimum labeling index	23%	20%	17%
Time after ^{3}H-thymidine application required to reach first minimum labeling index (h)	192	180	174
Labeling index at second curve peak	33%	36%	28%
Time after ^{3}H-thymidine application required to reach second curve peak (h)	216	204	198

Rabbit basophils according to our results are distinguished by the following kinetic criteria: the initial influx begins 24 to 30 h p.i. and ranges from 0.77 to 0.89% per h. The increase is relatively constant. The maximum is reached between the 63rd and 96th hours p.i. The subsequent fall in the labeling index is exponential. In agreement with the findings for neutrophil granulocytes, a fall of this type signifies a random disappearance of blood basophils from the circulation. Mean circulation time as measured on intensely labeled cells ranges from 11.6 to 14.5 h with a half-life of 8 to 9.6 h. The kinetic data obtained are summarized in Tables 19 and 20.

Table 20. Average circulation time and half-disappearance time of ^{3}H-thymidine labeled blood basophils in rabbits (K_{1-3})

Rabbit No.	K_1	K_2	K_3
Half-disappearance time (h)	9.6	8.0	9.9
Average circulation time (h)	13.9	11.6	14.5

In summary, the results show definitely that blood basophils are short-lived cells and that their kinetic behavior largely corresponds with that of neutrophil granulocytes. It can therefore be concluded that basophil granulopoiesis represents an active system with a high turnover rate. Further, the half-life determined rules out the much-discussed capability of blood basophils to restore their discharged granules. Each granulolysis apparently initiates the process of necrobiosis or cell death.

3. Kinetics of Human Blood Basophils

The rarity of human blood basophils and the solubility of their specific granules have hampered autoradiographic processing. Thus, the cytokinetics of these cells long resisted clarification. Fixatives and stains otherwise suitable for the preservation of human blood basophils (PARWARESCH and LENNERT, 1967) produce chemographic artifacts, which make a quantiative analysis of the results impossible. Salts, such as basic lead acetate, or quaternary ammonium compounds, such as N-cetylpyridinium chloride or N-cetyltrimethylammonium bromide, which are potent fixatives for human blood basophils, produce a high background. The same proved to be true of such panoptic stains as WRIGHT, LEICHMAN, MAY-GRÜNWALD and GIEMSA, and dyes such as toluidine blue, methylene blue, thionine and alcian blue. Subsequent staining of autoradiographs also proved unsuccessful.

Rabbit basophils have many features in common with human basophils, yet the technique used for autoradiography of rabbit basophils failed with human blood. Attempts to prevent direct contact between the blood smears and the sensitive emulsion by coating the slides with collodium, Vinalak, or Formvar gave poor results. Formvar dissolved in ethylene dichloride (STUB-

BLEFIELD, 1965), for instance, severely reduced labeling intensity (KOPRIWA and LEBLOND, 1962), but did not similarly reduce background; this made it difficult to exclude nonspecifically marked cellular elements.

The problem of autoradiographic tracing of labeled human basophils remained unsolved until the introduction of 5-aminoacridine (PARWARESCH and ARNDT, 1975). The compound 5-aminoacridine hydrochloride is mainly used in chemistry to effect a selective precipitation of glycosaminoglycans; it proved to be the only compound in the acridine group that does not induce chemographic effects. The bonding to glycosaminoglycans is fairly stable, insoluble in water, and resistant to variations in pH within a reasonable range. With 5-aminoacridine hydrochloride a technique was developed which permits both the clear distinction of labeled human blood basophils in autoradiographs and a quantitative analysis of the experimental results. The kinetics of human blood basophils was studied on the basis of this new method.

Isotopic labeling. Three male patients, two with circumscribed carcinoma of esophagus (0=71 years and M=65 years of age) and one with papillary carcinoma of urinary bladder (K=71 years), each received a single intravenous injection of 0.1 μ Ci ^{3}H-thymidine (Radiochemical Centre, Amersham; specific activity 1.9 Ci/mM) per gram body weight. Blood samples were taken for the first time after 12 h and then 2 to 4 times per day for the next 17 days, or about 40 times during the course of the experiment. Fresh blood samples were immediately subjected to total leukocyte and direct basophil determination (COOPER and CRUICKSHANK, 1966), and smears of leukocyte concentrates were prepared according to DESAGA and PARWARESCH (1971). Differential blood picture, platelet, and erythrocyte counts were performed regularly to exclude hematological abnormalities.

Fixation and staining. Air-dried smears of leukocyte concentrates were prefixed in methanol-formalin (9 : 1 v/v) for 5 min at 4° C according to KAPLOW (1955). For final fixation the slides were transferred to a 0.4% solution of 5-aminoacridine hydrochloride in 65% ethyl alcohol for 30 min at room temperature. They were then rinsed in methanol-formalin and stained for 30 min in a 0.5% solution of basic aldehyde fuchsin in 80% ethyl alcohol, to which 1 ml paraldehyde and 1 ml concentrated hydrochloric acid has been added (GOMORI, 1950) to bring it to pH 1. The slides were finally rinsed in a 0.5% borax solution ($Na_2B_4O_7 \times 10\ H_2O$) in 80% enthyl alcohol, differentiated in 70% ethyl alcohol and air-dried.

Autoradiography. Smears from leukocyte concentrates were fixed and stained as described above, dipped in the same batch of Kodak nuclear trace liquid emulsion NTB-2 at 43° C, cooled to 4° C in humified chambers, and exposed in lightproof boxes at 4° C for 60 days, developed in Kodak-D 19 for 3 min, rinsed in distilled water, fixed in an aqueous solution of 20% sodium thiosulfate and 2.5% potassium metabisulfide for 3 min at 20° C, and rinsed in tap water for 15 min. Hemalum was used for nuclear counterstaining, when required.

Determination of the background. The background is the sum total of the grains independent of the radioactivity of the applied isotope. This comprises grains induced by the chemographic activity of the different chemical agents used and those resulting from mostly undetectable causes.

To detect any chemographic grains produced by the various agents used, the grains over about 100 segmented nuclei per slide were counted and the values were compared with those of control slides. A random distribution was assumed in all

Table 21. $\bar{X}$ and $\pm S$ values of grains over 100 basophils as compared with corresponding values for 100 neutrophils

Treatment prior to autoradiography	Grain counts over Basophils	Neutrophils
Methanol-formalin	0.72 ± 0.73	0.62 ± 0.69
Methanol-formalin and 5-aminoacridine	0.61 ± 0.67	0.70 ± 0.71
Methanol-formalin, 5-aminoacridine, and borax	0.68 ± 0.71	0.66 ± 0.70
Methanol-formalin, 5-aminoacridine, borax, and aldehyde fuchsin	0.73 ± 0.73	0.71 ± 0.72

computations. All item rules were subjected to variance analysis with the F test as a general test for independent populations. Means were computed for a significant difference on the basis of a 95% p-level using the t-test. The control slides had been subjected to (a) methanol-formalin fixation, autoradiography and nuclear staining, (b) methanol-formalin and 5-aminoacridine fixation, (c) the same as (b) plus borax treatment, and (d) the same as (c) plus aldehyde-fuchsin staining. The results are listed in Table 21. The probability that 5-aminoacridine hydrochloride accumulates in the specific granules and so leads to an artificial elevation of grain production over the cytoplasm of the basophils was determined by comparing the mean cytoplasmic grain counts of 100 blood basophils with those of 100 other leukocytes.

Background irrespective of the chemography caused by the agents applied can be influenced by the thickness of the tracer emulsion, thickness of the cell layer, and the structural density of the cells under consideration. Variations in the thickness of the tracer film are negligible (Darlington and Rogers, 1966). Grain count dispersions resulting from variances in the thickness and density of the cells or smears to be coated by the tracer emulsion cause relevant differences (Tonna and Cronkite, 1958; Hale, 1958; Stillström, 1963; 1965). The dispersion of such grains is affected by a number of factors one of which (cell-thickness) follows a normal pattern of distribution.

Table 22. Means ($\bar{X}$) and standard deviations (S) of background-induced grain counts per surface unit (equal to the surface of one erythrocyte or that of a basophil nucleus).

Grains over:	n	$\bar{X}$	± S	Difference Factor
Cell-free areas	3,800	1.02	0.09	+ 1.4
Erythrocytes	4,800	0.74	0.08	+ 1.0
Cell-free areas equal to basophil nuclei	24,000	0.85	0.05	+ 1.2
Neutrophil nuclei	100	0.69	0.05	− 1.1
Basophil nuclei	100	0.68	0.04	− 1.1

In our study the mean grain count per surface unit over the cell-free areas exceeded the values over erythrocytes by a factor of 1.25 to 1.5 (Table 22). The difference proved by the t test to be statistically significant ($p < 0.05$). These results are in accordance with the findings reported by other authors (PERRY *et al.*, 1961; MARTIN and BENDER, 1963).

A further control test was administered to rule out background variations between the slides for the different sampling intervals. In each slide the mean grain count over a surface equal to that of 100 basophil nuclei in cell-free areas was determined and compared with the corresponding values from other slides. The total mean amounted to 0.85 grain with a range of 0.27 – 1.79. No statistically significant difference between the means of the variances could be found, as computed by the chi-square test. The maximum variability encountered remains within the limits given by the dispersion index according to the formula

$$\chi^2 = \sum \frac{(f - fc)^2}{fc}. \tag{1}$$

Assuming a mean background value of $\lambda = 0.85$ grains per basophil nucleus and on the basis of $n = 200$ basophils considered per slide, the probability (p) for the occurrence of background-induced grains over a basophil nucleus amounts to

$$p = \frac{\lambda}{n} = 0.04. \tag{2}$$

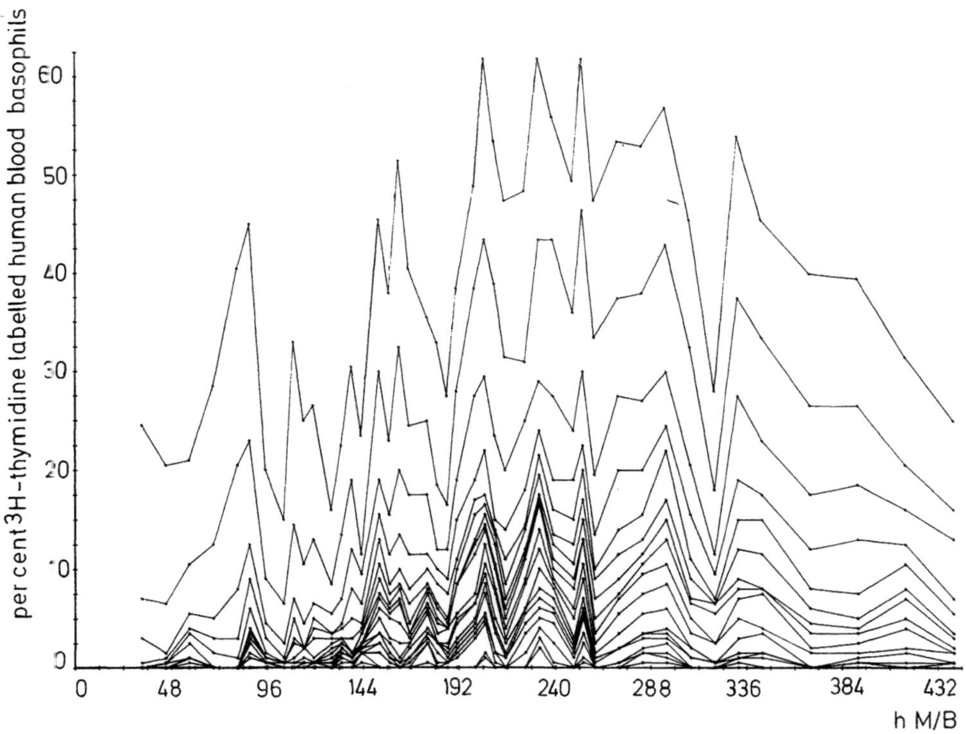

Fig. 36. Computer-drawn labeling curves of blood basophils (patient M) on the basis of continuously ascending grain counts (2 – 40 per nucleus) arranged in grain classes with grain counts > 2 > 3 > 4 . . . > 40 per basophil nucleus

The random distribution of background grains follows by virtue of the low *p* value and the large n value, or on the basis of the finite pn-value, a POISSON pattern

$$p(k) = \frac{\lambda^k : e^{-\lambda}}{k!}. \qquad (3)$$

Where $\lambda = 0.85$ represents the expected background value; $k=2$ is the grain level beyond which the cells will be regarded as genuinely labeled; and e is the basis of the natural logarithm. For $\lambda = 0.85$ the probability that 2 grains over a basophil nucleus will be induced by background is very small, amounting to 0.05%. Taking the difference factor for the cell-specific background distribution, the probability for every basophil nucleus to receive 2 artificial grains falls to $0.05 \times 1.4 = 0.03\%$. Hence it falls within the confidence limits.

Accordingly, the two-grain limit is here regarded as the justifiable level of discrimination above which all basophils are assumed to be genuinely labeled. In reality, this level is certainly lower. The level of the background is a function of the labeling index and the mean grain count per nucleus. With a high labeling index and a high mean grain count all necessary conditions seem to be fulfilled in the present study. The real background values lie well below the assumed values (SAWICKI *et al.*, 1971). The labeling index (% labeled basophils in blood) and the individually corrected labeling intensity (grain count per nucleus) were recorded for each sampling

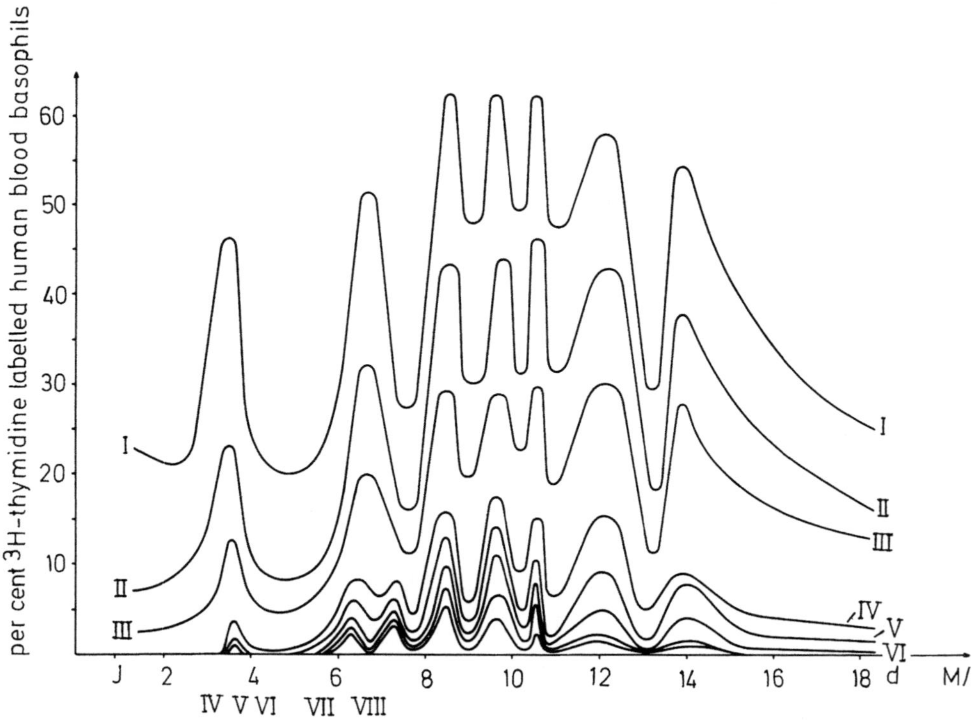

Fig. 37. Curves of blood basophils labeling indices for patient M following i. v. ^{3}H-thymidine (0.1 μ Ci/g b.w.) puls application (*J*). The curves (I – VIII) represent basophils of different labeling classes: I≧2; II≧3; III≧4; IV≧5; V≧8; VI≧15; VII≧25; VIII≧35 grains per nucleus. Fluctuations represent only statistically significant peaks selected following a polynomial approximation

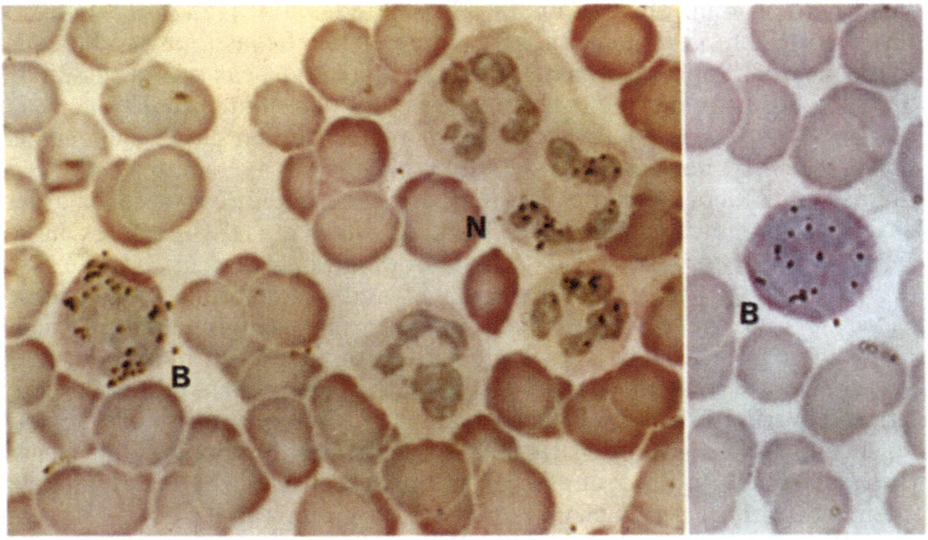

Fig. 38. Autoradiographs demonstrating ^{3}H-thymidine-labeled human leukocytes. Basophils (*B*) are easily discernable from neutrophils (*N*) by cytoplasmic metachromasia. 5-aminoacridine hydrochloride fixation and aldehyde fuchsin staining. ×1,270

interval. The curves of the labeling index for all labeling intensities were drawn by computer (Fig. 36). In a further step, all peaks resulting from the undulating course of the curves were subjected to the distribution-free WILCOXON test in modification of MANN-WHITNEY (KOLLER, 1969). Thus only peaks that exceeded the basic line by a significant height ($p < 0.01$), corresponding to a polynomial approximation, were expressed in the chart (Fig. 37).

Results. The staining technique described allows blood basophils to be clearly distinguished, as shown in Fig. 38. The cytoplasm of basophils is well preserved and light violet to pale purple in colour. Other leukocytes did not stain at this pH and were therefore easily distinguished from basophils even under low magnification. No evidence of the artificial destruction seen in most staining procedures due to the leaching of water-soluble basophil granules was observed.

Extensive control tests excluded chemographic activities. With the agents used in this procedure there was no significant difference between the background grain dispersion of the control slides and the smears subjected to the whole procedure (see Table 21). This was also true for grain counts over the cytoplasms.

In the slides from the samples taken 12 h p.i. 21% of basophils showed grain counts of up to 12 per nucleus. Within a period averaging 44.6 h p.i. the labeling index still amounted to 22.0 ± 3.7% and the labeling intensity reached values of around 18 grains. During the initial massive influx the mean inflow rate reached a value of 1.3 ± 0.3% basophils per hour. This initial peak of the labeling index comprised mainly basophils of low or medium labeling intensity and the maximum grain count in this phase amounted to 17 per basophil. The maximum labeling index averaged 43.7% and was observed 67.2 h p.i. The mean inflow time of 10.6 h was found to be equal to the mean disappearance time, when the first curve peak was considered.

The entire compartment-transit time (CTT) amounted to 21.2 h. Peaks occurring 5 to 7 days p.i. revealed approximately similar data. The mean labeling intensity, however, was definitely higher. On average over 43.1% of the basophils were labeled in this period of time. The inflow rate for different peaks amounted to 1.6% per h. Up to this stage the labeling index curves followed a more or less parallel course for all grain classes in all three cases (Fig. 37). At the beginning the maxima and the minima of the curves showed a more or less parallel course, which increasingly faded into complete asynchronism. The increasing fading of the synchronism observed among the progression courses of the index curves for continuous grain classes covering cells with 2 to 40 grains (Fig. 37) becomes more obvious when the continuous grain classes are rearranged into grain-count groups (Fig. 39). These grain groups (gg) comprise cells with a maximal grain count of 3 grains per nucleus (gg I); 4 to 8 grains (gg II); 9 to 15 grains (gg III); and more than 16 grains (gg IV).

The rearrangement was performed on the basis of the following observations. Charts demonstrating the semilogarithmic course of the disappearance rate of labeled basophils, prepared for the purpose of calculating t/2, showed a common trend in their course within certain grain classes (Fig. 40). Further, the frequency distribution of grain counts during the entire course of the experiment in all 3 cases presented certain central tendencies, so that particular grain counts were shared by a considerable bulk

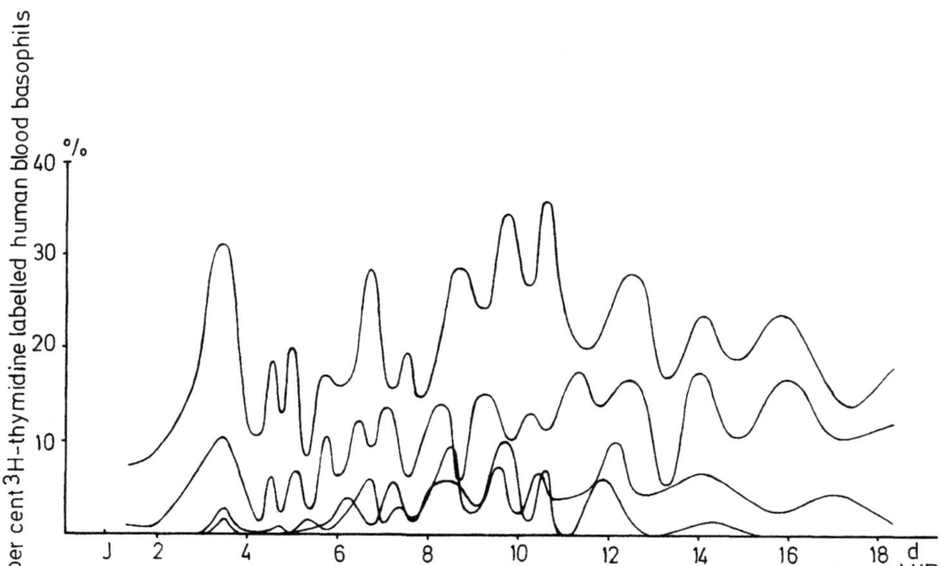

Fig. 39. Curves of labeling indices of human blood basophils in patient M after ^{3}H-thymidine application (*J*), arranged in groups (gg I – IV) according to grain counts: ggI = 2 – 3, ggII = 4 – 8, ggIII = 9 – 15, ggIV > 16 grains per nucleus

of cell numbers. These distribution patterns corresponded to the grain groups chosen above.

In estimating further kinetic parameters, namely half-life (t/2), mean circulation time (MCT), and compartment-transit time (CTT), we took the following considerations into account: t/2 values estimated on the basis of the rearranged grain groups reflect the kinetic situation more accurately

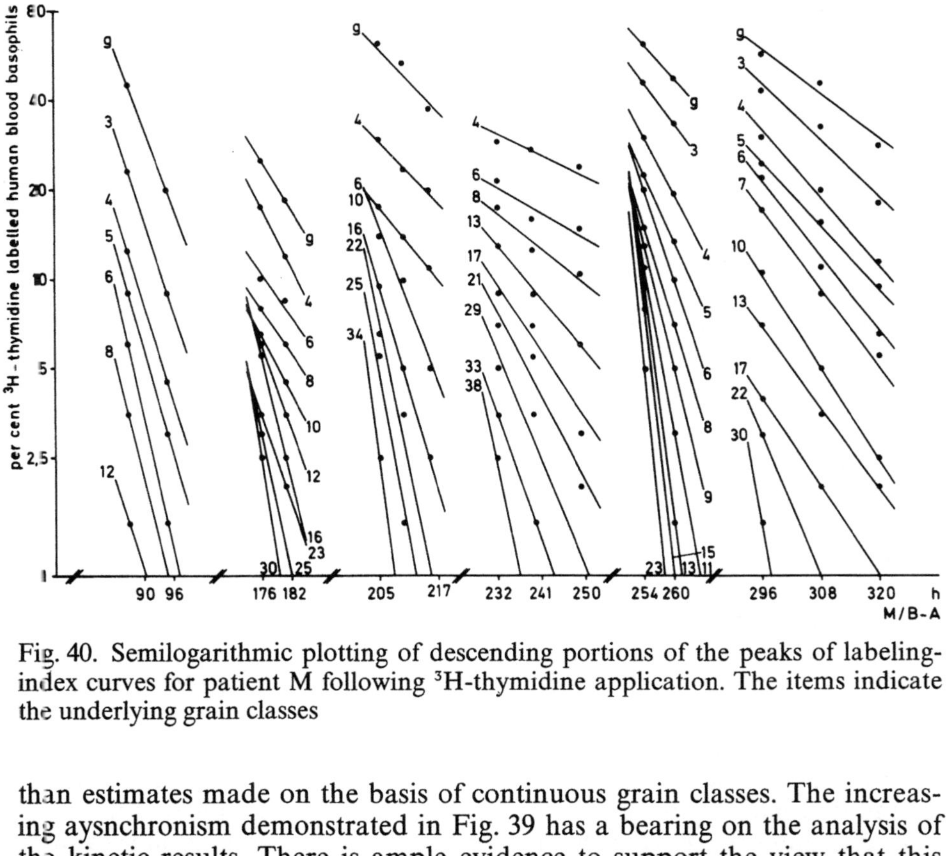

Fig. 40. Semilogarithmic plotting of descending portions of the peaks of labeling-index curves for patient M following ^{3}H-thymidine application. The items indicate the underlying grain classes

than estimates made on the basis of continuous grain classes. The increasing aysnchronism demonstrated in Fig. 39 has a bearing on the analysis of the kinetic results. There is ample evidence to support the view that this asynchronism arises from increasing mingling of cellular pools with different proliferation rates.

The half-circulation time (t/2), i.e. the period of time beginning at t_0 in the course of which the circulating count of a certain cell population (n labeled basophils) is reduced by 50% (n/2), is expressed by the differential equation

$$\frac{dn\,(t)}{dt} = -\,cn\,(t). \tag{4}$$

where (c) represents a factor indicating the proportionality between the time-dependent reduction of the cell number and the total cell count. On inserting c_1 as an integral constant, the equation becomes

$$\ln n(t) = -ct + c_1 \quad (5)$$

or

$$n(t) = c_1 \cdot e^{-c \cdot t/2} \quad (6)$$

Solving for t/2, we obtain

$$\frac{t}{2} = \frac{\ln 2}{c}. \quad (7)$$

The mean circulation time (MCT) is by definition

$$\text{MCT} \; \frac{\int_0^\infty t \cdot e^{-c}\, dt}{\int_0^\infty e^{-ct}\, dt}. \quad (8)$$

Partial integration of (8) gives

$$\text{MCT} = \frac{1}{c}. \quad (9)$$

Inserting t, we obtain

$$\text{MCT} = \frac{\frac{t}{2}}{\ln 2}. \quad (10)$$

The compartment transit time (CTT) under the condition of normal equilibration was obtained from the equation: CTT = 4 t/2 or calculated independently from t/2 on the basis of the mean inflow time (MIT) and the mean disappearance time (MDT): CTT = MIT + MDT. A check is provided when both calculations are performed.

For the purpose of estimating t/2 in the current studies, we took as a basis the descending portions of the peaks of the labeling-index curves arranged in grain classes (Fig. 40; Tables 23 and 24) and grain groups (Tables 25 and 26), as previously explained. The e-functional (exponential) curve was straightened by semilogarithmic plotting (Fig. 40). The half-circulation time averaged 5.7 h (range 7.3 – 2.9) when estimated on the basis of the charts for all grain groups. Assuming t/2 = 5.7 h, the corresponding MCT amounts to 8.3 h. CTT as calculated from the inflow and disappearance times is on average 21.0 h. The same parameter worked out on the basis of CTT = 4 t/2 gives a value of 22.6 h. The reasonable agreement of the values indicates the reliability of the results.

Intensely labeled basophils (gg IV) could be detected up to day 16th p.i. and made up about 5% of the total peripheral basophil count (Fig. 37). The kinetic data calculated on the basis of this percentage of labeled cells agree well with the values mentioned above (Tables 23 and 25). As previously

Table 23. Means ($\bar{X}$) and standard deviations (S) of different kinetic parameters of human blood basophils estimated on the basis of grain classes in three patients, O, M and K. OMK represents the mean values of all three subjects. ET = Emergence time, GT = Generation time, MIR = Mean inflow rate, MIT = Mean inflow time, LI = Labeling index, LIT = Labeling-index time, t/2 = Half-life, MCT = Mean circulation time, MDT = Mean disappearance time, CTT = Compartment-transit time

Patient	0		M		K		OMK
	$\bar{X}$	S	$\bar{X}$	S	$\bar{X}$	S	$\bar{X}$
ET (h)	12.0		12.0		12.0		12.0
GT (h)	51.9	4.0	45.8	4.8	36.0	0.0	44.6
MIR (%/h)	1.4		0.9		1.5		1.3
MIT (h)	12.6	2.5	8.3	4.8	11.0	0.0	10.6
LI (%)	45.5		45.0		40.5		43.7
LIT (h)	75.0	0.0	66.0	0.0	59.0	0.0	66.7
t/2 (h)	7.3	1.4	6.8	2.7	2.9	0.6	5.7
MCT (h)	10.5	2.1	9.7	3.9	4.4	0.7	8.2
MDT (h)	14.2	3.5	10.8	4.3	6.6	2.7	10.6
CTT (h)	28.4	5.8	26.3	10.7	12.8	1.91	22.5
MIT + MDT	28.0	5.7	19.1	8.5	16.8	2.5	21.3
MIR (%/h)	1.7		2.4		1.6		1.9
MIT (h)	9.7	1.2	8.1	3.5	17.7	5.7	11.8
LI (%)	45.0		51.5		42.5		46.3
LIT (h)	144.5	2.5	127.9	5.8	156.4	10.2	142.9
t/2 (h)	5.9	1.6	5.9	5.2	5.4	0.1	5.8
MCT (h)	8.6	2.3	8.5	7.1	7.8	5.2	8.3
MDT (h)	11.6	1.6	8.9	4.8	5.3	1.1	8.6
CTT (h)	24.6	2.9	23.5	8.8	21.6	5.2	23.2
MIT + MDT	21.8	1.5	17.4	4.1	21.4	3.4	20.2
MIR (%/h)	2.3		1.8		2.1		2.1
MIT (h)	16.1	5.3	15.5	4.5	9.0	0.0	13.5
LI (%)	60.5		62.0		47.0		56.5
LIT (h)	178.1	5.2	184.0	0.0	179.0	0.0	180.4
t/2 (h)	5.9	3.2	6.3	4.7	4.2	1.9	5.5
MCT (h)	8.5	5.7	9.4	6.8	6.1	2.8	8.0
MDT (h)	9.9	0.5	8.7	2.1	5.9	1.2	8.2
CTT (h)	23.6	12.9	26.1	14.2	16.8	7.7	22.2
MIT + MDT	25.4	4.7	24.2	8.1	15.0	1.2	21.5

Table 24. Different kinetic parameters of human blood basophils on the basis of grain classes (mean values of 3 subjects)

Emergence time	12.0 h
Generation time	44.6 h
Mean inflow rate	1.8%/h
Mean inflow time	12.0 h
Half-life	5.7 h
Mean circulation time	8.2 h
Mean disappearance time	9.1 h
Compartment-transit time	22.6 h
Turnover	21.0 h

Table 25. Means ($\bar{X}$) and standard deviations (S) of basophil t/2 values arranged according to grain groups: ggI = 2 – 3 grains per nucleus; ggII = 4 – 8; ggIII = 9 – 15; and ggIV = over 15. T p.i. = Time in hours after ^{3}H-thymidine injection. The values are specified as follows: t/2 < 10 h no brackets; t/2 ≦ 15 h in ( ), t/2 ≦ 20 h in { }, t/2 > 20 h in [ ]

Patient 0

T p.i.	75 – 89	142 – 156 – 169	179 – 203 – 217 – 227 – 234		263 – 299 – 347		$\bar{X}_1$t/2 T	S_1t/2 T
t/2 gg I	(11.0)	(12.0)	8.7	–	–	–	10.6	1.7
t/2 gg II	6.0	5.7	8.0	(13.8)	[24.5]	{15.5}	6.6	1.3
t/2 gg III	5.7	4.8	4.6	4.5	(10.0)	[25.0]	4.9	0.6
t/2 gg IV		4.0	2.3	8.3	3.7	8.3	3.3	0.9
$\bar{X}_1$ t/2 gg	7.6	6.6	5.9	6.4	3.7	8.3		
S_1 t/2 gg	3.0	3.7	3.0	2.7				

Patient M

T p.i.	60 – 74	131 – 160	179 – 194	204 – 228	233 – 251	263 – 299	323 – 347	395 – 419	$\bar{X}_1$t/2 T	S_1t/2 T
t/2 gg I	10.5	{18.0}	–	–	[22.2]	[26.3]	–	–	10.5	
t/2 gg II	7.4	(15.0)	5.5	[24.5]	–	(11.5)	–	–	8.1	3.1
t/2 gg III	3.5	3.3	4.5	5.0	(10.3)	(12.0)	[26.7]	(15.0)	4.1	0.8
t/2 gg IV	3.7	6.1	5.8	(10.5)	2.4	(12.2)	6.3	–	4.9	1.7
$\bar{X}_1$ t/2 gg	6.3	4.7	5.3	5.0	2.4		6.3			
S_1 t/2 gg	3.3	2.0	0.7							

Patient K

T p.i.	59 – 64	107 – 135	155 – 170	179 – 189 – 194 – 204		212 – 218	228 – 252	264 – 276	360 – 385	$\bar{X}_1$t/2T	S_1t/2 T
t/2 gg I	3.2	{17.0}	5.6	8.3	–	{17.4}	[28.0]		8.8	6.5	2.6
t/2 gg II	2.0	5.0	9.6	(11.6)	9.5	–	(10.8)	(13.5)	7.4	6.7	3.2
t/2 gg III	2.2	(11.4)	–	2.0	(12.4)	–	[25.6]	–	5.6	3.3	2.0
t/2 gg IV	–	3.0	3.2	4.0	5.5	(13.0)	–	–	3.0	3.8	1.1
$\bar{X}_1$ t/2 gg	2.5	4.0	7.0	4.8	7.5				6.2		
S_1 t/2 gg		0.6	1.4	3.2	2.8				2.5		

Table 26. Means ($\bar{X}$) and standard deviations (S) of all t/2 values estimated on the basis of grain groups in three patients (O, M, and K). The different t/2 ranges are X_1 t/2 = 10 h, X_2 t/2 = 15 h, X_3 t/2 = 20 h, X_4 t/2 = 20 h

Patient	O		M		K		OMK	
	$\bar{X}$	S	$\bar{X}$	S	$\bar{X}$	S	$\bar{X}$	S
$\bar{X}_1$ t/2	6.4	2.16	5.8	2.2	5.2	1.8	5.8	0.9
$\bar{X}_2$ t/2	11.7	1.6	11.2	0.9	12.1	1.0	11.7	1.1
$\bar{X}_3$ t/2	15.5	–	17.2	0.3	16.0	1.7	16.3	1.3
$\bar{X}_4$ t/2	24.8	0.4	24.9	2.1	26.8	1.7	25.4	1.7

pointed out, the kinetics of human blood basophils has long resisted clarification because of the technical difficulties. Kinetic data obtained for rabbit basophils, however, resemble those of other granulocytes (PARWARESCH *et al.*, 1973). The t/2 values averaged 9.2 h and circulation time 13.2 h. These data are in agreement with the values obtained during the regeneration time following basopenia experimentally induced by cortisone or compound 48/80.

In the current studies, labeled human blood basophils first appeared in the peripheral blood 12 h after ^{3}H-thymidine application. The relatively short initial emergence time is highly suggestive of a correspondingly short turnover time. This was substantiated by the values obtained for t/2 and compartment-transit time. The labeling-index curves for human blood basophils were characterized by clear and long-lasting undulations with statistically significant peaks. A second maximum was also observed in the labeling-index curves of rabbit basophils. Similar findings were reported by PATT and MALONEY (1959), FLIEDNER *et al.* (1964 a; 1966), and HERION *et al.* (1970). The phenomenon of a cyclic fluctuation was interpreted as the expression of a synchronism in the generation cycle (FLIEDNER *et al.*, 1964 a). It was suggested that such fluctuations approximately reflect the generation time of myelocytes. In an asynchronously proliferating population, the period of the generation cycle would far exceed the availability of the injected ^{3}H-thymidine for the proliferation pool in the bone marrow (HERION *et al.*, 1970). In an equilibrated system, cyclic fluctuations appear in the labeling curves in the presence of undisturbed cell transit in the bone marrow pool. The magnitude of the amplitude represents a function of the transit time of the peripheral compartment and the mode of the peripheral disappearance. This may imply that the proliferating basophilic marrow compartment has a particularly short generation cycle, which seems improbable. For instance, the observation of a high incidence of mitoses in the basophilic cell line of human bone marrow (PARWARESCH and NOTTBOHM, 1975) contradicts this view. In this study 50% of the total basophil population of the human bone marrow was found to comprise precursors capable of proliferation. Finally, we must consider the objection that such fluctuations might result from a direct toxic effect of ^{3}H-thymidine or from a reutilization of labeled DNA fragments. Both possibilities seem improbable. On the one hand, the fluctuations occur regularly and the curve peaks are detectable at all labeling levels, as indicated in a different context by FLIEDNER *et al.* (1961). On the other hand, PARWARESCH *et al.* (1973) were ablé to demonstrate the chronological coincidence of the mean grain count halftime and of a clearcut second peak in the labeling curves of rabbit basophils. Furthermore, a similar pattern of labeling curves was found in the present study for labeled neutrophils and eosinophils.

The majority of the reports on this subject make no mention of a labeling curve with multiple maxima. This could well be due to the fact that such deviations from a smooth curve often fall within the margins of error. Furthermore, in the majority of studies no continuous statistical computation of the labeling indices at the various sampling intervals had been accomplished. Again, if the time intervals were too long, peaks or minima might easily escape attention. Small sampling intervals as well as large sample values make apparently minor fluctuations in the curve more obvious.

The compilation of multiple curve peaks enables us to make more accurate statements on the kinetic data, especially the turnover rate and t/2 values. The semilogarithmic plotting of the descending peak sides at various sampling intervals (Fig. 40) reveals an obvious parallelism between the curves of the same grain groups. This parallelism indicates the close association in the proliferation cycle of these populations, approximating to a kinetic synchronism of their proliferation pools. The synchronism in the generation cycle of the labeled basophils within each group, however, vanishes as time progresses. This is expressed in the increasing slope of the labeling-index curves, which becomes obvious in the course of the experimental time (Figs. 39 and 40). The slope peaks, in our opinion, cover a different number of overlapping labeling peaks of cells with similar grain counts (identical grain groups). These populations differ in their proliferative stages. It is evident that basophils within the same grain group might stem from different kinetic populations, as the emergence of the cells occurs at different times relative to ^{3}H-thymidine application. Within this period of time promyelocytes and myelocytes, (a) take up different quantities of the isotope, and (b) undergo different numbers of mitoses. These events cause major differences in the labeling intensities of the mature basophils. In other words, basophils from the same grain group might derive from precursor populations at different kinetic stages. The t/2 values estimated on the basis of the slope efflux rates were found to be clustered around the values: 11.7 ± 1.1, 16.3 ± 1.3, or 25.4 ± 1.7 h and thus represented multiplication products by the factors 2, 3 and 5 of the basic t/2 value (estimated on the basis of a homogeneous basophil population with steep labeling peaks) averaging 5.7 h. Consequently, the increasing slope of the labeling curves reflects the asynchronism taking place among the proliferating basophil strains, resulting in an artificial prolongation of t/2 to cover multiplication products of the basic t/2 values.

The individual kinetic data obtained in the present work seem to diverge from the results reported for other granulocytes (Table 27). Thus, the

Table 27. Survey of kinetic data of myelogenous leukocytes in human blood. Values in brackets are calculated on the basis of basic data reported by each author. ET = emergence time (h), t/2 = half-life (h) MCT = mean circulation time (h), CTT = compartment-transit time (h)
1. BOND and CRONKITE (1957), 2. FLIEDNER *et al.* (1961), 3. MURAKAMI *et al.* (1969), 4. FLIEDNER, *et al.* (1969)

Myelogenous Leukocytes		ET	t/2	MCT	CTT
Neutrophil	(1,2)	96	6.9 – (14)	10 – (20)	(28) – 55
Eosinophil	(3)	60 – 72	17 – 33	24 – 48	(68 – 132)
Basophil		12	6	8.5	2.4
Monocyte	(4)	24	8	32 – 39	144

emergence time of 12 h is much shorter than those of neutrophils, which average 96 h (BOND and CRONKITE, 1957; FLIEDNER *et al.,* 1961), and of eosinophils, which ranges from 60 to 72 h (MURAKAMI *et a.,* 1969). The emergence time is a function of the grain count level, above which the cells are regarded as being genuinely labeled. This level is fairly low in these experiments, which explains the rather short emergence time. At this stage only low-labeled basophils could be detected in the peripheral blood. The labeling index averaged 21%. The short emergence time of low-labeled cells and the fact that the labeled cells comprise 21% of blood basophils favor the view that these cells are derived from a homogeneous myelocyte population. At the time of ^{3}H-thymidine incorporation they should have been in a late stage of the S phase. This view is fairly consistent with the finding that the general ^{3}H-thymidine uptake capacity of myelocytes is considerably lower than that of promyelocytes (FLIEDNER *et al.,* 1962). Moreover, the initial labeling index of 21% accords well with the finding that $24.5 \pm 6.4\%$ of the whole basophil population of human bone marrow consists of myelocytes (PARWARESCH and NOTTBOHM, 1975). This implies that about 45% of all basophil myelocytes in human bone marrow mature and turn directly into polymorphonucleated basophils and are released from the marrow without further division after labeling and single division.

Such a short emergence time is further evidence for the magnitude of the proliferative capacity of basophil granulopoiesis, as expected on the basis of the relatively large proportion of dividing precursors in the marrow. If the hypothesis that heparin and histamine released from basophil granules exert a singnificant physiological influence is true, then basophils must be short-lived cells. In addition, the low peripheral count and the relative scarcity of basophils in the bone marrow imply a high turnover if their complex physiological role is to be properly accomplished.

Particular inferences can be drawn from the initial phase of the labeling curves. The S phase, for instance, may be approximately calculated on the basis of inflow time and disappearance time. This amounts to 10.6 h and agrees well with the value of 11 h presented by STRYCKMANS *et al.* (1966) for neutrophils.

The time intervals between the curve peaks averaged 44.6 h. This period is believed to express the generation time. Assuming identical values for the subcycle phases (mitosis, presynthetic rest period, and premitotic rest period) for basophils and neutrophils (BOLL, 1966) and inserting the value for the S phase as estimated above, the generation time for basophils will amount to 43 ± 6 h, which is fairly consistent with the measured time interval between the curve peaks.

The apparent discrepancy between the mean turnover time of about 21 h and the generation time of 44.6 h with a ratio of 1 : 2 may be explained by the assumption of two pools proliferating in parallel at different proliferative velocities, hence rapidly and slowly proliferating compartments. This was also proposed by BOLL (1966) for neutrophils. Some evidence might be provided by the observation that heavily labeled basophils appear in the blood at a relatively late phase of the experimental period. No information, however, is available on the magnitude and proliferation velocity of each pool. The possibility, however, exists that the low-velocity compartment might serve as a basic proliferative reserve.

Blood basophils derive from nonspecific promyelocytes in bone marrow. They represent short-lived, nondividing 'end'-cells with a half-circulation time of about 6 h. Their precursors in bone marrow comprise less than 0.5% of the total marrow leukopoietic cells. Nevertheless, over 50% of this population represents promyelocytes or myelocytes, which are capable of division. These properties support the view that basophils of the peripheral blood, like other granulocytes, also represent functional 'end'-cells whose granule discharge is closely associated with cell necrobiosis. The evidence presented excludes the possibility of regranulation of blood basophils and is also consistent with the ultrastructural features of these cells, basophils being poor in ergastoplasm, microsomes, Golgi structures, and mitochondria.

The close specification of human basophil kinetics with a half-renewal rate of about 17×10^6 cells per hour substantiates their functional significance. It further refutes the objection that the quantity of heparin and histamine they contain would not suffice for effective action.

4. The Effect of Compound 48/80 on Rabbit Basophils

Thirty noninbred rabbits, about 6 months old and weighing on average 3,500 g, were examined in two groups of 15 animals. In the experimental group, both ears of each rabbit were carefully depilated and after injection of compound 48/80 (2 mg/kg body weight in 0.5 ml saline solution) the blood basophil count and the total leukocyte count were directly determined, initially at 2 min intervals and after 30 min at 3 h intervals up to the 18th hour p.i. The control group received a single injection of 0.5 ml saline solution; blood samples were taken at the same intervals.

To test the hypothesis that blood basophils resynthesize their granules after degranulation, we carried out similar experiments *in vitro*. Fifteen 10 ml, freshly obtained blood samples were mixed with compound 48/80 in the same concentration as in the *in vivo* experiment (0.5 mg) and incubated at 37° C under aseptic culture conditions. Fifteen other samples served as controls and were examined after addition of 0.5 ml RINGER solution under the same conditions. The glassware was siliconized. Sedimentation of the blood cells was prevented by light shaking and mild air insufflation. In the first 20 min the total leukocyte and basophil counts were determined at 2-min intervals. After 30 min this was done every 3 h.

a) In-vivo Tests

No significant variation of the total leukocyte count was observed in either control or test animals during the entire *in-vivo* investigations. The injection of compound 48/80, however, led to a massive fall in blood basophils within 4 to 6 min. Subsequently, the blood basophil count rose again to the initial value, the highest values being reached 30 min after the injection. This swift rise was followed by a continuous decrease of the basophil count to 20 to 30% of the initial values. After 9 h, a gradual increase began. The basophil count still lay, after 12 h, well below normal values and the initial values were reached only after 18 h (Fig. 41). Morphological examinations of the blood basophils in the various test phases revealed no alteration of the granules in the intact cells. At each test phase, an average of 50 blood basophils chosen at random from different areas of the blood smear were photographed and compared with each other and with the corresponding cells from the control group. We used the semiquantitative grading method of SHEL-

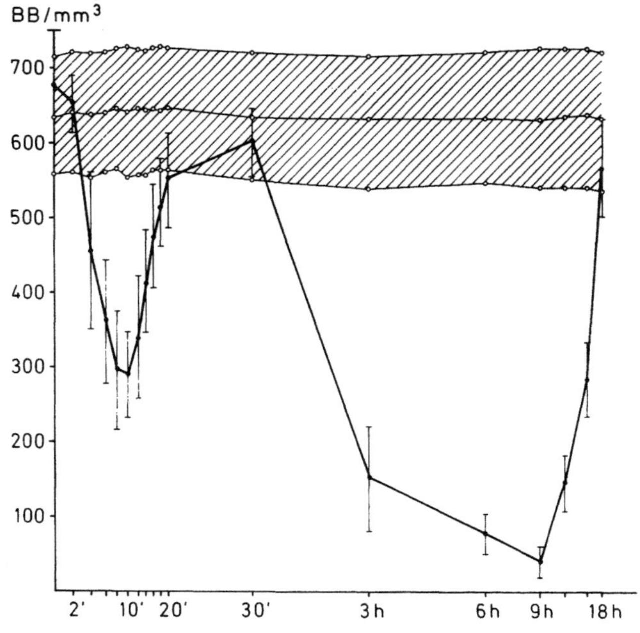

Fig. 41. Basophil count after a single intravenous injection of compound 48/80 (2 mg per kg body weight in 0.5 ml saline) and 0.5 ml saline for controls (hatched area). n = 15 rabbits in each group

LEY and attempted to quantitatively determine the granule content in the basophils. These examinations have shown that blood basophils from the same blood samples display very different distribution patterns of their metachromatic granules and possess varying granule contents. It was not possible, however, to ascertain a significant difference between the granule content of treated and untreated blood basophils.

b) In-vitro Tests

The in-vitro test results are quite different from those obtained *in vivo.* After 3 h the control samples show a steady decrease of blood basophils, whereas in the test samples a drop occurs only 6 min after addition of compound 48/80. The rest of the curve runs almost parallel with that of the control (Fig. 42). The prepared smears show considerable morphological alterations in the blood basophils. Along with pyknotic forms, distinct signs of an intracytoplasmatic granulolysis with diffuse metachromatic staining of the entire cytoplasm were consistently observed. All stages of 'degranulation', as described by SHELLEY, were detectable (Fig. 43). Many blood basophils displayed large intracytoplasmic vacuoles, like those often observed in tissue mast cells after addition of compound 48/80, or following an antigen-antibody reaction.

The investigations afford an insight into the kinetics of basophil granules. Compound 48/80 leads to a rapid destruction of blood basophils in rabbits. Under *in-vitro* conditions, the decrease in blood basophils is continuous, and it is possible to observe all morphological 'disintegration' stages of blood basophils. *In vivo,* compound 48/80 first produces a primary basophil fall, apparently as a direct effect of the applied noxa (compound 48/80).

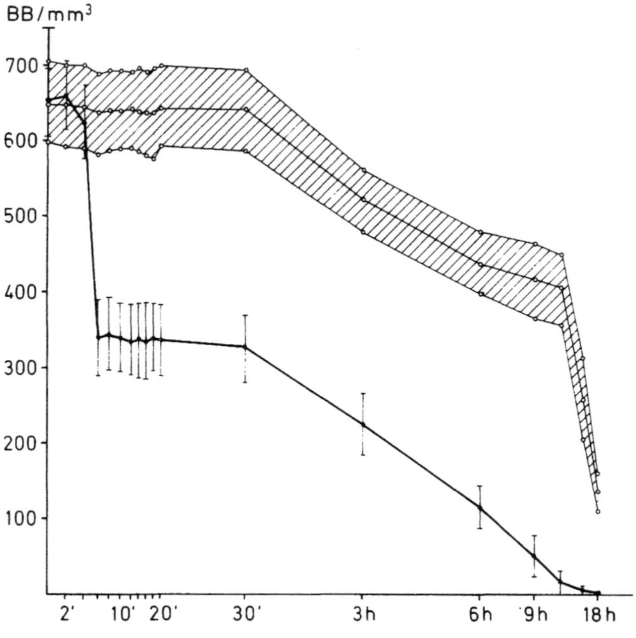

Fig. 42. The influence of compund 48/80 (0.5 mg in 0.5 ml saline) upon the number of blood basophils incubated *in vitro.* For controls (hatched area) 0.5 ml of saline was added to equal blood volumes (10 ml)

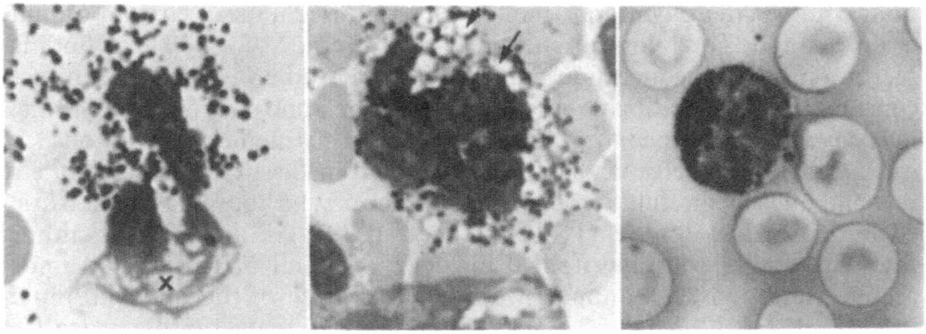

Fig. 43. "Degranulation" forms of rabbit basophils after incubation *in vitro* with compound 48/80 (50μg per ml blood at 37° C for 15 min). An intact untreated blood basophil to the right. Note the vacuoles in treated cells (arrow) and the evident karyolysis (*x*). 5-amino-acridine prefixation; aldehyde fuchsin-hemalum stain. ×1,380

The swift, primary basophil fall is soon largely compensated for by activation of a basophil pool system (peripheral or in the bone marrow), leading to accelerated emergence. The further action of the histamine liberator and/or the activation of some other serum factors lead to a renewed fall in the basophil count; this depression lasts longer and the count very slowly returns to normal over the next 12 to 18 h. The behavior of basophils after addition of compound 48/80 is basically the same under in-vitro and in vivo-conditions. *In vitro* there was no recovery of the basophil granules and therefore no interruption of the steadily falling basophil count. If the degranulated blood basophils were indeed reconstituted by regranulation of the degranulated cells circulating in the blood, one would expect the *in-vitro* basophil curve to be similar to that observed *in vivo.* Clearly, blood basophils react to compound 48/80 in much the same way under *in-vivo* and *in-vitro* conditions, except that *in vivo* the initial steep basophil fall stimulates accelerated emergence of blood basophils out of their pools.

Our investigations do not, however, shed any light upon the origin of these cells. It is quite possible that there is an extramedullary pool for blood basophils as well, although sound evidence for this has not yet been found. We have occasionally observed numerous relatively well preserved blood basophils in smears of the pleural aspirate and of lung punctures. The count of these cells was higher than that of the blood. This finding could indicate the existence of a peripheral pool for blood basophils. It seems, however, that blood basophils after a basophil fall are mainly replaced by the emergence of more or less mature cells from the bone marrow (in man, always naphthol AS-D chloroacetate esterase-negative). The results obtained from the kinetic studies with ^{3}H-thymidine also clearly support the view stated above. The blood basophil count falls sharply in the 9 h following the administration of compound 48/80 to rabbits, after which there is a gradual return to the initial values within 18 h. The basophil count is observed to double within the last three sampling intervals, i.e. within 3 h. In the investigations with tritiated thymidine, the basophils showed a mean circulation time of 13.3 h, and the biological half-life (t 1/2) averaged 9.1 h. These findings seem to justify the conclusion that increasing peripheral utilization induces considerable acceleration of emergence from the bone marrow. Similar findings have been obtained for other myeloid cells in kinetic investigations.

In tissue mast cells, which are best studied in the peritoneal exudate of rats and mice, degranulation also leads to complete cytolysis, as demonstrated by PARWARESCH *et al.* (1971). We treated 30 CAP and 30 CDF inbred rats with a single intraperitoneal injection of 10 ml of paraffin oil under aseptic conditions. Six animals were killed in each of the following intervals: 0.5, 1, 2, 4, 12, 24, 48, 72, 96, 120 h p.i. The peritoneal cavity was washed with saline solution to which 0.02 g% of disodium EDTA had been added. The suspension was centrifuged and the total cell count and tissue mast cell count were determined. Smears from the cell concentrates were prepared at

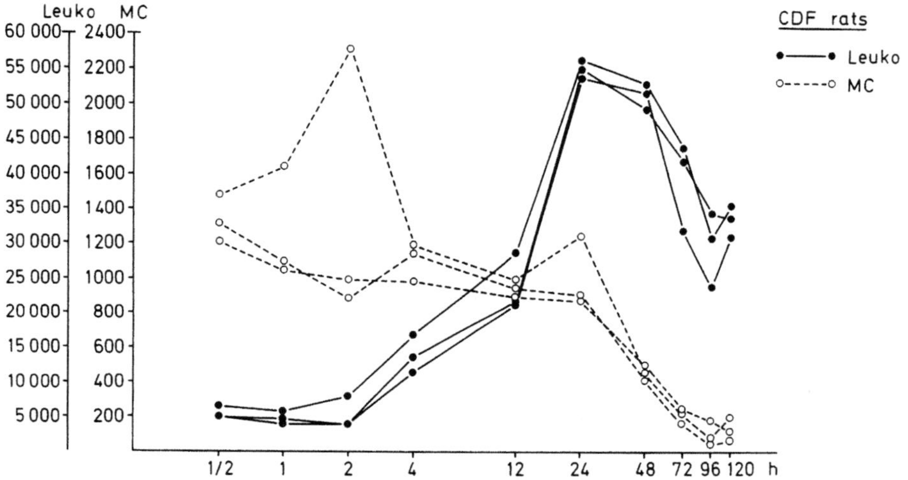

Fig. 44. Total leukocyte and tissue mast cell count (*MC*) in 30 CDF rats at various time intervals after intraperitoneal injection of paraffin oil.

the same time and a differential blood count was taken. The results are shown in Figs. 44 and 45. The total leukocyte count increases steadily and reaches its maximum 24 h p.i. in both animal strains. This increase is an expression of activated phagocytosis and the result of sterile peritonitis. On the other hand, in both strains the tissue mast cell count falls steadily to less than 0.5% of total cells 96 h p.i. Since any degranulated cells which may be present can be clearly identified both in the chamber countings and the leukocyte concentrate smears, it seems reasonable to conclude that paraffin injection leads to degranulation of tissue mast cells. Degranulated tissue mast cells can be clearly identified as such, but their count decreases steadily, which indicates the swift disappearance of these cells from the peritoneal cavity. In addition to these investigations, studies with compound 48/80 and adenosine triphosphate have also shown that degranulation is accompanied by explosive destruction of the whole cell. Less strongly influenced or only slighlty degranulated tissue mast cells quickly progress to necrosis.

The findings up to now have clearly shown the close similarity between tissue mast cells and blood basophils in both mode of degranulation and the morphological alterations associated with the course of granule discharge. More parallels between tissue mast cells and blood basophils are illustrated by experiments with metabolic inhibitors. The similarity of the effects of antimetabolites on the degranulation of blood basophils and mast cells points to their functional similarity, and hence to the participation of identical or very similar enzymes in mast cell and basophil granulolysis. Immunological mast cell degranulation can be prevented by application of a variety of substances, including antipyretics, nicotinic acid derivatives, chymotrypsin substrate, and chymotrypsin inhibitors (MOTA *et al.*, 1960; AUSTEN and

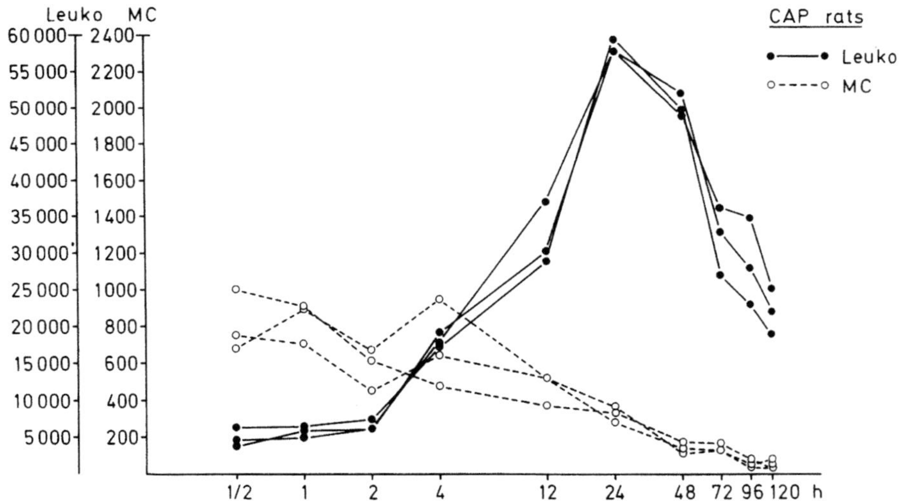

Fig. 45. Total leukocyte and tissue mast cell count (*MC*) in 30 CAP rats at various time intervals after intrapertitoneal injection of paraffin oil

BROCKLEHURST, 1960; 1961). Similarly, basophil degranulation can be inhibited by the addition of sodium phenylbutazol, paraaminomethylbenzoic acid, pyridylcarbinol, pyridostigmine bromide, and nicotinic acid derivatives (FRICK and FRICK, 1966, 1968; STARR and WEINSTOCK, 1970). Substances such as phenol, 2,4 dinitrophenol, fluoride ions, and imidazole in millimolar concentrations inhibit anaphylactic histamine liberation from blood basophils. The compound 2,4 dinitrophenol in a final concentration of 50 mM proved to be especially effective in preventing basophil granulolysis.

The work of LICHTENSTEIN and MARGOLIS (1968) is of interest in this connection. They were able to prevent IgE-induced histamine liberation from human blood basophils by applying isoproterenol, noradrenaline, cyclic AMP, diethylcarbamazine (hetrazan) and theophylline. These findings provide further proof of the close similarity between blood basophils and tissue mast cells (MONGAR and SCHILD, 1958; LICHTENSTEIN and OSSLER, 1964; STARR and WEINSTOCK, 1970; ISHIZAKA and ISHIZAKA, 1970; LICHTENSTEIN *et al.*, 1970).

In conclusion, up till now only a very few of the biochemical steps in basophil degranulation have been clarified. The papers so far available have displayed many contradictory results, due to the limited number of studies made and methodological difficulties. In contrast, many steps in the degranulation mechanism of tissue mast cells are supported by good experimental data, so that the scattered bits of information hitherto available can be brought together to form the basis for a sound working hypothesis. A corresponding hypothesis for the degranulation mechanisms of blood basophils assuming an enzymatically controlled chain of reactions with partici-

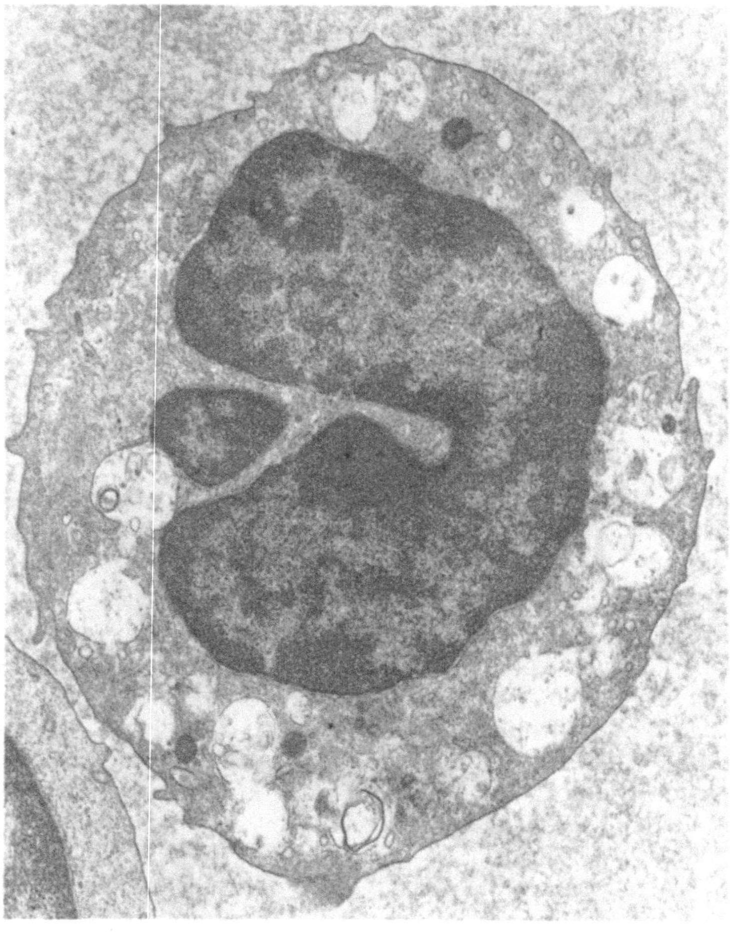

Fig. 46. Electronmicrograph of a human blood basophil following inadequate fixation. The vacuoles represent empty spaces left by the dissolved granules. ×24,000

pation of membrane-bound enzymes and phospholipases, is only possible by analogy with tissue mast cells.

Research to date has definitely shown that blood basophils, under certain cirucumstances, liberate biologically active substances from their granules. It can further be maintained that the granule contents are made available to the organism by enzymatically induced and controlled disintegration of the total cell. Each degranulation appears to lead to cell necrobiosis. With sufficient intensity of stimulation, explosive destruction of the blood basophils occurs, accompanied by a rapid fall in the basophil count in the peripheral blood. It seems highly likely that disintegrated blood basophils are quickly removed from the circulation by the macrophage system. The basophil granulocytes, as well as the other elements of the myeloid system, are short-lived blood cells whose peripheral utilization is balanced by acceleration of their random energence from the bone marrow.

On the basis of our present state of knowledge, it seems improbable that blood basophils are capable of merocrine secretion. If one desires to retain the term 'secretion', the expression 'holocrine secretion' seems more justified. The optically empty vacuoles often observed in intact blood basophils in smear preparations are mostly artifacts due to the method employed. Such artifactual vacuoles can be particularly well demonstrated in the commonly used electron-microscopic preparation techniques (Fig. 46). They should not be interpreted as morphological correlates for certain functional phases of granule discharge, but rather as empty sites where granules have dissoluted.

References

AUSTEN, K. F., BROCKLEHURST, W. E.: Inhibition of the anaphylactic release of histamine from chopped guinea pig lung by chymotrypsin substrates and inhibitors. Nature (Lond.) **186,** 866 – 868 (1960).

AUSTEN, K. F., BROCKLEHURST, W. E.: Anaphylaxis in chopped guinea pig lung. J. exp. Med. **113,** 521 – 539 (1961).

BOBITT, J. R., SCHLECHTER, H., POLLAK, V. E.: A critical evaluation of the indirect basophil degranulation test. Proc. Soc. exp. Biol. Med. **117,** 608 – 610 (1964).

BOLL, I.: see page 96.

BOND, V. P., CRONKITE, E. P.: Effects of radiation on mammals. Ann. Rev. Physiol. **19,** 299 – 328 (1957).

BOSEILA, A.-W. A.: Influence of histamine liberator substance 48/80 on basophil leukocytes of rabbit blood. Proc. Soc. exp. Biol. Med. **98,** 184 – 186 (1958).

COOPER, J. R., CRUICKSHANK, C. N. D.: see page 22.

DARLINGTON, D., ROGERS, A. W.: Epithelial lymphocytes in the small intestine of the mouse. J. Anat. (Lond.) **100,** 813 – 830 (1966).

DESAGA, J. F., PARWARESCH, M. R.: Eine Methode zur Darstellung der basophilen Granulopoese beim Kaninchen in autoradiographischen Präparaten. Blut **23,** 139 – 142 (1971).

FAWCETT, D. W.: An experimental study of mast cell degranulation and regeneration. Anat. Rec. **121,** 25 – 51 (1955).

FELDBERG, H., TALESNIK, J.: Reduction of tissue histamine by compound 48/80. J. Physiol. **120,** 550 – 568 (1953).

FLIEDNER, F. M., CRONKITE, E. P., BOND, V. P.: Das Studium der Proliferationsdynamik der Myelopoese unter Verwendung der Einzelzellautoradiographie. Fol. haemat., N. F. **6,** 210 – 228 (1961).

FLIEDNER, T. M., CRONKITE, E. P., BOND, V. P.: Studies on myelocytic cell turnover in bone marrow and blood . In: W. KEIDERLING, G. HOFFMANN: Radio-Isotope in der Hämatologie, p. 279. Schattauer: Stuttgart 1962.

FLIEDNER, T. M., CRONKITE, E. P., KILLMANN, S. A., BOND, V. P.: Granulocytopoiesis II. Emergence and pattern of labeling of neutrophilic granulocytes in human blood. Blood **24,** 683 – 700 (1964 a).

FLIEDNER, T. M., FACHE, I., ADOLPHI, C.: Über die Umsatzkinetik der Leukocyten bei keimfreien Mäusen. Schweiz. med. Wschr. **96,** 1236 – 1238 (1966).

FLIEDNER, T. M., LAEGER, F., CRONKITE, E. P.: Zytokinetische Untersuchungen am menschlichen Blutmonozyten. Haemat. Bluttransfus. **7,** 39 – 51 (1969).

FRICK, G., KONRAD, H.: see page 23.

FRICK, G., FRICK, U.: see page 23.

FRICK, G., FRICK, U.: see page 23.

FRICK, G., FRICK, U.: Zur Rolle der basophilen Leukocyten und Mastzellen in Fibrinolyse und Allergie. III. Wirkung einer allergischen Sofortreaktion ohne und mit Vorbehandlung durch ε-Aminocapronsäure oder p-aminomethylbenzolsäure auf Zahl und Degranulierung von basophilen Leukocyten. Folia haemat. **88,** 1 – 16 (1967).

FRICK, G., FRICK, U.: Comparative study of the effect of fibrinolysin inhibitors on the degranulation grade of basophilic granulocytes. Z. ges. inn. Med. **23,** 321 – 325 (1968).

FRIEDLAENDER, S., FRIEDLAENDER, A. S.: Studies on basophil degranulation as an indicator of hypersensitivity. Sinai Hosp. J. (Baltimore) **12,** 59 – 65 (1964).

GOMORI, G.: see page 23.

GREAVES, M. W., BURDIS, B. D.: see page 158.

HALE, A. J.: The interference Microscope in Biological Research. E. and S. LIVINGSTONE, Edinburgh, 1958.

HAYE, K. R., SCHNEIDER, R.: The difference in behaviour of basophil leukocytes and mast cells towards compound 48/80. Brit. J. Pharmacol. **28,** 282 – 288 (1966).

HAYE, K. R., COOPER, F. K., CRUICKSHANK, C. N. D.: Studies on the degranulation of human basophil leukocytes in vitro. Brit. J. Derm. **80,** 811 – 821 (1968).

HERION, J. C., GLASSER, R. M., WALKER, R., PALMER, J. G.: Eosinophil kinetics in two patients with eosinophilia. Blood **36,** 361 – 370 (1970).

HÖGBERG, B., UVNÄS, B.: The mechanism of the disruption of mast cells produced by compound 48/80. Acta physiol. scand. **41,** 345 – 369 (1957).

HÖGBERG, B., UVNÄS, B.: 1959. Cited in: Further observations on the disruption of rat mesentery mast cells caused by compound 48/80, lecithinase A, decylamine and antigen-antibody reaction. Acta physiol. scand. **48,** 133 – 145 (1960).

HÖGBERG, B., UVNÄS, B.: Further observations on the disruption of rat mesentery mast cells caused by compound 48/80, lecithinase A, decylamine and antigen-antibody reaction. Acta physiol. scand. **48,** 133 – 145 (1960).

HUBSCHER, T., GOODFRIEND, L.: see page 159.

HUNT, T. E., HUNT, E. A.: Mitotic activity of mast cells. Proc. Soc. exp. Biol. Med. **94,** 166 – 169 (1957).

HUNT, T. E., HUNT, E. A.: The effect of 48/80 on the blood basophils of cockerels. Anat. Rec. **130,** 419 – 420 (1958).

HUNT, T. E., HUNT, E. A.: Blood basophils of cockerels before and after intravenous injection of compound 48/80. Anat. Rec. **133**, 19 – 31 (1959).
ISHIZAKA, K., ISHIZAKA, T.: see page 159.
JUHLIN, L.: see page 160.
JUHLIN, L., SHELLEY, W. B.: see page 160.
JUHLIN, L., SHELLEY, W. B.: see page 160.
JUHLIN, L., WESTPHAL, O.: see page 160.
KAPLOW, L. S.: A histochemical procedure for localizing and evaluating leukocyte alkaline phosphatase activity in smears of blood and bone marrow. Blood **10**, 1023 – 1029 (1955).
KATZ, H., GILE, K., BAXTER, D., MOSCHELLA, S.: Indirect basophil degranulation test in penicillin allergy. J. Amer. med. Ass. **188**, 351 – 358 (1964).
KOLLER, S.: Neue graphische Tafeln zur Beurteilung statistischer Zahlen. Darmstadt: Dr. Dietrich Steinkopff Verlag 1969.
KOPRIWA, B. M., LEBLOND, C. P.: Improvements in the coating technique of radioautography. J. Histochem. Cytochem. **10**, 269 – 284 (1962).
KRAVIS, L. P., LECKS, H. J., WHITNEY, T.: Basophil degranulation tests in atopic allergic states: a pilot study of ragweed pollen-sensitive patients. J. Allergy **36**, 23 – 28 (1965).
LANGNER, R., STEIGLEDER, G. K.: see page 61.
LEVI, L., MENEGHINI, C. L.: Liveratori d'istamina, istaminemia e mastociti circolanti in alcune dermatosi allergiche. G. ital. Derm. **6**, 613 – 619 (1959).
LICHTENSTEIN, L. M., OSLER, A. G.: see page 161.
LICHTENSTEIN, L. M., MARGOLIS, S.: see page 161.
LICHTENSTEIN, L. M., LEVI, D. A., ISHIZAKA, K.: In vitro reversed anaphylaxis: characteristics of anti-IgE mediated histamine release. Immunology **19**, 831 – 841 (1970).
MARKS, B. H., SORGEN, R., GINSBURG, H.: Histamine-liberator 48/80 and basophilic leukocytes. Biochem. Pharmacol. **2**, 200 – 205 (1959).
MARKS, B. H., OBERER, D.: Effects of snake venom on rabbit basophil leukocytes. Biochem. Pharmacol. **11**, 9 – 15 (1962).
MARTIN, G., BENDER, M. A.: A comparison of mammalian cell killing by incorporated ^{3}H-thymidine and ^{3}H-uridine. Int. J. Radiat. Biol. **7**, 235 – 244 (1963).
MONGAR, J. L., SCHILD, H. O.: The effect of calcium and pH on the anaphylactic reaction. J. Physiol. (Lond.) **140**, 272 – 284 (1958).
MONGAR, J. L., SCHILD, H. O.: Cellular mechanisms in anaphylaxis. Physiol. Rev. **42**, 226 – 270 (1962).
MOORE, J. E., JAMES, G. W.: see page 25.
MORELLE, L.: see page 25.
MOTA, J., DIAS DA SILVA, W., FERNANDES, J. F.: The inhibition of mast cell damage and histamine release in anaphylaxis by pyridine and diphosphopyridine nucleotidase inhibitors. Comparison with compound 48/80. Brit. J. Pharmacol. **15**, 406 – 409 (1960).
MURAKAMI, I., OGAWA, M., AMO, H., OTA, K.: see page 98.
NORDLANDER, N. B.: The use of a new histamine liberating substance, compound 48/80 in human subjects. Acta med. scand. **157**, 235 – 240 (1957).
PARWARESCH, M. R., LENNERT, K.: see page 25.
PARWARESCH, M. R., MÜLLER-HERMELINK, H. K., DESAGA, J. F., ZAKARI, V., LENNERT, K.: see page 131.
PARWARESCH, M. R., DESAGA, J. F., NEBELIN, K.: Die Kinetik der basophilen Granulocyten im peripheren Blut beim Kaninchen. Blut **27**, 33 – 43 (1973).

PARWARESCH, M. R., ARNDT, D.: An autoradiographic study of human blood basophils. Histochemical J. **7**, 357 – 360 (1975).

PATT, H. M., MALONEY, M. A.: Kinetics of neutrophil balance. In: F. SOHLMAN: The Kinetics of Cellular Proliferation, pp. 201 – 207. New York and London: Grune and Stratton 1959.

PERRY, R. P., ERRERA, M., HELL, E. A., DURWALD, H.: Kinetics of nucleoside incorporation into nuclear and cytoplasmic RNA. J. biophys. biochem. Cytol. **11**, 1 – 13 (1961).

REYNOLDS, R. D., SMITH, R. E.: The indirect basophil degranulation test. Ann. Allergy **25**, 318 – 323 (1967).

RILEY, J. F., WEST, G. B.: see page 66.

RILEY, J. F., WEST, G. B.: see page 66.

SAMPSON, D., ARCHER, G. T.: see page 26.

SAWICKI, W., BLATON, O., ROWINSKI, J.: Correction of autoradiographic grain count in respect to precisely calculated background. Histochemie **26**, 67 – 73 (1971).

SCHÖNHERR, D., HERMANN, F.: Basophilendegranulation bei anaphylaktoiden Reaktionen insbesonderer erworbener Kälteurticaria. Arch. klin. exp. Derm. **220**, 362 – 373 (1964).

SCHWARTZ, J., KLOPSTOCK, A., VARDINON, N.: The role of the complement in the basophil cells test. Int. Arch. Allergy **26**, 142 – 152 (1965).

SHELLEY, W. B., JUHLIN, L.: see page 132.

SHELLEY, W. B.: New serologic test for allergy in man. Nature (Lond.) **195**, 1181 – 1183 (1962).

SHELLEY, W. B., CARO, W. A.: Detection of anaphylactic sensitivity by basophil degranulation response. An experimental study. J. Amer. med. Ass. **182**, 172 – 178 (1962).

SHELLEY, W. B., JUHLIN, L.: Functional cytology of the human basophil in allergic and physiologic reactions: technic and atlas. Blood **19**, 208 – 216 (1962).

SHELLEY, W. B.: Indirect basophil degranulation test for allergy to penicillin and other drugs. J. Amer. med. Ass. **184**, 171 – 178 (1963 a).

SHELLEY, W. B.: Indirect basophil degranulation test for allergy to penicillin and other drugs. J. Amer. med. Ass. **184**, 105 – 112 (1963 b).

STARR, M. S., WEINSTOCK, M.: Studies in pollen allergy. I. A method for estimating histamine release from sensitized leukocytes in the presence of serum. Int. Arch. Allergy **37**, 239 – 247 (1970).

STILLSTRÖM, J.: Grain count corrections in autoradiography. Intern. J. appl. Radiation Isotopes, **14**, 113 – 118 (1963).

STILLSTRÖM, J.: Grain count corrections in autoradiography II. Int. J. appl. Radiat. **16**, 357 – 363 (1965).

STRYCKMANS, P., CRONKITE, E. P., FACHE, J., FLIEDNER, T. M., RAMOS, I.: DNA synthesis time of erythropoietic and granulopoietic cells in human beings. Nature (Lond.) **211**, 717 – 720 (1966).

STUBBLEFIELD, E.: Quantitative tritium autoradiography of mammalian chromosomes. I. The basic method. J. Cell. Biol. **25**, 109 – 119 (1965).

TONNA, E. A., CRONKITE, E. P.: Factors which influence the latent image in autoradiography. Stain Technol. **33**, 255 – 260 (1958).

UVNÄS, B.: Release processes in mast cells and their activation by injury. Ann. N. Y. Acad. Sci. **116**, 880 – 890 (1964).

D. The So-Called Basophilic Leukemias

I. Review of the Literature

It is noteworthy that the first discovery of blood basophils ensued from a case of myeloid leukemia (EHRLICH, 1879). EHRLICH and LAZARUS (1898) as well as LEVADITI (1901) already knew that myeloid leukemias might be accompanied by an elevated basophil count.

A systematic investigation of blood basophils in connection with leukemias was conducted by JOACHIM (1906). He reported on two patients, 33 and 52 years of age, both suffering from chronic myeloid leukemia with an excessive (53.6 and 56%) level of blood basophils. Both cases showed considerable enlargement of the lymph nodes, the liver and the spleen; hemorrhagic diathesis, and high-grade anemia with erythropoietic precursors in the peripheral blood were also mentioned. TOMASZEWSKI (1911) reported another case with markedly elevated (28%) blood basophils. SARZISARTORI (1927) described a case with a basophil count of 45% of total leukocytes. The following years brought more reports on basophilic leukemias (VASATURO, 1925 a, b; MASSA and MARINONI, 1926; SABRAZES, 1926; ELLIOT and YOUNG, 1931; GROAT *et al.*, 1936).

Although most authors viewed what was called basophilic leukemia as a special form of mature-celled myeloid leukemia, the 'Italian School' ascribed special properties to these cells. For example, FRANCO and FERRATE (1919) and DI GUGLIELMO (1925) described these cells as histiocytic mast cells and regarded them as hemohistioblasts of reticulo-endothelial origin.

In a detailed work, DOAN and RINEHART (1941) reported on 4 especially interesting cases of basophilic leukemia out of a total of 107 myeloid leukemias. They distingushed between a primary and a secondary form. In the primary form, which they called blood mast cell leukemia, basophils attain large numbers form the onset of the disease on. Secondary basophilic leukemia includes, according to these authors, typical, mature-celled myeloid leukemias, with a massive increase in predominantly immature basophils. They also emphasized that such cases are very resistant to therapy. The cases described by JOACHIM (1906) and DOAN and RINEHART (1941) are especially interesting, as the clinical course is minutely described along with the hematological findings, and except in JOCHAIM's second case, the relevant post-mortem findings are given.

CHEVALLIER and MARINONI (1948, 1951) examined the 10 published cases and added one of their own. They adopted the classification of DOAN and RINEHART (1941) into primary and secondary forms, and set up new but arbitrary criteria for their differentiation. The elevated basophil count in cases of chronic myeloid leukemia has been frequently noted. Basophils have been claimed to reach values up to 10% (ALDER, 1923; HOLMGREN and WOHLFART, 1941) or 20% (NAEGELI, 1923) of the total leukocytes.

It has sometimes been suggested that the term 'primary' basophilic leukemia should be applied to cases with blood basophil counts of over 20% of total leukocytes. DOAN and RINEHART suggested a minimum of one third of the total leukocytes. CHEVALLIER and MARINONI (1948, 1951) defined primary basophilic leukemia as when (a) atypical immature basophils occur in the peripheral blood and (b) basophil counts in excess of one third of the total leukocytes persist throughout the whole course of the disease. KYLE and PEASE (1966) speak in terms of values over 50% of total leukocytes as making up the primary form of basophilic leukemia, with persistent or constant elevation of the blood basophil count.

LENNERT *et al.* (1956), in a systematic investigation, reviewed all published cases of basophilic leukemia. Their classification comprised primary basophilic leukemia, corresponding to the basocytic leukemia of CHEVALLIER and MARINONI, and secondary basophilic leukemia, corresponding to these authors' 'temporary' basocytic leukemia. In addition, they described another case of basophilic leukemia which was, due to its chronic course, markedly different from the cases known up until then. QUATTRIN *et al.* (1959) reviewed 32 published cases, of which 8 were their own. KYLE and PEASE (1966) reported upon an American collection in the Mayo Clinic. In 1968, SCHUBERT and MARTIN published a review of their observations; on the basis of an exhaustive study of the literature and their own experience, they suggested the possibility of a cytologic separation of normal and neoplastic basophils by means of the toluidine-blue pH series, PAS staining, the peroxidase and leucine aminopeptidase reactions. With regard to the possible therapeutic consequences, they advocated strict separation of basophilic leukemias from other types of myeloid leukemia. MITRAKUL *et al.* (1969) reported a case of acute basophilic leukemia in a 6-year-old boy, leading to death within 8 weeks. The ultrastructural abnormalities of leukemic basophils were studied by CECIO *et al.* (1970).

A survey of the available case reports shows that basophilic leukemia has generally been regarded as a special, but not rare form of granulocytic leukemia. The majority of authors agree that basophilic leukemia is a nosological entity and should be distinguished from the other types of well-differentiated myeloid leukemias (DOAN *et al.*, 1941; CHEVALLIER and MARINONI, 1948; ASTALDI *et al.*, 1953; QUATTRIN *et al.*, 1959; STORN and MAURI, 1963; SCHUBERT and MARTIN, 1968). A second group of authors reject the idea that basophilic leukemia is a nosological entity, claiming that there are no reasonable grounds for separating granulocytic leukemias with high basophil counts from those with low basophil counts (GROAT *et al.*, 1936; HAYHOE, 1960; KYLE and PEASE, 1966; LEDER, 1970; PARWARESCH *et al.*, 1970). They emphasize the regular increase in blood basophils so often observed during the course of typical chronic myeloid leukemias, which can reach high levels in the terminal phase of the disease. They claim that, if a sufficiently large number of cases is reviewed, all gradual transitions can be observed, from classic chronic myeloid leukemia with a moderate increase in basophil counts, to full-blown basophilic leukemia.

II. Clinical and Pathoanatomical Features

In this section we cover the clinical course, hematologic diagnosis, prognosis, and pathoanatomical findings of the basophilic leukemias.

Classification of the Basophilic leukemias. Taking into account the cases of basophilic leukemia published up to 1970, it appears sensible to keep the usual terminology in order to facilitate comparison of the results described. In addition, this classification can be useful for the clinical distinction between various courses run by the disease. The following classification is widely accepted in the literature.

1. Primary Basophilic Leukemia
   a) per-acute form
   b) acute form
   c) chronic form
2. Secondary Basophilic Leukemia
   a) temporary blood basophil involvement
   b) terminal basophil crisis

1. Primary Basophilic Leukemia

Primary basophilic leukemia, first described by DOAN *et al.* (1941) and later more exactly defined by CHEVALLIER *et al.* (1948), and LENNERT *et al.* (1956), is a special form of myeloid leukemia, generally showing an extremely high leukocyte count of 100,000/mm^3 or more. In typical cases, the blood basophil count, which is extremely high right from the beginning of the disease, hovers between 40% and 80%. Primary basophilic leukemia appears in two clinically distinct forms, the 'acute' form being by far the more common. The 'chronic' forms are very rare and represent a relatively benign variation of the disease. The acute form leads to death within a matter of months. Table 28 presents all the cases of acute primary basophilic leukemia accessible to us from the literature. Figure 47 gives the frequency distribution of the duration of the disease; in the majority of cases (16 out of 28) duration was less than 4 months and in some cases even less than one week. DOAN *et al.* (1941) reported two cases which broke out from a previous state of complete good health and terminated in death within a few days. QUATTRIN (1959) named this 'per-acute primary basophilic leukemia'.

Chronic primary basophilic leukemia is one of the rarities of hematology; so far, only 8 definite cases have been described. The longest duration of 6 years was reported by LENNERT *et al.* (1956). The main symptom is an excessive rise in the total leukocyte count with a blood basophil count of up to

80% or 90%. Although most cases present with an increase of leukocytes and blood basophils, myelo-aplastic forms have also been reported by QUATTRIN *et al.* (1959).

The clinical features of primary basophilic leukemia are very similar to those of a well-differentiated myeloid leukemia. They begin abruptly or insidiously with fatigue, weakness and progressive prostration. Fever sometimes appears in typical cases. The extremely pronounced splenomegaly is occasionally noticed by the patient. There is almost always considerable hepatomegaly. The course can be complicated by bacterial infections or, rarely, by fungal infections. An increased tendency to bleeding generally appears at a late stage, along with other complications. Though in some cases extreme hemorrhagic diathesis with massive hemorrhages may be attributed to the heparin content of the proliferating blood basophils, most hemorrhages are due to thrombocytopenia. It appears that the polyanions of the basophil granules hardly reach even the degree of maturity necessary for effective anticoagulant activity. Among the initial hemorrhagic manifestations, purpura is by far the most common, but is not often of striking degree.

The rare forms associated with circulatory failure have an extremely bad prognosis and have been repeatedly described in the literature. The circulatory failure leading to shock seems to be caused by the biogenic amines abundantly present in the basophil granules. The histamine and glycosaminoglycan content may be raised in both serum and urine. SHIBATA *et al.*

Table 28. Survey of Reports on Primary Basophilic Leukemia

Author (Year)	Age	Sex	Total Leukocytes	Basophil Count %	Duration of the Disease in Weeks
JOACHIM (1906)	52	m	189,000	53.6	40
JOACHIM (1906)	33	m	237,000	56	28
TOMASZEWSKI (1911)	50	f	303,000	46	about 2 years
SABRAZES (1924)	68	f	155,000	43	12
MANA *et al.* (1926)	35	m	35,000	43	
TINTI (1926)	40	f	120,000	33	8
VASATURO (1926)	40	f	550,000	55	32
SARZI-SARTORI (1927)	25	f	56,000	45	12
GROAT *et al.* (1936)	40	m	61,000	61	about 3 years
ELLIOT *et al.* (1939)	57	f	18,000	64	24
DOAN *et al.* (1941)	12	f	380,000	26	48
DOAN *et al.* (1941)	45	m	300,000	43	0.5
DOAN *et al.* (1941)	47	m	79,000	65	0.5
CASEY *et al.* (1946)					3
CHEVALLIER *et al.* (1947)	51	m			12
CATTANEO (1950)	50	f	118,000	29	6
HULE (1950)	27	m	3,800	28	3
CHEVALLIER *et al.* (1951)	23	m	404,000	44	20

Table 28 (continued)

Author (Year)	Age	Sex	Total Leukocytes	Basophil Count	Duration of the Disease in Weeks
FERRARA (1952)	40		11,600	30	5 years
NATALE (1952)	22	m	8,000	32	2
FERRARA (1953)	24	f	450,000	35	52
BAREAS (1954)	52	m	265,000	79	32
QUATTRIN *et al.* (1954)	49	f	10,000	61.5	8
QUATTRIN *et al.* (1954)	39	m	1,100		8
QUATTRIN *et al.* (1955)	62	m	171,000	54	12
LENNERT *et al.* (1956)	16	m	36,500	35	6 years
QUATTRIN *et al.* (1956)	49	m	97,000	32	20
QUATTRIN *et al.* (1957)	68	m	Leukopenia		12
QUATTRIN *et al.* (1957)	12	m	33,800	34	4
HIRAKI *et al.* (1958)	10	m	384,000	95	24
HIRAKI *et al.* (1958)	18	f	2,700	43	20
QUATTRIN *et al.* (1959)	50	m	350,000	84.5	5.5 years
QUATTRIN *et al.* (1959)	32	f	23,100	62.5	chron.
KYLE *et al.* (1966)	45	m	223,000	78	44
SCHUBERT *et al.* (1968)	50	f	55,000	about 100	3
MITRAKUL *et al.* (1969)	7	m	474,000	about 52	14

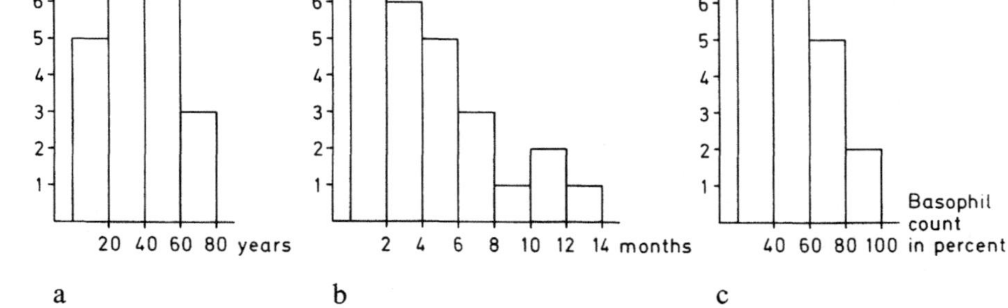

Fig. 47 a – c. (a) Distribution of the patients' ages in cases of basophilic leukemia. (b) Frequency distribution curve of the duration (from the appearance of the first symptoms till death) of primary basophilic leukemia. (c) Distribution of basophil counts

(1966) found the histamine level in serum and urine to be 10 to 50 times the norm, at the same time showing a marked rise in glycoprotein. In contrast, values for 5-hydroxytryptamine were found to be normal.

When the typical changes in blood count are present, the diagnosis of basophilic leukemia is not difficult. In the majority of cases, the extremely high leukocytosis can readily be detected even in smears. The high basophil count can be well demonstrated with the usual panchromatic stains. The borderline points of 20% and 30% should be regarded as reference points and not as absolute criteria. The cytomorphologic findings seem to us to be of far more importance. Neoplastic blood basophils can be distinguished from normal basophils by several cytochemical features. In addition, there are the typical clinical and hematological symptoms of myelosis, which facilitate the diagnosis. Basophil precursor cells, as well as mature but highly atypical cells, are regularly observed in the peripheral blood. They are distinguished by their fine uniform granulation, which either partly or completely covers both the cytoplasm and nucleus. The granules are less sharply defined and show a more limited optical density than normal granules. They are further distinguished by their extreme water solubility. Occasionally, however, they are, like the granules of tissue mast cells, water-insoluble and show a high optical density. Careful observation sometimes reveals basophils with round or oval nuclei without any recognizable segmentation tendency; in such cases, distinguishing between typical blood basophils and tissue mast cells can be very problematical. Atypical blood basophils are one of the criteria for the diagnosis of acute basophilic leukemia, since they rarely appear in chronic forms. Because of their increased vulnerability, abundant damaged, but still easily recognizable blood basophils occur in smears. In leukocyte concentrates they outweigh the intact basophils. Atypical forms of neutrophils, eosinophils, and monocytes almost always occur at the same time. Granulopoietic precursors are also often observed in the peripheral blood.

The pathoanatomical findings correspond to those of well-differentiated chronic myeloid leukemia; post-mortem examination reveals rapid generalized autolysis and heterolysis of the corpse. It is possible that post-mortem spreading of putrefactive agents proceeds with particular speed in cases of basophilic leukemia. This can be explained by post-mortem cytolysis of the blood basophils, causing the body to be flooded with biogenic amines, which in turn activate the tissue hyaluronidase, thereby aiding in the spreading of putrefactive agents.

The hematopoietic bone marrow of the long cylindrical and flat bones is usually a diffuse grey-red in color. Sometimes a patchy deep red is observed, which is due to hemorrhages. The spleen is always enlarged and has a rather firm consistency. The follicular and trabecular structures are hardly recognizable against the grey-red cut surface. The spleen can, especially in chronic cases, outweigh a normal liver. Ischemic spleen infarction indicates a disordered blood circulation or infiltration of a blood-vessel wall. In most cases the enlargement of the liver is already clinically manifest. In post-mortem examination the liver capsule is found to be under tension. The leukemic infiltrates are rarely visible to the naked eye. In some cases, scarring indicates the existence of an induration caused by a more or less diffuse fibrosis of the organ. In these instances, the liver can weigh five or more times the norm. The lymph nodes present the usual picture of myeloid leukemia, usually without generalized swelling. Lymph node infiltrates do, however, occur.

Leukemic infiltrates can also appear in the kidneys, skin, and mucous membranes. These often show secondary ulceration. Ulcerated tonsilitis or infiltration of the gingivae and the mucosa of the gastrointestinal tract have occasionally been observed. As indication of the anemia that is practically always present, pallid organs are observed. Hemorrhagic diathesis with petechial or ecchymotic bleeding is not rare. Suppurative or necrotic inflammatory foci are also observed. These, as well as the otherwise rare fungus infections, are common with hemoblastosis in general.

Massive bleeding, heart failure following bronchopneumonia, or intra-alveolar hemorrhage and cachexia are often cited as the cause of death. Irreversible histamine shock with fatal outcome has been also reported to follow massive cytostatic therapy.

The histologic pattern seen in the hematopoietic bone marrow is the same as in other cases of myeloid leukemia. There is a decrease in fat cells. The displacement of erythrocytopoiesis and thrombocytopoiesis varies from case to case. The preponderance of myeloid precursors is especially noticeable. With proper techniques, slightly segmented mature blood basophils can be observed in large quantities. There are many cases described in the literature of a large increase in argyrophil fibers, usually appearing as fibrotic patches (Fig. 48). LENNERT *et al.* (1956) were the first to call attention to this, and since then many other authors (RAPPAPORT, 1966) have also observed them in connection with basophil leukemia. In most bone areas, the histologic pattern is almost isomorphous. Attenuation of trabeculae, which become slender with irregular borders, is very common but erosion of the cortex is much less often seen in histologic examinations.

The spleen appears to be especially rich in cells. The pre-existing structures are largely destroyed. The follicles are much diminished in size. Coarse, patchy leukemic infiltrates are found in the broadened pulp cords. In good preparations metachromatic structures can be clearly observed in many cells. The infiltrates can also be observed near or within the trabeculae (LENNERT *et al.*, 1956).

The liver displays periportal infiltrates. Myeloid precursors and their mitotic forms may be present in the dilated sinusoids. Precursors of erythropoiesis and thrombopoiesis may occur with a patchy or diffuse distribution.

In cases with enlargement of the lymph nodes, as in other myeloid leukemias, the structure of the lymphatic tissue is largely destroyed. Uncharacteristic and optionally occurring infiltrates in the rest of the organs behave largely as in myeloid leukemias. Further description is therefore superfluous.

In summary, it has been shown that both the clinical and morphologic features of basophil leukemia correspond to those of typical myeloid leuke-

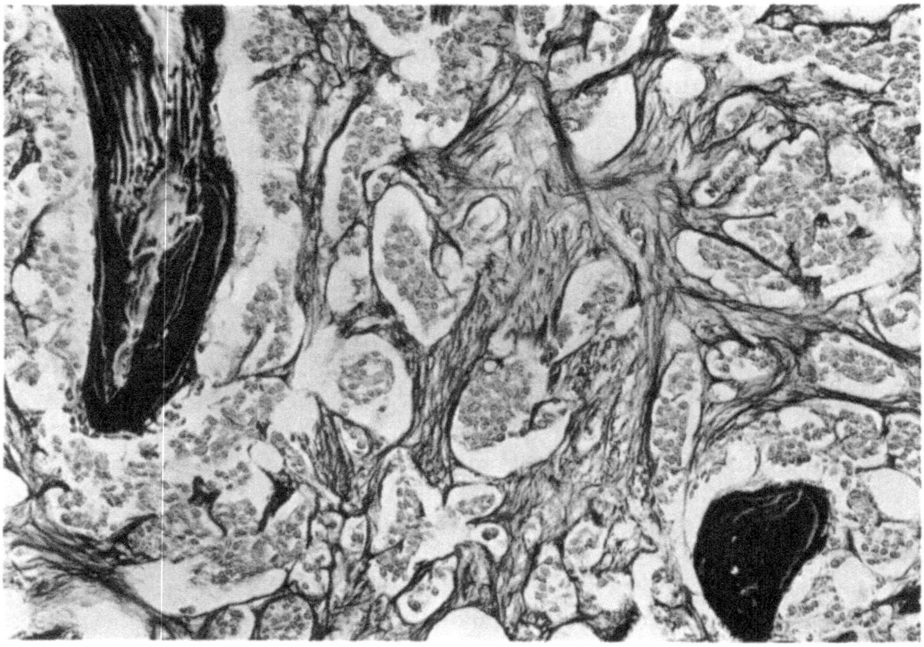

Fig. 48. Bone marrow fibrosis in a case of primary basophilic leukemia, resembling the alterations characteristic of myelofibrosis. Vertebra. Silver impregnation. ×150

mia. There have been hardly any findings reported that have not also been found in other myeloid leukemias. The intense involvement of the spleen and liver is characteristic for myeloid leukemia. Skin and mucous membrane infiltrates, especially in the oral region, which are occasionally viewed as typical of basophilic leukemias, have also been described in the literature (DOAN and WISEMAN, 1934; EVANS, 1942; HITTMAIR, 1963; LEDER, 1967) as accompanying myelomonocytic leukemia and so-called eosinophilic leukemia (GERHARD and HENSCHEL, 1958). Even the histotopography of infiltrates within the organs is not distinguished from the rest of the myeloid leukemias by any peculiarity. The typical structure of the spleen is largely destroyed due to infiltrates. Bone marrow usually shows diffuse involvement. The lymph nodes are infiltrated in the pulp cords, but myeloid cells may also appear in the trabecular and intratrabecular regions. Infiltrates in other organs, for example in the lungs and kidneys, show the same distribution as in myeloid leukemia. Nor should the organ fibrosis described by LENNERT *et al.* (1956) and RAPPAPORT (1966) be viewed as peculiar to basophilic leukemia, as it is often observed in other forms of chronic myeloid leukemia (CHIBA *et al.*, 1964).

2. Secondary Basophilic Leukemia

Primary basophilic leukemia as defined above is at least differentiated from other forms of myeloid leukemia by the fact that the leukemic basophils are dominant from the onset of the disease. It is therefore not as difficult to differentiate from other types of myeloid leukemia as is secondary basophilic leukemia.

Involvement of blood basophils can occur in the terminal stage of chronic, mature-celled myeloid leukemia. Analogous to the myeloblast crisis, this is called the terminal basophil crisis. There may also be a temporary basophil increase in the peripheral blood in the course of myeloid leukemia. This type of intercurrent basophilia is distinguished by its short duration. Because of this, the term 'temporary basophilic leukemia' is used.

SCHUBERT and MARTIN (1968) emphasized the clinical importance of such forms and therefore felt justified in regarding them as a nosologic entity. If the literature is carefully reviewed, numerous cases which have been described as primary basophilic leukemia can be interpreted as actually being myeloid leukemias with an intercurrent or terminal involvement of blood basophils.

A classification into primary and secondary basophilic leukemia seems especially questionable, since a rise in basophils occurs in practically every mature-celled myeloid leukemia. It is not rare in the literature for a mild basophil increase in cases of chronic myeloid leukemia, polycythemia rubra vera, and myelomonocytic leukemia to be interpreted as a paraneoplastic 'reaction' to the current proliferative process. Only if in the course of the disease the basophil count exceeds the more or less arbitrary borderline of 20% or over is the case designated as 'temporary basophilic leukemia', 'secondary terminal basophilic leukemia', or even 'primary basophilic leukemia and regarded as a separate nosologic entity'.

III. Cytomorphology and Cytogenesis of Leukemic Blood Basophils

Most leukemic blood basophils, when studied in the usual panoptically stained blood or bone marrow smears, are difficult to distinguish from normal basophils. Among the variety of cytomorphologic criteria, few are sufficiently indicative of the neoplastic process when taken singly. A combination of the different morphological and cytochemical features strengthens the evidence of the suspected condition. Leukemic blood basophils are highly susceptible to mechanical injury; this is best seen in smears of leukocyte concentrates (buffy coat) prepared by centrifugation (Fig. 49).

Correct fixation and selective staining of blood basophils are of special significance in detecting cellular atypias. In nearly all cases some definitely abnormal and morphologically unusual basophil granulocytes can be detected in smears of the peripheral blood.

Blood basophils that are cytochemically and morphologically very similar to immature or small tissue mast cells are especially suggestive of neoplasia (Fig. 50). Such atypical blood basophils are only observed in connection with myeloproliferative diseases. Small, round blood basophils with

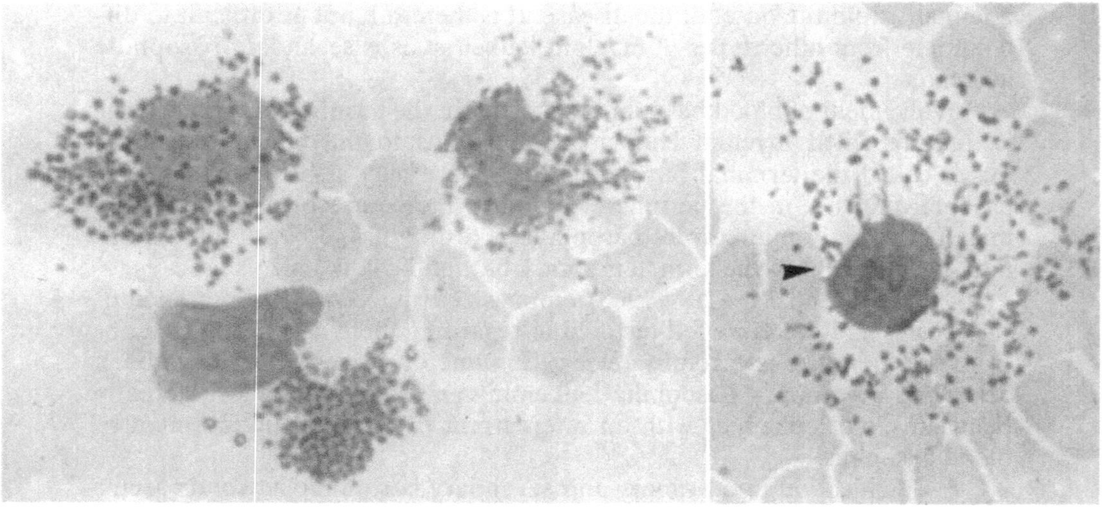

Fig. 49. Blood smear from a case of primary basophilic leukemia with four damaged blood basophils. Note the abundance and isomorphism of the granules and the round nucleus (arrow). Pappenheim stain. × 1,400

diffuse or extremely finely granulated metachromatic coloration of the entire cytoplasm (Fig. 50) are of similar diagnostic significance. Along with the atypical cells, the occurrence of basophil precursors is especially pathognomonic for the basophilic leukemias.

Metachromasia is less marked in leukemic blood basophils than in normal ones. The reddish-violet metachromasia of normal basophils tends in leukemic basophils to become dark blue-violet. Leukemic basophils often have far more granules than normal ones, and such granules are very readily water-soluble (HULE, 1950; LENNERT, 1955; BENDITT, 1963; SCHUBERT, 1968). In addition, a few basophils can be observed that contain relatively water-resistant granules. These granules remind of the granules of tissue mast cells due to their typical ultrastructure as well as to their insolubility (PARWARESCH, 1976).

While normal blood basophils, due to their rarity in the peripheral blood, have only occasionally been investigated, several authors have studied the cytochemical properties of blood basophils in cases of myeloproliferative disease with abundance of basophils. Detailed investigations of blood basophils in leukemia were undertaken by ASTALDI (1953), SHIBATA *et al.* (1966) and, in particular, by SCHUBERT and MARTIN (1968).

SCHUBERT ascribed special importance to the toluidine-blue pH series. While most normal basophils stain metachromatically with basic dyes in the pH range 2.8 to 4.0, the affinity of leukemic blood basophils for basic dyes shows a marked shift to the more alkaline region within the range pH 4 to 7. SCHUBERT found that this 'shift-to-the-right' was most pronounced in cases of basophilic leukemia. From pH 2 up to pH 4.93, no blood basophils could be detected; at pH 7, 100% of the blood basophils were stained.

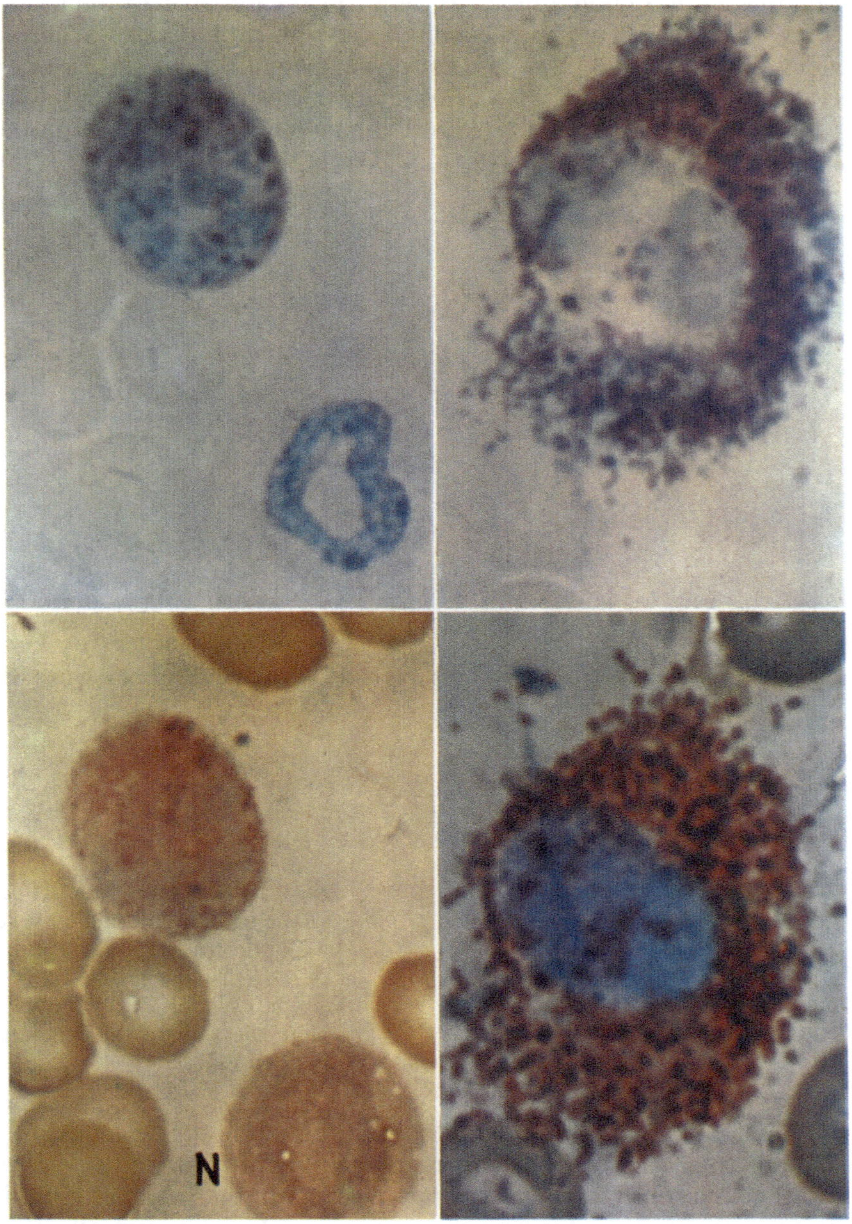

Fig. 50. Blood smear from a case of primary basophilic leukemia. Above: Toluidine blue at pH 6.4. Below: The same cells subjected to the naphthol AS-D chloroacetate esterase reaction. On the right, a tissue mast cell-like blood basophil; on the left, a small, rounded blood basophil with diffuse metachromasia of the cytoplasm. Both cells are enzyme-positive. Note the enzyme defect in a neutrophil (*N*). ×2,000

To test the specificity of SCHUBERT's finding for basophilic leukemia, we examined the toluidine-blue pH series in 5 cases of basophilic leukemia (Figs. 51 and 52). The same technique was applied to 5 cases of chronic myeloid leukemia (Fig. 53), 3 cases of polycythemia rubra vera, 3 cases of myelomonocytic leukemia, 3 cases of myelosclerosis with myeloid metaplasia (Fig. 54), and one case each of eosinophilic leukemia, essential thrombocytemia, and mixed-granule myeloid leukemia.

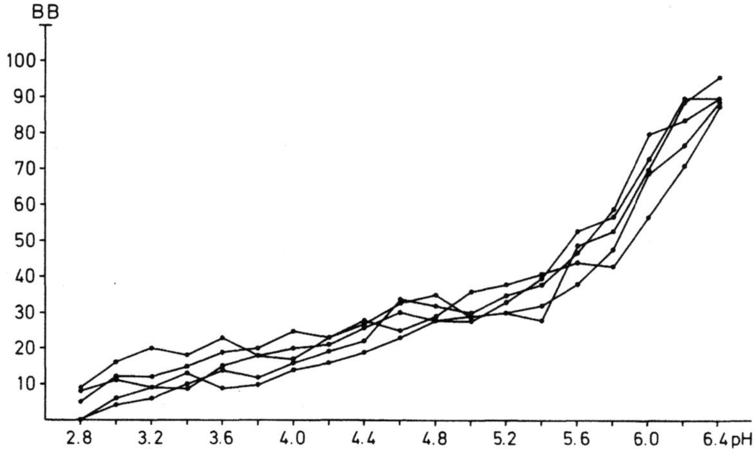

Fig. 51. Toluidine-blue pH curves for five cases of primary basophil leukemia

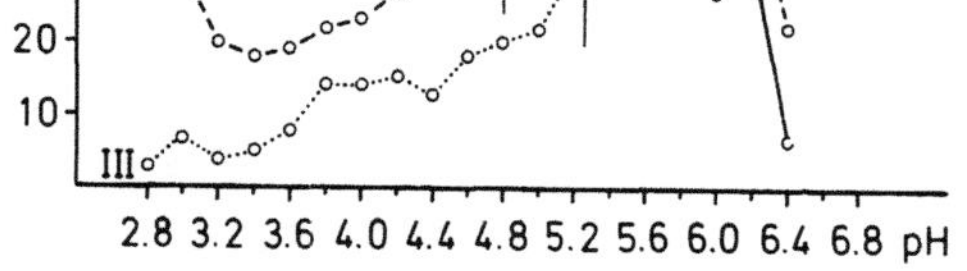

Fig. 52. Toluidine-blue pH curves in a case of basophil leukemia taken at 6-month intervals from the onset: O —— O at the beginning, O - - - - O 6 months later, O · · · · · O prefinal. Note the shift of the median values to the right

We found in all cases a definite right shift of the staining maxima on the toluidine-blue pH scale, so confirming that the shift is an indication of a deficit of acidic substances (glycosaminoglycans) in the basophil granules and by no means specific for basophilic leukemia. Our findings also show that blood basophils are altered in the same manner in practically all myeloproliferative diseases. The toluidine-blue pH series was counducted on chronic lymphatic leukemias as a control; the results obtained with these were identical with those of normal findings.

While the extreme shift of the 'staining maxima' of blood basophils in cases of basophilic leukemia is typical, it cannot be regarded as specific, since it occurs in many other myeloproliferative disorders. The extent of shift shows great fluctuations. In cases with predominance of undifferentiated cells, extreme divergences from the norm are observed. Cases with well-differentiated basophils show a much milder, yet still statistically significant shift. With increasing cytological features of dedifferentiation, the shift becomes more accentuated. This is best seen in cases with a terminal basophil crisis.

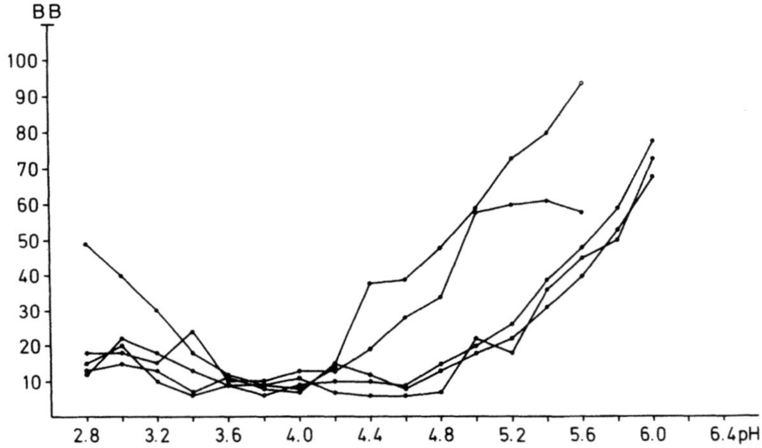

Fig. 53. Toluidine-blue pH curves for five cases of chronic myeloid leukemia with considerably raised blood basophil count

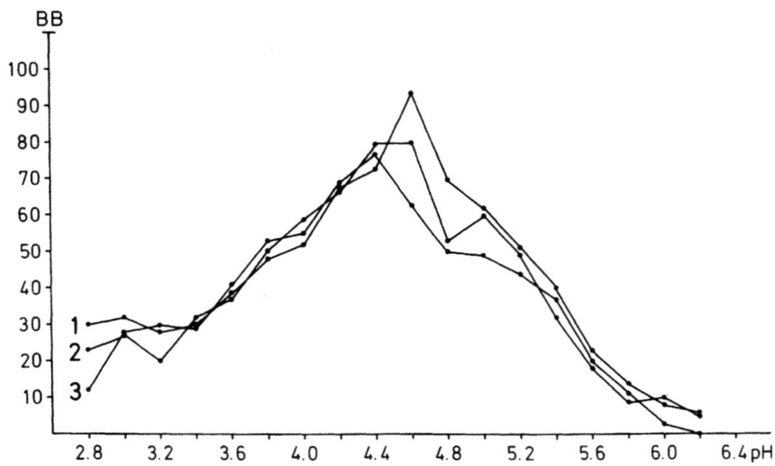

Fig. 54. Toluidine-blue pH curves (mean values) for three cases of myelofibrosis (1), three cases of polycythemia rubra vera (2), and three cases of myelomonocytic leukemia (3)

With the PAS reaction, normal blood basophils show a diastase-labile, weak and diffuse coloration of the cytoplasm. Leukemic blood basophils sometimes form a coarsely granular pattern which can be attributed to a local accumulation of glycogen. Similar findings have been observed with other forms of leukemia (LÖFFLER, 1969; LEDER, 1971). The coarsely granular PAS reaction indicates a disturbance in glycogenolysis with consequent retention and deposition of glycogen in the cytoplasm. This fundamental disturbance in the basic mechanisms of cell metabolism is highly typical and suggestive of neoplastic growth. A similar disordered cell metabolism has been found in other neoplastic diseases.

Myeloperoxidase activity in blood basophils has been studied in most cases on leukemic basophils. Although GRAHAM (1920), TOKUÉ (1929), and

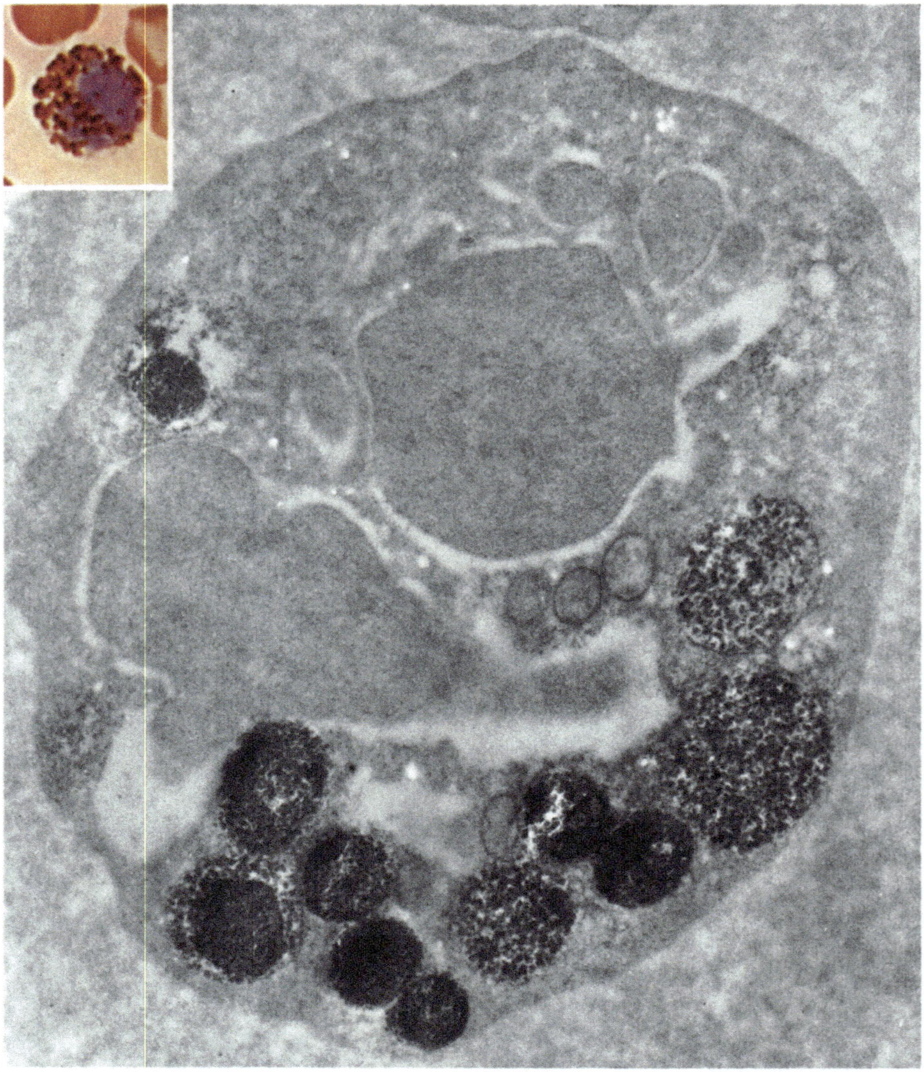

Fig. 55. Leukemic blood basophils. Myeloperoxidase reaction. The reaction product is localized exclusively within the specific granules. ×25,000, Inset ×1,400

Doan and Rinehart (1941) could detect no peroxidase activity in leukemic blood basophils, Kreibich (1910), Naegeli (1931), and Shibata *et al.* (1966) reported markedly peroxidase-positive blood basophils. In our experience, most of the normal blood basophils reveal a weak and some a negative peroxidase reaction. In contrast, in basophilic leukemia and other myeloproliferative diseases with basophil involvement, most of the blood basophils are peroxidase-positive and the reaction displays a coarse granular pattern (Fig. 55).

The increased and block-like myeloperoxidase activity seen in some basophils in different myeloproliferative diseases is confined to the specific granules as detected by electron microscope (Fig. 55). On the other hand, a loss in activity to leucine aminopeptidase has been reported to occur in leukemic basophils (Schubert *et al.*, 1968). Like normal basophils, leukemic blood basophils give a positive acid phosphatase and unspecific esterase reaction. Adenosine triphosphatase does not occur in either normal or leukemic basophils (Schubert and Martin, 1968) as studied by cytochemical methods.

Alkaline phosphatase has never been seen in normal basophils. In one case of basophilia associated with osteomyelofibrosis without myeloid metaplasia, we noted a positive reaction in basophils along with enhanced activity in neutrophils. Conclusive results were obtained with Leder's esterase (naphthol AS-D chloroacetate esterase) in blood basophils. Normal blood basophils present no activity to this enzyme, even in cases of reactive leukocytosis. To facilitate identification of the enzyme-negative basophils, the slides were first stained with dilute toluidine-blue solutions and basophils positive to this dye were photographed. Then the enzyme reaction was performed on the same cells, which were readjusted and photographed for a second time. In contrast to the behavior of normal basophils, some of the

Table 29. Incidence of naphthol AS-D chloroacetate esterase (Leder's esterase)-positive mature basophils in different myeloproliferative disorders

Myeloproliferative Disorders	Number of Cases	Mean Incidence of Basophils Positive to Leder's esterase %
1. Basophilic leukemia	7	60%
2. Eosinophilic leukemia	2	2%
3. Myelomonocytic leukemia	4	0.5%
4. Myelofibrosis with myeloid metaplasia	3	20%
5. Chronic myeloid leukemia	7	30%
6. Thrombocythemia	2	40%
7. Polycythemia vera	3	18%
8. Tissue mast cell leukemia	1	100%
9. Erythroleukemia	2	5%

Table 30. Typical cytochemical pattern of normal and leukemic blood basophils (BB). Φ = negative, (+) = positive but rare, + = positive

Cytochemical Reactions	Normal BB	Leukemic BB or BB in Myeloproliferative Disorders
Acid phosphatase	+ +	+ +
Alkaline phosphatase	Φ	Φ/(+)
Adenosine triphosphatase	+	Φ
Naphthol AS-D acetate esterase	+	+
Naphthol AS-D chloroacetate esterase (LEDER's esterase)	Φ	Φ/+ + +
Myeloperoxidase	Φ/+	Φ/+ + +
Leucine aminopeptidase	+	Φ
PAS reaction	+	+ +
Sudan black	+	+ +
Toluidine blue		
pH 2 to 4	+ + +	Φ/+
pH 4 to 7	Φ/+	+ + +

blood basophils in myeloproliferative diseases were identified as chloroacetate esterase-positive (Fig. 50). The percentage of enzyme-positive cells varies from case to case in the same disease. There appears to be a correlation between the number of basophils reacting positively to LEDER's esterase and the total basophil count. Enzyme-positive basophils were observed in tissue mast cell leukemia, basophilic and eosinophilic leukemias, myelomonocytic and chronic myeloid leukemias, and polycythemia rubra vera (Table 29). Positive basophils were also found in a case of essential thrombocythemia (megakaryocytic myelosis), and in cases of myelofibrosis with or without myeloid metaplasia.

Naphthol AS-D chloroacetate positivity of blood basophils in cases of myeloproliferative diseases may seem an unimportant feature relative to disordered proliferation, but considered in combination with numerous other findings, which we discuss later, this observation has a significant bearing on the nosologic interpretation of basophil leukemia and the genesis of the basophilia so often associated with myeloproliferative diseases. Table 30 lists the cytochemical properties of normal basophils as compared with basophils in myeloproliferative diseases.

IV. Nosology of the So-Called Basophilic Leukemia

We regard basophilic leukemia as a variant of myeloid leukemia. This conclusion is based upon the fact that blood basophils arise out of promyelocytes and represent a special type of granulocytes.

It is generally possible to distinguish basophilic leukemia from other leukemias on the basis of blood picture and to mark it off as an apparent entity. However, the complete spectrum of cytomorphologic variations seen in myeloid leukemia is taken into consideration, there seems to be no theoretical justification for regarding basophilic leukemia as a nosologic entity separate from other forms of myeloid leukemia. The close cytogenetic relationship between blood basophils and the other granulocytes strongly favors this view. Moreover, in most cases, the difference in basophil count between the myeloid leukemias and the classic basophilic leukemia is merely quantitative, with all transitional forms being seen. In our view, basophilic leukemia represents a myeloid leukemia with a special tendency to differentiate in the direction of the basophil cell line. Like the other granulopoietic cells, blood basophils show both neoplastic proliferation (Table 31) and, as in every myeloproliferative disorder 'atypias'. It is significant that in cases of basophilic leukemia neither the atypical cells nor the leukemic proliferation affect the blood basophils alone; there is also a simultaneous increase in neutrophils and eosinophils and/or monocytes. An equally rampant proliferation of eosinophils and their precursors in bone marrow can also be seen from time to time in cases of basophilic leukemia, and atypical forms of neutrophils, eosinophils, and monocytes do occur in typical cases of basophilic leukemia.

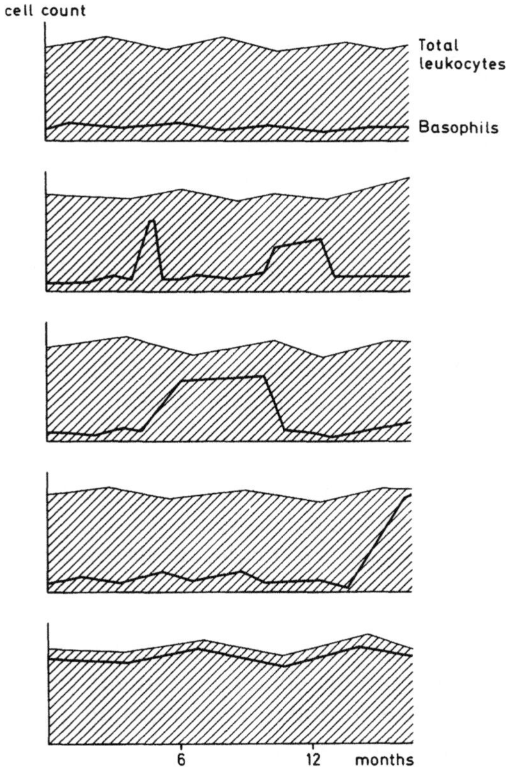

Fig. 56. Behavior of blood basophil counts in five cases of well – differentiated chronic myeloid leukemia

Obvious transitional forms occur between well-differentiated myeloid leukemia and 'primary' basophilic leukemia, distinguished only by the number of atypical elements. The qualitative alterations detectable in mature-celled myeloid leukemias are also found in typical cases of basophilic leukemia. Fig. 56 shows the wide variations in the quantitative involvement of blood basophils in 5 cases of well-differentiated myeloid leukemia. The basophil count in the peripheral blood is almost always elevated to between 2 and 20% of total leukocytes, sometimes accounting for 80% or more. Periods of severe peripheral basophilia may be of long or short duration; they occasionally occur preterminally and can then be compared with the terminal paramyeloblastic crisis.

To substantiate our views, we compared the differential blood count for 5 normal individuals, 5 cases of chronic myeloid leukemia and 5 cases of basophilic leukemia. The results are summarized in Table 31. Assuming a normal distribution, the quantitative statements are based upon a comparison of the means at the $p < 0.01$ level. In chronic myeloid leukemia, apart from the neutrophil count, the number of eosinophils, basophils and monocytes clearly exceeds normal values, whereas the number of lymphocytes in the peripheral blood remains within the normal range. The values for basophilic leukemia also show a considerable elevation of neutrophil, eosinophil, and monocyte counts without a corresponding increase in lymphocytes.

This comparison shows beyond doubt that not only in chronic myeloid leukemia, but also in typical cases of basophilic leukemia, the whole granulopoietic system – in which we must also include the cells of the monocytopoiesis – is affected by the leukemic disorder.

We arrive at similar conclusions when considering the qualitative alterations that are specific for leukemia. The 'atypias' being manifestations of malignant neoplasia (anaplasia) cover the following aberrations:

A. Nuclear Atypias

1. Pseudo-Pelger form (in neutrophils)
2. Rounded nuclei (in basophils and eosinophils)
3. Polyploidism
4. Hypersegmentation of the nucleus (in monocytes)
5. Nuclear folds (in monocytes)

B. Cytoplasmic Atypias

1. Naphthol AS-D chloroacetate esterase defect (of mature neutrophils and basophil precursors)
2. Naphthol AS-D chloroacetate esterase positivity (of basophils and eosinophils)
3. Peroxidase defect (of neutrophils)
4. Enhanced myeloperoxidase positivity (in basophils)
5. Alkaline-phosphatase positivity (in basophils)
6. Coarse granular PAS reaction (in basophils, eosinophils, neutrophils, and monocytes)

Table 31. Absolute count of total leukocytes and absolute differential leukocyte count in normal subjects, in chronic myeloid leukemia, and in basophilic leukemia

Normal Subjects:
(n=5)

	Total Leukocytes	Neutrophils	Eosinophils	Basophils	Monocytes	Lymphocytes
	8,800	5,104	176	35	528	2,957
	7,900	4,740	237	47	632	2,244
	7,200	3,960	288	21	288	2,642
	6,500	4,225	130	32	325	1,787
	6,000	4,140	180	36	480	1,164
Σ	36,400	22,169	1,011	171	2,253	10,794
$\bar{X}$	7,280.00	4,433.80	202.20	34.20	450.60	2,158.80
±S	1,112.21	473.64	61.17	9.31	143.16	708.12

Chronic Myeloid Leukemia:
(n=5)

	Total Leukocytes	Neutro	Eo	Baso	Mono	Lympho
	260,000	179,400	26,260	23,400	26,000	2,340
	180,000	104,400	21,600	15,120	21,960	2,520
	150,000	109,500	4,500	6,000	27,150	2,850
	98,000	64,680	10,780	5,390	14,406	2,744
	66,000	46,860	4,620	1,980	10,758	1,782
Σ	754,000	504,840	67,760	51,890	100,274	12,236
$\bar{X}$	150,800.00	100,968.00	13,552.00	10,378.00	20,054.80	2,447.20
±S	75,426.79	51,187.52	9,945.69	8,755.46	7,205.15	421.19

Basophilic Leukemia:
(n=5)

	Total Leukocytes	Neutro	Eo	Baso	Mono	Lympho
	180,000	47,900	12,600	109,800	7,200	2,500
	110,000	13,500	13,200	73,700	6,600	3,000
	96,000	34,660	10,560	43,200	5,760	1,820
	58,000	8,352	4,060	42,340	1,740	1,508
	35,000	12,020	1,050	16,330	2,800	2,800
Σ	479,000	116,432	41,470	285,370	24,100	11,628
$\bar{X}$	95,800.00	23,286.40	8,294.00	57,074.00	4,820.00	2,325.60
±S	55,715.35	17,182.33	5,434.78	35,798.41	2,412.63	639.22

C. Atypias of Specific Granules

1. Granule defect, overgranulation, and oversized granules (in basophils and eosinophils)
2. Basophil granules in eosinophils and vice versa (mixed-type granules) (Figs. 57 and 58)
3. Occurrence of water-insoluble granules (in basophils).

We compared the cytomorphologic properties of white blood cells from a group of 15 cases of severe reactive leukocytosis with those from 5 cases of chronic myeloid leukemia, and 5 cases of basophilic leukemia (Table 32).

The frequency of atypias was expressed as a percentage relative to over 1000 cells from each line in cases of reactive leukocytosis, chronic myeloid leukemia, and basophilic leukemia. The results are presented in Table 32. It

Table 32. Incidence of cellular atypias in chronic myeloid leukemia (CML) and basophilic leukemia (BL) compared to severe reactive leukocytosis.
Each item represents a percentage of 1000 leukocytes.
NASDCl = Naphthol AS-D Chloroacetate esterase reaction.

Atypias	Occurring in	Reactive Leukocytosis n = 15	CML n = 5 %	BL n = 5 %
A. *Nuclear Atypias*				
1. Pseudo-Pelger forms	Neutro, Baso	–	4	18
2. Rounded nuclei	Eos, Baso	–	8	22
3. Polyploidism	Neutro, Eos	–	0.7	0.9
4. Hypersegmentation	Mono	–	4	0.3
5. Nuclear folds	Mono	–	2	3
B. *Cytoplasmic Atypias*				
1. NASDCl-esterase defect	Neutro, Immature Baso	–	0.5	19
2. NASDCl-esterase positivity	Eos, Baso	–	11	63
3. Peroxidase defect	Neutro	–	0.2	0.8
4. Enhanced myeloperoxidase positivity	Baso	–	16	82
5. Alkaline-phosphatase positivity	Baso	–	rare	rare
6. Coarse granular PAS reaction	Baso, Eos Neutro, Mono	–	6	73
C. *Atypias of Specific Granules*				
1. Huge granules	Baso, Eos	–	2	32
2. Granule defect	Baso, Eos	–	2	18
3. Enhanced granules	Baso	–	5	16
4. Mixed-type granules	Baso, Eos	–	0.2	27

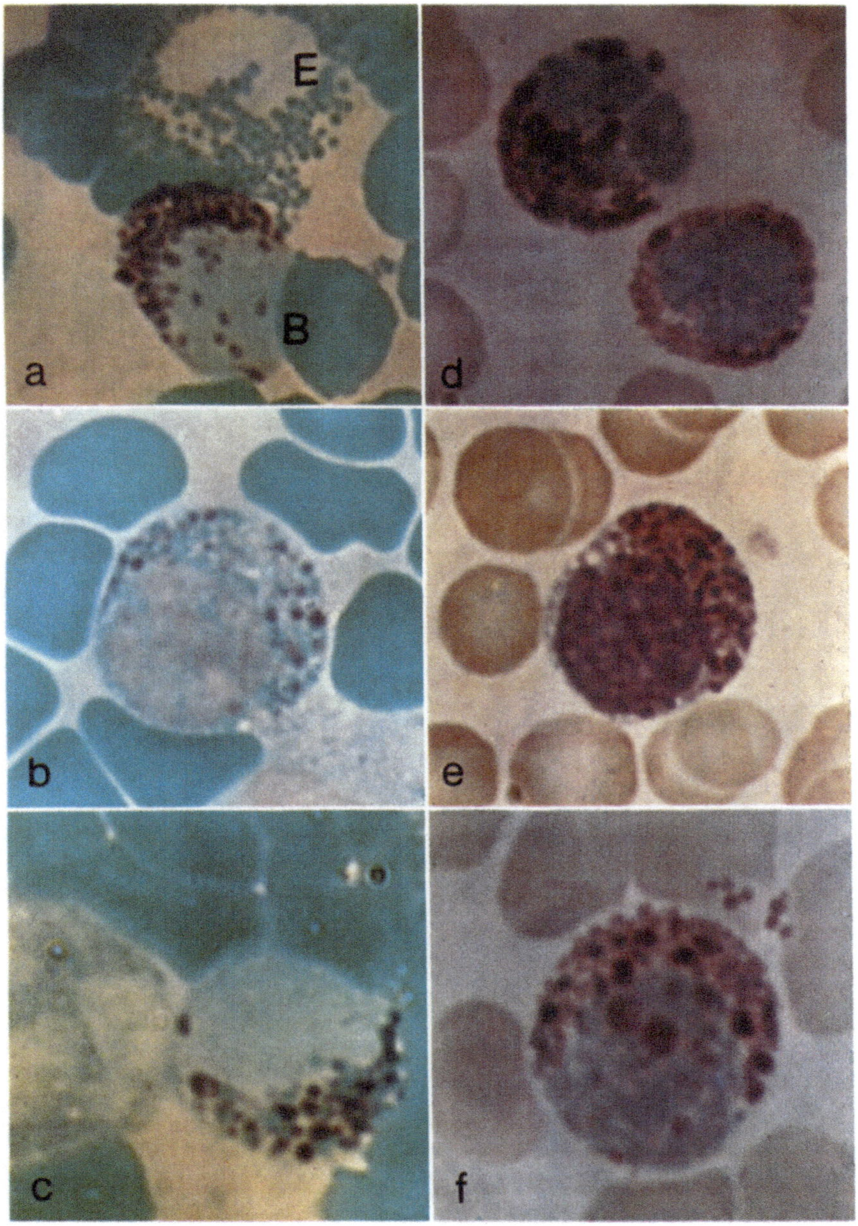

Fig. 57 a – f. Mixed-granule leukocytes from a case of chronic myeloid leukemia. (a): Above a normal eosinophil (*E*) and below a normal basophil (*B*) granulocyte; Light green aldehyde-fuchsin stain. (b) and (c): Mixed-granule leukocytes; Light green aldehyde-fuchsin stain. (d): A blood basophil (above) and a mixed-granule leukocyte (below); Aldehyde-fuchsin-eosin stain. (e): A mixed-granule leukocyte. Note the pseudo-Pelger form of the nucleus. Pappenheim stain. (f): A mixed-granule cell stained with aldehyde-fuchsin-eosin. Note the rounded nuclear form. Blood smears (a) to (e) × 1,800, (f) × 2,000

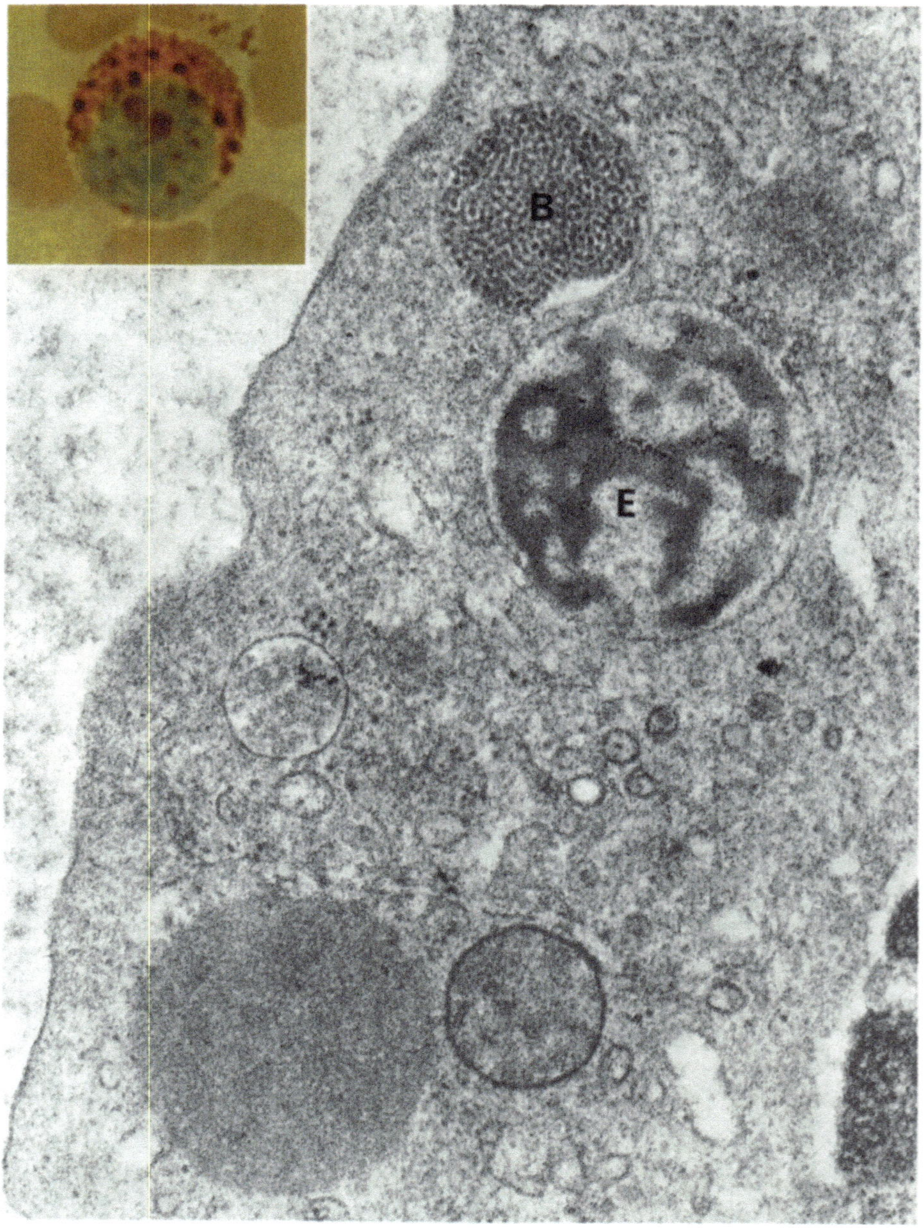

Fig. 58. Fine structure of a mixed-granule leukocyte with a basophil (*B*) granule and an atypical eosinophil granule (*E*). × 100,000. *Inset:* A mixed-granule leukocyte (yellow-green filter). × 1,500

is clear that nuclear atypias and cytoplasmic abnormalities regularly occur in both forms of leukemia, the difference being purely quantitative. For example, in cases of basophilic leukemia the coarse pattern of peroxidase reaction appears in 73% of blood basophils but in only 11% of total blood basophils in the 5 cases of chronic myeloid leukemia. Chromosomal aberrations, such as the presence of the Philadelphia-1 chromosome typical of mature-celled myeloid leukemia, were observed by us in 2 of the 5 cases of basophilic leukemia. This chromosomal aberration has also been reported by KYLE (1966) and MITRAKUL (1969) in cases of basophilic leukemia.

All these considerations, especially the results of our quantitative and qualitative comparisons of chronic myeloid and basophilic leukemia, indicate the existence of smooth transitional stages. Almost all chronic myeloid leukemias are accompanied by a considerable elevation in the basophil count. This phenomenon was earlier regarded as a concomitant reaction of basophils (HULE, 1950). We believe that the atypias among the increased blood basophils are obvious signs of leukemic anaplasia and prove the neoplastic nature of such basophils occurring in cases of myeloid leukemia. This view is further supported by the fact that the basophilia associated with chronic myeloid leukemia is accompanied by marked hyperhistaminemia and that the blood histamine does not fall upon administration of corticosteroids. During the course of chronic myeloid leukemia the blood basophils sometimes rise to 80% and more of the total leukocyte count. The occasionally observed terminal rise in blood basophils, which, by analogy with the 'paramyeloblast crisis' that occurs in chronic myeloid leukemia, is called 'terminal basophil crisis', may be regarded as a further indication that the entire granulocytic system is involved in the neoplastic process.

With regard to both cell atypias and the quantitative increase in the various types of granulocytes, it is highly suggestive that basophilic, eosinophilic, neutrophilic and monocytic leukemias all represent extreme forms of well-differentiated myeloid leukemia, and indeed, all theoretically possible transitional forms between well-differentiated myeloid leukemia and such extreme variants may be expected to occur. The criteria hitherto considered 'specific' for this or that type of leukemia can also be seen in intermediate forms, for example, in secondary basophilic leukemia or terminal basophil crisis.

Consequently, we may say that all these disorders represent the various forms of myeloproliferative disease, in the broad sense of the word, and of myeloid leukemia in a narrower sense. If we question the existence of basophilic leukemia as an independent entity, in spite of its relatively typical clinical course, we also maintain the same reservations with respect to the terms monocytic, eosinophilic, and neutrophilic leukemia. For instance, an increase in eosinophil granulocytes is often observed in well-differentiated cases of myeloid leukemia and basophilic leukemia, while markedly atypical eosinophils are observed in both types of leukemia. Such atypias appear only in neoplastic eosinophils and are pathognomonic for them. Mild eosinophilia can accompany the entire course of chronic myeloid leukemia or it can occur in crisis, making up the majority of granulocytes in either bone marrow or blood. The transition from myeloid leukemia to more or less pure 'eosinophilic' leukemia has often been observed, and in the same way both acute and chronic forms of eosinophilic leukemia may occur as with the predominantly 'neutrophilic' leukemia, 'basophilic' leukemia. Cases with an aleukemic course have also been reported (STILLMAN, 1912; HAY and EVANS, 1929; BARONE, 1930; MCCOWEN and PARKER, 1932; STEPHENS, 1935; REYE, 1940; HODGSON *et al.,* 1945). Other manifestations of 'eosinophilic' leukemia also display similarities with 'basophilic' leukemia. The duration of the disease, for instance, from the first symptoms until death, closely resembles that of 'basophilic' leukemia.

BENVENISTI and ULTMANN (1969) reported 3 cases of eosinophilic leukemia with distinct myelofibrosis. This finding is of interest because it can be observed not only in cases of basophilic leukemia but also in typical myeloid leukemia and other less common forms of myeloproliferative disease. The presence of myelofibrosis was first reported for basophilic leukemia by LENNERT *et al.* (1956) and confirmed by RAPPAPORT (1966). One of our cases of basophilic leukemia also developed extensive bone-marrow fibrosis. The development of myelofibrosis in the course of chronic myeloid leukemia has frequently been reported (KASARA, 1964; CHIBA *et al.,* 1964). Conversely, patients with initial myelofibrosis occasionally develop myeloid leukemia, and in such cases the 'increase' in leukocyte count and the 'atypias' can be especially prominent in one or all four types of granulocytes. In these cases the activity of neutrophils to alkaline phosphatase diminishes as blood cellularity increases.

There appears to be a mechanism similar to that of myelofibrosis at work in cases where bone marrow fibrosis accompanies myeloid leukemia. Whether or not this can be ascribed to monocytes cannot be determined at our present stage of knowledge. Indications that a transformation of monocytes into fibroblasts really can take place have often been noted. Organ fibrosis, however, has not been observed in cases of 'monocytic' leukemia. However, there is hardly any doubt that monocytopoiesis is involved in typical cases of myeloid leukemia. Like basophils, monocytes can be affected to varying degrees by the leukogenic stimulant. Apart from the fact that almost all cases of chronic myeloid leukemia are accompanied by a simultaneous rise in the absolute monocyte count, transitional stages from well-differentiated myeloid leukemia into myelomonocytic or almost pure monocytic leukemia have often been described. When we carefully searched for cell atypias, we also found atypical monocytes in cases of basophilic leukemia.

Transitions may be expected to occur from chronic myeloid leukemia to basophilic, eosinophilic, or monocytic leukemia, because all these cells represent mature forms of the morphologically, cytochemically, and enzyme-cytochemically uniform population of promyelocytes. It thus seems unlikely that neoplasia would affect a single myeloid series exclusively. This view is supported not only by the occurrence of arbitrary transitions between myeloid variants, but also by specific cytochemical findings and by chromosomal analysis. The occurrence of Philadelphia chromosomes is a characteristic of chronic myeloid leukemia. KYLE (1966), MITRAKUL (1969) and we ourselves have observed this aberration in cases of basophilic leukemia. It has also been observed in eosinophilic leukemia by KAUER and ENGLE (1964), GRUENWALD *et al.* (1965), and BENVENISTI and ULTMANN (1969).

When all these facts are taken into consideration, myeloid leukemia can be understood as being a generalized leukemic condition of the entire granulocytic system. Thus it is natural that the clinical course and the differential blood count (in accordance with the law of probabilities) should be dominated in the majority of cases by neutrophil granulocytes and to a lesser extent by monocytes, basophils, and eosinophils. The frequency of the various forms of myeloid leukemia as distinguished by the type of cells involved is determined primarily by the leukocyte precursor count (in bone marrow) and by the turnover rate, or by the generative capacity of the various types of granulocytes.

Therefore, we regard myeloid leukemia as a biological entity having special variants of monocytic, eosinophilic and basophilic leukemia. The variants differ from typical, well differentiated myeloid leukemia in that one particular type of granulocyte is present in numbers far in excess of the normal ratio. Hence, the monocytic, eosinophilic, and basophilic variants are somewhat less differentiated forms of myeloid leukemia than is the typical chronic myeloid leukemia, in which the normal ratio between the four myelogenous types of leukocyte is still to some extent preserved. Theoretically, such cases would be expected to run a much more malignant course, and this is in fact the case.

A strict demarcation of basophilic, eosinophilic, and monocytic leukemias from myeloid leukemia cannot be imposed simpley because of the heterogeneous phenotype of myeloid leukemia. However, although a simplification of this kind has theoretical significance, it need not exclude a purely pragmatic subdivision of myeloid leukemia to enable the clinician to distinguish the different courses of the disease for clinical or therapeutical purposes. The proliferating cell types that give rise to a special clinical picture, are, after all, cells with different biological features, and different therapeutic treatments may well be required in order to influence their apparently disordered metabolism and growth. In practice, a division on the basis of the response of different cell types to specific treatments is entirely admissible. However, the adoption of a nosological classification on the basis of response to symptomatic therapy can be valid only for clinical practice. It was not our intention to simplify the terminology. A simplification does ensue, however, if cytogenetic criteria are accepted as a basis for a nosologic classification rather than such phenotypic secondary features like clinical course and therapeutic particularities.

In summary: transitional stages occur between chronic myeloid leukemia and basophilic leukemia. Basophilic leukemia, in our view, represents a special form of myeloid leukemia with a tendency to differentiate preferentially toward blood basophils. A leukemic aberration of the total granulocytic system is present in basophilic leukemia as it is in the other forms of myeloid leukemia. Our opinion is based primarily upon two observations: (1) in both forms of leukemia turnover of all four elements of the granulocytic system is disturbed; (2) cell atypias specific for malignant neoplasia are found in all four cell series of the granulocytopoiesis in both chronic myeloid leukemia and basophilic leukemia. Furthermore, mixed forms between chronic myeloid leukemia and basophil leukemia exist, as well as transitional stages from one form to the other. This view enables otherwise anomalous observations, such as the presence of a myeloid leukemia with mixed-granule cells and the simultaneous proliferation of basophils and eosinophils in cases of chronic myeloid leukemia, to be explained without the need for additional hypotheses. A sharp distinction between basophilic leukemia and other types of myeloid leukemia is no longer justified, although it is accepted that the different forms can run a clinically 'special' course and may therefore require 'special therapy'.

References

ALDER, A.: Über abnorme Zellformen und ihre Häufigkeit bei akuter Myelose. Folia haemat. (Lpz.) **29**, 105 – 120 (1923).

ASTALDI, G., RONDANELLI, E. G., BERNADELLI, E.: see page 56.

BARONE, V. G.: Mielosi aleucemia eosinofila. Haematologica **11**, 437 – 447 (1930).

BENDITT, E. P.: Round table discussion. Ann. N. Y. Acad. Sci. **103**, 453 (1963).

BENVENISTI, D. S., ULTMANN, J. E.: Eosinophilic leukemia. Report of five cases and review of literature. Ann. intern. Med. **71**, 731 – 745 (1969).

CECIO, A., DINI, E., QUATTRIN, N.: Preliminary observations with the electron microscope of two cases of acute basophilic leukemia. Boll. Soc. ital. Biol. sper. **46/9**, 459 – 462 (1970).

CHEVALLIER, P., MARINONI, G.: La leucémie à basocytes. Sang **19**, 193 – 217 (1948).

CHEVALLIER, P., MARINONI, G.: La leucose aigüe à basoblastes. Sang **22**, 374 (1951).

CHIBA, K., UEDA, H., KOMIYA, M., KITAHAMA, K., YAMAGUCHI, H., NOMURA, T.: Two cases of myelofibrosis secondary to chronic myelogenous leukemia. Acta haemat. (Basel) **27**, 280 – 281 (1964).

DI GUGLIELMO, G.: Emoistioblasti in orientamento granulocitico basofilo. Haematologica **2**, 245 (1925).

DOAN, C. A., REINHART, H. L.: The basophil granulocyte, basophilicytosis and myeloid leukemia, basophil and mixed granule types; an experimental, clinical and pathological study, with the report of a new syndrome. Amer. J. clin. Path. **11**, 1 – 39 (1941).

DOAN, C. A., WISEMAN, B. K.: Monocytes, monocytosis, and monocytic leukosis: clinical and pathological study. Ann. intern. Med. **8**, 383 – 416 (1934).

EHRLICH, P.: see page 23.

EHRLICH, P., LAZARUS, A.: Die Anaemie. I. Abt. Die normale und pathologische Histologie des Blutes. In: Nothnagel: Spezielle Pathologie und Therapie, Bd. 8. Wien: Hoelder 1898.

ELLIOT, A., YOUNG, R.: Myelogenous leukemia. Med. Clin. N. Amer. **15**, 579 – 587 (1931).

EVANS, T. S.: Moncytic leukemia (General review of the subject). Medicine (Baltimore) **21**, 421 – 456 (1942).

FRANCO, E. M., FERRATA, A.: Cellule istioidi (emoistioblasti) e porco derivati nel sangue circolante. Arch. Sci. med. **43**, 109 – 122 (1919).

GERHARD, J., HENSCHEL, E.: Sogenannte eosinophile Leukaemie mit Hautinfiltraten. Folia haemat. **75**, 643 – 653 (1958).

GRAHAM, G. S.: see page 59.

GROAT, W. A., WYATTE, T. C., ZIMMER, S. M., FIELD, R. E.: Acute basophilic leukemia. Amer. J. med. Sci. **191**, 457 – 466 (1936).

GRUENWALD, H., KIOSSOGLOU, K. A., MITUS, W. J., DAMESHEK, W.: Philadelphia chromosome in eosinophilic leukemia. Amer. J. Med. **39**, 1003 – 1010 (1965).

HAY, J., EVANS, W. H.: Acute eosinophilic leukemia and eosinophilic erythro-leukemia. Quart. J. Med. **22**, 167 – 189 (1929).

HAYHOE, F. G. J.: Leukemia. Research and Clinical Practice. London: J. & A. Churchill Ltd. 1960.

HITTMAIR, A.: Die myeloische Monocytenleukaemie (Monocytenmyelose). In:- Handbuch der ges. Haematologie, Bd. IV/2, München-Berlin: Urban & Schwarzenberg 1963.

HODGSON, J. R., KAUMP, D. H., STEINER, G., BOVILL, J.: Myeloid leukemia probably eosinophilic in character. Amer. J. clin. Path. **15**, 389 – 394 (1945).

HOLMGREN, H., WOHLFART, G.: Om de basofilia levkocyternas diagnosticas betydelse. Nord. Med. **11**, 2771 – 2775 (1941).

HULE, V.: Die akuten basophilen und eosinophilen Leukosen. Sang **30**, 423 – 436 (1950).

JOACHIM, G.: Über Mastzellenleukaemien. Dtsch. Arch. klin. Med. **87**, 437 – 455 (1906).

KASARA, K., OTAKE, Y., TSUCHIYA, J., MATSUMOTO, S., SHIRAKURA, T., OKA, K., MAEKAWA, T., SHIGIYA, R., FUKAI, K.: Report of an autopsy case with myelofibrosis showing an atypical clinical course. Acta haem. jap. **27**, 281 (1964).

KAUER, G. L., ENGLE, R. L.: Eosinophilic leukemia with Ph_1 – positive cells. Lancet **1964 II**, 1340.

KREIBICH, C.: see page 61.

KYLE, R. A., PEASE, G. L.: Basophilic leukemia. Arch. intern. Med. **118**, 205 – 210 (1966).

LEDER, L.-D.: see page 62.

LEDER, L.-D.: A case of acute leukemia with pseudo-Pelger cells containing Auer bodies. Acta haemat. (Basel) **42**, 58 – 63 (1969).

LEDER, L.-D.: see page 97.

LENNERT, K.: see page 62.

LENNERT, K., KÖSTER, E., MARTIN, H.: Über die Mastzellenleukaemie. Acta haemat. (Basel) **16**, 255 – 272 (1956).

LEVADITI, C.: Un cas de leucémie myélogène; considérations sur la mastzellen-leucocytose et sur l'étérochromasie des granulations leucocytaires. J. Physiol. Path. gén. 424 – 438 (1901).

MCCOWEN, G. R., PARKER, H. B.: A case of acute eosinophilic leukemia. J. roy. nav. med. Serv. **18**, 131 (1932).

MASSA, M., MARINONI, E.: Rilievi su una forma vara di mielosi leucemica e piastrinemica con emoistoblasti in orientamento basofilo. Clin. med. ital. **57**, 487 – 503 (1926).

MITRAKUL, C., OTHAGANONDA, B.-O., MANOTHAL, P., BHANICHAYA-BHONGSA, S.: Basophilic leukemia. Report of a case. Clin. Pediat. (Philad.) **8**, 178 – 180 (1969).

NAEGELI, O.: Blutkrankheiten und Blutdiagnostik, 4th Ed. Berlin: Springer 1923.

NAEGELI, O.: Lehrbuch der Blutkrankheiten und Blutdiagnostik. Berlin: Springer 1931.

PARWARESCH, M. R., DANNENBERG, K., LEDER, L.-D.: see page 64.

PARWARESCH, M. R.: Ultrastruktur und Zytochemie der Leukämischen Blutbasophilen. STACHER, A., u. P. HÖCKER (Hrsg.) Erkrankungen der Myelopoese. Leukämien, Myeloproliferatives Syndrom, Polyzythämie. Urban und Schwarzenberg 1976.

QUATTRIN, N., DINI, E., PALUMBO, E.: Basophile Leukaemien. Blut **5**, 166 – 187 (1959).

RAPPAPORT, H.: Tumors of the hematopoietic system. Washington: Armed Forces Institute of Pathology 1966.

REYE, D.: A case of acute eosinophilic leukemia. Med. J. Aust. **2**, 156 – 157 (1940).

SABRAZÈS, J.: Leucémie à mastzellen et à cellules de Ferrata radiorésistantes (poussée aigüe terminale). Arch. Mal. Coeur **19**, 453 – 455 (1926).

SARZI-SARTORI, P.: Emoistioblasti a granulazione basofila in un caso de leucemia basogranulocitica (Mastzellen-leucemia). G. clin. med. **8**, 784 – 789 (1927).

SCHUBERT, J. F. C., MARTIN, H.: Beobachtungen bei Blutmastzell-Leukaemien. Blut **18**, 35 – 39 (1968).

SCHUBERT, J. F. C., MARTIN, H.: Observations on 7 patients with "blood mast cell leukemia". Klin. Wschr. **46**, 929 – 936 (1968).

SHIBATA, A., TAKASE, S., ONODERA, S., MIURA, A. B., SUZUKI, A., SAKAMOTO, S., OIKAWA, A., SATO, T.: Cytological studies on basophil leucocytes. Acta haemat. jap. **29**, 879 – 889 (1966).

STEPHENS, D. J.: Acute eosinophilic leukemia. Amer. J. med. Sci. **189**, 387 – 392 (1935).

STILLMAN, R. G.: A case of myeloid leukemia with predominance of eosinophile cells. Med. Rec. (N. Y.) **81**, 594 – 597 (1912).

STORTI, E., MAURI, C.: Die chronischen Myelosen. In: Handbuch der gesamten Haematologie. Eds. L. HEILMEYER und A. HITTMAIR, Bd. 4, Teil 2, S. 147 – 176. München und Berlin: Urban und Schwarzenberg 1963.

TOKUÉ, K.: see page 27.

TOMASZEWSKI, Z.: Über einen Fall von Mastzellenleukaemie. Folia haemat. (Lpz.) **12**, 115 – 124 (1911).

VASATURO, A.: La Mastzellenleucemia. Studium **15**, 172 – 176 (1925 a).

VASATURO, A.: Megacariociti ed emoistioblasti in circolo nella leukemia mastgranulocitaria. Folia Med. (Napoli) **11**, 561 – 584 (1925 b).

Subject Index

H. Begemann, J. Rastetter

Atlas of Clinical Haematology

Initiated by L. Heilmeyer, H. Begemann
With an Appendix on Tropical Diseases
by W. Mohr
Translated from the 2nd completely revised German edition by H. J. Hirsch
191 figures in color and 17 in black and white. XV, 324 pages. 1972

M. Bessis

Corpuscles

Atlas of Red Blood Cell Shapes
121 figures. 147 pages. 1974

M. Bessis

Living Blood Cells and their Ultrastructure

Translated by R. I. Weed
521 figures, 2 color plates. XXIII, 767 pages. 1973

M. Bessis

Blood Smears Reinterpreted
Red Cell Shape

Physiology, Pathology, Ultrastructure
Proceedings of a Symposium held June 20 and 21, 1972 at the Institute of Cell Pathology, Hôpital de Bicêtre (as part of the scientific exchange program between N.I.H., USA, and I.N.S.E.R.M., France
Editors: M. Bessis, R. I. Weed, P. F. Leblond
147 figures. VIII, 180 pages. 1973

R. Burkhardt

Bone Marrow and Bone Tissue

Color Atlas of Clinical Histopathology
Foreword by W. Stich
Translator: H. J. Hirsch
721 colored figures. XII, 115 pages. 1971

Springer-Verlag Berlin Heidelberg New York

GPSR Compliance

The European Union's (EU) General Product Safety Regulation (GPSR) is a set of rules that requires consumer products to be safe and our obligations to ensure this.

If you have any concerns about our products, you can contact us on ProductSafety@springernature.com

In case Publisher is established outside the EU, the EU authorized representative is:

Springer Nature Customer Service Center GmbH
Europaplatz 3
69115 Heidelberg, Germany

Batch number: 10620854

Printed by Printforce, the Netherlands